FOOT AND ANKLE SECRETS

FOOT AND ANKLE SECRETS

LAWRENCE B. HARKLESS, DPM

Professor
Podiatry Service
Director, Podiatry Residency Training Program
Department of Orthopaedics
University of Texas Health Science Center at San Antonio
San Antonio, Texas

KIM FELDER-JOHNSON, DPM

Assistant Professor
Podiatry Service
Department of Orthopaedics
University of Texas Health Science Center at San Antonio
San Antonio, Texas

HANLEY & BELFUS, INC./Philadelphia

Publisher: HANLEY & BELFUS, INC.
              Medical Publishers
              210 South 13th Street
              Philadelphia, PA 19107
              (215) 546-7293; 800-962-1892
              FAX (215) 790-9330
              Web site: http://www.hanleyandbelfus.com

Note to the reader: Although the information in this book has been carefully reviewed for correctness of dosage and indications, neither the authors nor the editors nor the publisher can accept any legal responsibility for any errors or omissions that may be made. Neither the publisher nor the editors make any warranty, expressed or implied, with respect to the material contained herein. Experimental compounds and off-label uses of approved products are discussed. Before prescribing any drug, the reader must review the manufacturer's current product information (package inserts) for accepted indications, absolute dosage recommendations, and other information pertinent to the safe and effective use of the product described. This is especially important when drugs are given in combination or as an adjunct to other forms of therapy.

Library of Congress Cataloging-in-Publication Data

Harkless, Lawrence B.
     Foot and ankle secrets / Lawrence B. Harkless, Kim Felder-Johnson.
        p.   cm. — (The Secrets Series)
     Includes bibliographical references and index.
     ISBN 1-56053-211-4 (alk. paper)
     1. Podiatry—Examinations, questions, etc.   I. Felder-Johnson, Kim.
II. Title.   III. Series.
     [DNLM: 1. Foot Diseases—examination questions.   2. Foot Injuries—
examination questions.   3. Ankle Injuries—examination questions.
4. Ankle—physiopathology—examination questions.   WE 18.2 H282f 1997]
RD563.H287   1997
617.5'85'0076—dc21
DNLM/DLC
for Library of Congress   97-19922
                                                                 CIP

FOOT AND ANKLE SECRETS   ISBN 1-56053-211-4

Last digit is the print number: 9   8   7   6   5   4   3   2

CONTENTS

CONTRIBUTORS

Stephen F. Albert, D.P.M.
Associate Professor and Chief, Podiatric Section, Department of Surgery, University of Colorado School of Medicine; Chief, Podiatric Section, Surgery Service, Veterans Affairs Medical Center, Denver, Colorado

Richard A. Bellacosa, D.P.M.
Clinical Assistant Professor, Podiatry Service, Department of Orthopaedics, University of Texas Health Science Center at San Antonio; Private practice of podiatry, San Antonio, Texas

Paul S. Bishop, D.P.M.
Morris Hospital, Morris, Illinois; Sandwich Community Hospital, Sandwich, Illinois

Maureen L. Caldwell, R.N., D.P.M.
Podiatry Service, Department of Orthopaedics, University of Texas Health Science Center at San Antonio, San Antonio, Texas

Thomas J. Chang, D.P.M.
Associate Professor, Department of Podiatric Surgery, Director of Surgical Residency Training, California College of Podiatric Medicine; Faculty, The Podiatry Institute; Mt. Zion/UCSF Hospital; Pacific Coast Hospital, San Francisco, California

Major Mary A. Cook, D.P.M.
Staff Podiatrist, Keesler Medical Center, Keesler Air Force Base, Biloxi, Mississippi

Mardon R. Day, D.P.M.
Assistant Instructor, Podiatry Service, Department of Orthopaedics, University of Texas Health Science Center at San Antonio; University Hospital System, Audie L. Murphy Memorial Veterans Hospital, San Antonio, Texas

Richelle D. Day, D.P.M.
Clinical Instructor, Podiatry Service, Department of Orthopaedics, University of Texas Health Science Center at San Antonio, San Antonio, Texas

Thomas M. DeLauro, D.P.M.
Professor, Divisions of Medical Surgical Sciences, New York College of Podiatric Medicine, New York, New York

Kenrick Johnson Dennis, D.P.M.
Associate Clinical Professor, Department of Family Practice, University of Texas Medical School at Houston, Houston, Texas

Kim Felder-Johnson, D.P.M.
Assistant Professor, Podiatry Service, Department of Orthopaedics, University of Texas Health Science Center at San Antonio, San Antonio, Texas

Jennifer Fung-Schwartz, D.P.M.
Clinical Supervisor, Podiatry Department, St. Clare's Hospital and Health Center, New York, New York

Vincent F. Giacalone, D.P.M.
Medical Director, Diabetic Foot Care Center, Westwood, New Jersey

L. V. Grant, D.P.M.
Private practice of podiatry; Staff, Summit Medical Center, Oakland, California

Jimmy L. Gregory, D.P.M.
Clinical Instructor, Department of Orthopaedics, Emory University, Atlanta, Georgia

Lawrence B. Harkless, D.P.M.
Professor and Director, Podiatry Residency Training Program, Podiatry Service, Department of Orthopaedics, University of Texas Health Science Center at San Antonio, San Antonio, Texas

Edwin J. Harris, D.P.M.
Associate Clinical Professor of Orthopaedics, Section of Pediatrics, Loyola University of Chicago, Stritch School of Medicine; Staff, Foster G. McGaw Hospital, Maywood, Illinois

Kevin R. Higgins, D.P.M.
Clinical Associate Professor, Podiatry Service, Department of Orthopaedics, University of Texas Health Science Center at San Antonio; Active Staff, Baptist Health System and Methodist Healthcare System, San Antonio, Texas

Bruce Elliot Hirsch, Ph.D.
Associate Professor of Anatomy, Department of Biomedical Sciences, Pennsylvania College of Podiatric Medicine; Adjunct Assistant Professor, Department of Radiology, University of Pennsylvania School of Medicine, Philadelphia, Pennsylvania

Richard Martin Jay, D.P.M.
Professor of Orthopaedics, Director of Pediatrics, Pennsylvania College of Podiatric Medicine; Director of Surgical Residency Program, The Graduate Hospital, Philadelphia, Pennsylvania

Richard O. Jones, D.P.M., M.P.H.
Private practice of podiatry, Victoria, British Columbia, Canada

Anthony S. Kidawa, B.S., D.P.M.
Professor, Department of Medicine; Section Chief, Vascular Diseases, Pennsylvania College of Podiatric Medicine, Philadelphia, Pennsylvania

Lisa G. Latham, P.T.
Chairperson, Physical Therapist Assistant Program, Hinds Community College, Raymond, Mississippi

Thomas B. Leecost, D.P.M., M.S.
Adjunct Professor, New York College of Podiatric Medicine, New York, New York; St. Mary's, Richmond Metropolitan, Richmond Community, and Richmond Memorial Hospitals, Richmond, Virginia

James Michael Losito, D.P.M.
Professor of Podiatric Biomechanics, Barry University School of Podiatric Medicine; Cedars Medical Center; Mercy Hospital, Miami, Florida

Richard O. Lundeen, D.P.M.
Director, Residency Training, Winona Memorial Hospital, Indianapolis, Indiana

Kelly Matthew-Gil, D.P.M.
Podiatry Service, Department of Orthopaedics, University of Texas Health Science Center at San Antonio, San Antonio, Texas

Thomas F. McCloskey, D.P.M.
East Texas Medical Center, Mother Francis Hospital, University of Texas Health Center at Tyler, Tyler, Texas

Gerit Mulder, D.P.M.
Department of Geriatrics, Center on Aging, University of Colorado Health Sciences Center, Denver, Colorado; Faculty, Wound Clinic, Regional Burn Center, University of California at San Diego, San Diego, California

Simon Nzuzi, D.P.M.
Professor, Primary Care Department; Director, Primary Podiatric Medical Residency Program, New York College of Podiatric Medicine, New York, New York

R. Daryl Phillips, D.P.M.
Professor and Clinical Faculty Member, College of Podiatric Medicine and Surgery, University of Osteopathic Medicine and Health Sciences, Des Moines, Iowa

Melvin B. Price, D.P.M., P.T.
Clinical Faculty, Department of Physical Medicine and Rehabilitation, Medical College of Wisconsin, Milwaukee, Wisconsin; Rankin Medical Center, Brandon, Mississippi; Medical Surgical Foot Institute, Jackson, Mississippi

Alex Reyzelman, D.P.M.
Podiatry Service, Department of Orthopaedics, University of Texas Health Science Center at San Antonio, San Antonio, Texas

Jeffrey A. Ross, D.P.M.
Assistant Clinical Professor, Baylor College of Medicine; Associate Chief, St. Luke's Hospital; Staff, Methodist Hospital, Houston, Texas

Lee J. Sanders, D.P.H.
Adjunct Clinical Associate Professor, Pennsylvania College of Podiatric Medicine, Philadelphia, Pennsylvania; Chief, Podiatry Service, Veterans Affairs Medical Center, Lebanon, Pennsylvania

Samuel J. Spadone, D.P.M.
Instructor, Pennsylvania College of Podiatric Medicine, Philadelphia, Pennsylvania

Morris A. Stribling, D.P.M.
Clinical Instructor, Podiatry Service, Department of Orthopaedics, University of Texas Health Science Center at San Antonio, Texas

Larry A. Suecof, D.P.M.
Assistant Clinical Professor in Orthopaedics, University of Connecticut School of Medicine; John Dempsey Hospital, Farmington, Connecticut; Director, Neuropathic Foot Clinic, Hartford Hospital, Hartford, Connecticut

Mary Yvonne Tobar, D.P.M., B.S.
Podiatry Service, Department of Orthopaedics, University of Texas Health Science Center at San Antonio, San Antonio, Texas

George F. Wallace, D.P.M.
Director, Podiatry Service, University Hospital, University of Medicine and Dentistry of New Jersey, Newark, New Jersey

Stephen C. Wan, D.P.M.
West Torrance Podiatrists Group, Inc., Torrance, California

Susan C. Warner, B.A.
Biomechanics Research Fellow, College of Podiatric Medicine and Surgery, University of Osteopathic Medicine and Health Sciences, Des Moines, Iowa

Alan Kendrick Whitney, A.B., D.P.M.
Professor Emeritus, Department of Podiatric Orthopaedics, Pennsylvania College of Podiatric Medicine, Philadelphia, Pennsylvania

Kendrick Alan Whitney, D.P.M.
Assistant Professor, Department of Podiatric Orthopaedics, Pennsylvania College of Podiatric Medicine, Philadelphia, Pennsylvania

Peter J. Williams, D.P.M.
Clinical Faculty, Podiatry Section, Department of Orthopaedics, University of Texas Health Science Center at San Antonio; Private practice of podiatry, San Antonio, Texas

Jeanean Denise Willis, D.P.M.
Clinical Assistant Professor, Pennsylvania College of Podiatric Medicine; Director of EMG/NCV Laboratory, Pennsylvania Hospital, Philadelphia, Pennsylvania

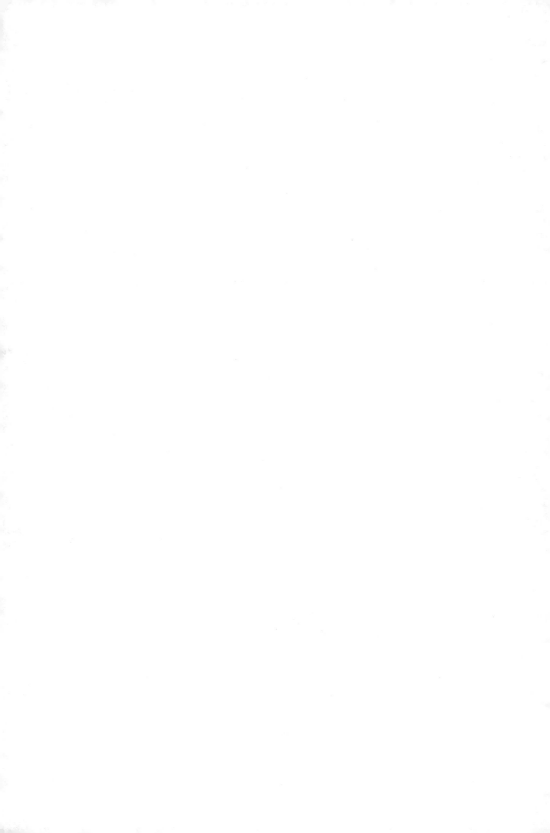

PREFACE

I feel you know what I am supposed to know
but you can't tell me what it is
because you don't know that I don't know what it is.
You may know what I don't know, but not
that I don't know it.
And I can't tell you. So you will have to
tell me everything.

R.D. Laing, 1970

Wisdom is supreme; therefore get wisdom. Though it cost all
you have, get understanding.

Proverbs 4:7

Wisdom is indeed supreme. Learning should never end, and striving for greater knowledge and understanding should be a priority. Learning is a challenging process for both the student and the teacher and involves many levels of growth.

However, there is a major obstacle to the teaching-learning process called the "pretend-to-know game." Neal Whitman, an educator in creative medical teaching at the University of Utah, listed three rules to this game that most of us know and have played during our learning process. The first rule is to avoid eye contact with the attending physician when he asks the ward team a question and you do not know the answer. The second rule is to nod in agreement when someone else answers a question and sounds like he knows what he is talking about. The final rule is to answer a question with a question if you do not know the answer. There is a penalty for successfully playing this game. The students and residents miss out on the understanding and knowledge that may have been gained from the teacher who was fooled by the successful player.

Many excellent podiatric textbooks and references are available and are frequently read by students, residents, and practitioners to supplement what they have been taught (or perhaps to learn what they missed while playing the "pretend-to-know game"). Without the clinical correlation, critical thinking skills, and experience, though, it can be difficult to review texts and journal articles and pull out the key information. There is a gap in the available references for a book that can readily provide key questions and answers and thus facilitate critical thought. The goal of this text is to provide that link between the standard reference text and the critical thought process. We hope this reference will serve as a source for the key topics discussed in the clinical situation and during medical rounds. It is not meant to be a complete source of information for any one topic. It will, however, provide a basis for preparation for rounds and presentations. It will stimulate and provide direction for the critical thought process and will serve as a guide for key information on topics encountered in clinical and practical situations.

The contributors to *Foot and Ankle Secrets* are to be commended and thanked for their outstanding contributions to this reference and to the profession. May your learning and quest for knowledge and understanding be constant with the ultimate reward of wisdom.

Lawrence B. Harkless, DPM
Kim Felder-Johnson, DPM

1. ANATOMY

Bruce Elliot Hirsch, Ph.D.

1. What is the blood supply of the talus?

Short bones typically receive much of their blood through the muscles attaching to them, but the talus does not have this source available. It relies on small vessels derived from each of the main arteries running near it, the anterior tibial/dorsalis pedis, posterior tibial, and peroneal.

A small twig splits off from the anterior tibial artery near the ankle joint and enters the superior surface of the talar neck. The artery of the sinus tarsi comes off the lateral tarsal artery, a branch of the dorsalis pedis, and enters the sinus tarsi to supply the talus as well as the calcaneus and soft tissues within the space.

The artery of the canalis tarsi arises from the posterior tibial artery, just before it splits into the plantar branches. This small vessel first sends deltoid branches to the medial side of the talus, then enters the canalis tarsi to supply the talus, calcaneus, and soft tissues. It anastomoses with the artery of the sinus tarsi.

Branches from the peroneal artery (or from the posterior lateral malleolar or lateral calcaneal arteries) anastomose with branches of the medial calcaneal to supply the part of the talus near the lateral tubercle.

The head of the talus receives all of its blood from the small arteries entering the bone through the neck, sinus tarsi, and tarsal canal, so it is at risk whenever those vessels are damaged. The body has a more widely distributed supply.

2. What are the components of the sesamoid apparatus?

Two small bones, the medial and lateral sesamoid bones of flexor hallucis brevis, articulate with the plantar aspect of the first metatarsal head. Although these bones, like all other sesamoids, are located within a tendon, they are intimately related to other structures as well. That is because the tendon itself blends with other muscles and with components of the first MTP joint. The sesamoids, tendon fibers, and various articular structures make up the sesamoid apparatus.

3. How are the sesamoids arranged?

The tendons of the two heads of flexor hallucis brevis, medial and lateral, enter into the plantar MTP ligament (plantar plate or pad). The tendon fibers contribute to the fibrous component of that fibrocartilaginous structure. As a result, the two sesamoid bones are almost completely embedded in the ligament. Only their superior surfaces, which are coated with hyaline cartilage, are free; they articulate with the first metatarsal head.

The medial head of flexor hallucis brevis is joined, near its insertion, by the tendon of abductor hallucis. On the other side, the transverse head of adductor hallucis joins the oblique head, and this combined tendon, in turn, blends with the lateral head of flexor hallucis brevis. Therefore, the fibrous component of the plantar ligament includes contributions from those two muscles.

Various ligaments attach to the sesamoids and help stabilize and maintain their position. They are at least partly blended with the plantar ligament. These include the medial and lateral metatarsosesamoid ligaments, medial and lateral phalangeosesamoid ligaments, and intersesamoid ligament.

4. What structures are located on and around the lateral side of the ankle and may be involved in a sprain?

There are three ligaments on the lateral side of the ankle, connecting the fibula to the talus and calcaneus. Together, they are called the **lateral ligament**. Unlike the deltoid ligament on the medial side of the ankle, the lateral ligament's components are distinct and separate from each other. They are the anterior and posterior talofibular (or fibulotalar) ligaments and the calcaneofibular ligament (see figure).

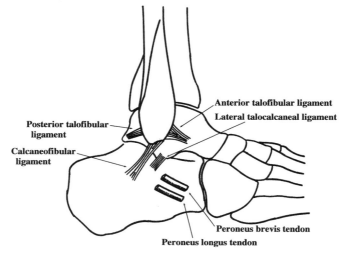

Lateral ankle ligaments.

Both the anterior and posterior talofibular ligaments lie almost horizontally. The anterior runs from the anterior border of the lateral malleolus to the rough area anterior to the facet on the lateral malleolar surface of the talus. The posterior ligament connects the lateral malleolar fossa to the posterior rough strip on the lateral malleolar surface and to the lateral talar tubercle.

The calcaneofibular ligament attaches to the summit of the lateral malleolus, and from there passes inferiorly and slightly posteriorly to the lateral surface of the calcaneus, where its attachment is marked by a small tubercle. This ligament crosses the subtalar as well as the ankle joint. It is, in fact, parallel and immediately superficial to a ligament of the subtalar joint. the lateral talocalcaneal ligament.

The origin of **extensor digitorum brevis** lies slightly anterior and inferior to the ankle joint and is actually rather extensive. The bony origin spreads from the lateral edge of the sulcus calcanei onto the lateral surface of the calcaneus as far as the sulcus for peroneus brevis. Thus, the extensor digitorum brevis takes up a large part of the sinus tarsi. The soft tissue origin includes the stem of the inferior extensor retinaculum and perhaps the lateral talocalcaneal ligament as well.

The stem of the **inferior extensor retinaculum** has an expansive attachment to the calcaneus and within the sinus tarsi. As it approaches its attachment to bone, the stem splits into three roots. The lateral root remains superficial, crossing over extensor digitorum brevis and attaching to the lateral surface of the calcaneus. The intermediate root attaches to the sulcus calcanei, just medial to the extensor digitorum brevis origin. The medial root has the most complicated attachment. It passes into the sinus tarsi and continues into the tarsal canal, where it is bound to both the talus and calcaneus. Some of its fibers, however, bend back on themselves before entering the sinus tarsi and remain superficial, surrounding the extensor digitorum longus and peroneus tertius tendons. They form the **fundiform ligament**.

A branch of the lateral tarsal artery, the artery of the sinus tarsi, enters the sinus and continues medially to anastomose with the artery of the tarsal canal. The remaining space in the sinus tarsi is occupied by a plug of fat, which is malleable and able to fill the variably changing space as other structures move. It is sometimes called "Hoke's tonsil."

5. How are the layers of the plantar muscles arranged?

In dissection of the foot, the plantar muscles are typically exposed sequentially, going from the most superficial to the deepest muscles. These muscles can be separated into four layers:

The first layer consists of, from medial to lateral, the abductor hallucis, flexor digitorum brevis, and abductor digiti minimi. All take partial origin from the calcaneal tuberosity.

The second layer includes five muscles, which all attach in some way to the flexor digitorum longus (FDL) tendon: the quadratus plantae (flexor accessorius) and the four lumbrical muscles.

The third layer is made of muscles that act on the hallux and little toe and include the flexor hallucis brevis, adductor hallucis, and flexor digiti minimi brevis.

The fourth layer comprises the plantar and dorsal interossei. These muscles arise from the bases and shafts of the metatarsals, soft tissues of the tarsometatarsal region, and the fasciae which separate the muscles.

6. Can the intrinsic muscles of the sole be grouped into functional compartments?

There are three osteofascial compartments in the foot. The large space enclosed by the tarsal bones, intertarsal joints, and plantar aponeurosis is subdivided into three smaller spaces by two intermuscular septa.

The medial intermuscular septum lies in an approximately sagittal plane, connecting the plantar aponeurosis to the plantar aspects of the calcaneus, navicular, intermediate cuneiform, and first metatarsal. The part of the aponeurosis medial to this septum attaches to the medial side of the tarsus. This forms the **medial osteofascial compartment**.

The lateral intermuscular septum also lies in an approximately sagittal plane. Its deep edge is attached to the calcaneus, cuboid, and fifth metatarsal, and its superficial edge to the plantar aponeurosis. The part of the aponeurosis lateral to the septum is attached to the lateral side of the tarsus, forming the **lateral osteofascial compartment**.

The remaining space, between the two septa, is the **central compartment**.

7. Which muscles are included within each of these compartments?

The muscles within the medial compartment are abductor hallucis and flexor hallucis brevis. They act on the hallux.

The muscles in the lateral compartment, both acting on the little toe, are abductor digiti minimi and flexor digiti minimi brevis.

All of the muscles of the central compartment, with one exception, act on the second, third, and fourth toes. They are the flexor digitorum brevis, quadratus plantae, the four lumbricals, and the interosseous muscles. The exception is the adductor hallucis, both of whose heads act on the hallux.

8. What is the "master knot of Henry"?

The tendons of flexor hallucis longus and flexor digitorum longus cross as they enter the central compartment of the foot, where fibers usually pass from the long hallucal flexor to flexor digitorum longus. In the 1940s, A.K. Henry observed that a band of connective tissue (actually a thickening of the medial intermuscular septum of the foot) loops across the two tendons at that point, strapping them to the plantar surface of the navicular. He found that reflecting abductor hallucis and cutting this strap, which he called the "master knot," allowed the plantar musculature to drop away from the bones and provide access to structures deep within the sole.

9. Is there such a muscle as extensor hallucis capsularis?

Strictly speaking, no. Some podiatrists use this term for a thin slip of the extensor hallucis longus tendon, which appears to serve a special function at the first MTP joint. This slip separates from the medial side of the main tendon, somewhere in the tarsal or metatarsal region, and inserts onto the joint capsule. It can insert either into the fibrous or synovial parts of the capsule, where it appears to function as a capsular retractor during extension of the hallux.

Extensor hallucis capsularis is an unofficial term and not really a good one. Although it has the form of a muscular name, it doesn't refer to a muscle, for no special belly is attached to this slip of tendon.

10. How is the sural nerve formed? What are its branches?

The sural nerve is strictly cutaneous, forming in the leg by the combination of branches of the tibial and common peroneal nerves. The **medial sural cutaneous nerve** is a branch of the tibial nerve, separating from it in the popliteal fossa. The **sural communicating branch** of the peroneal nerve appears near the head of the fibula, either as an independent branch or from the lateral sural cutaneous nerve. These two nerves join, usually in the upper part of the calf but variably from the popliteal fossa to the ankle. The sural nerve pierces the deep fascia at or below midcalf and then travels with the small saphenous vein. It runs first along the midline of the calf, then veers laterally to pass behind the lateral malleolus and enter the foot. In the leg, it supplies the posterolateral skin of at least the distal third of the calf and may extend somewhat onto the anterior surface.

As it enters the foot, the name of the sural nerve changes to **lateral dorsal cutaneous nerve**. This nerve supplies at least the heel (via lateral calcaneal branches), the lateral edge of the foot, and the lateral side of the fifth toe. It also sends a branch to join with the intermediate dorsal cutaneous nerve, extending its area of coverage to the fourth interspace.

11. Describe the source and path of the saphenous nerve.

The saphenous nerve is a branch of the femoral nerve, the only branch, in fact, to extend past the region of the knee. It is derived from the posterior division of the femoral nerve, travels in the adductor canal to just above the knee, and then becomes superficial. In the thigh and around the knee, it gives off several branches.

The **saphenous nerve** parallels the great saphenous vein along the medial side of the leg, supplying the skin. It gives off a number of small branches which are known collectively as the **medial crural nerves**. About two-thirds of the way down the leg, it splits into two branches. One travels along the medial border of the tibia to the ankle, which it may innervate. The other continues, in company with the vein, into the foot. It supplies skin on the medial edge of the foot, rarely reaching as far as the first MTP joint.

12. Which nerves supply the ankle?

The common peroneal and tibial nerves both send branches to the ankle, and the saphenous nerve may also innervate the joint.

Articular branches of the **deep peroneal** nerve branch off just proximal to the ankle. Others may come off the lateral and medial terminal branches of the deep peroneal nerve.

The articular branches from the **tibial** nerve generally appear before it divides into the medial and lateral plantar nerves, although sometimes twigs may come from them.

13. What is the distribution of the superficial peroneal nerve?

The common peroneal nerve ends within a tunnel between peroneus longus and the neck of the fibula, where it divides into its terminal branches. One of those branches is the superficial peroneal nerve which, in the upper part of the leg, innervates peroneus longus and peroneus brevis. About two-thirds of the way down the leg, the superficial peroneal nerve passes through the crural fascia, soon dividing into the medial and intermediate dorsal cutaneous nerves.

These two branches of the superficial peroneal supply most of the skin anterior to the ankle and on the dorsum of the foot. They remain in the superficial fascia, crossing superficial to the extensor retinacula and innervating the skin along their paths out to the toes. The following branching pattern is typical, but variations are fairly common.

At the level of the ankle joint, the medial dorsal cutaneous nerve divides into two dorsal digital nerves. The more medial is the proper dorsal digital nerve to the hallux, supplying the skin on the medial side of the great toe. The common dorsal digital nerve innervates the skin of the interspace between the second and third toes. The intermediate dorsal cutaneous nerve splits into two common dorsal digital nerves, going to the third and fourth interspaces.

It should be noted that the dorsal digital nerves do not innervate the skin out to the tips of the toes. The tips of the toes and at least the distal halves of the nail beds are supplied by the plantar nerves.

14. Describe the structures found in the first intermetatarsal space.

The space between the first and second metatarsals contains a number of structures which have varying functions and affect different parts of the foot. A sheet of connective tissue extends from one metatarsal to the next, placed so that the shafts of the bones are in the plantar compartment. Therefore, except for some of the joint structures, everything described here is located in the sole.

Structures related to joints. Parts of the MTP joint capsules bound the space. At the hallucal joint, they include the lateral metatarsosesamoid, phalangeosesamoid, and collateral ligaments. The medial collateral and suspensory ligaments of the second MTP joint can also be found. Very importantly, the first part of the deep transverse metatarsal ligament connects the plantar ligaments (plantar pads) of the two joints.

Intrinsic plantar muscles. Muscles lying in three of the four plantar layers can be found in the space. The first dorsal interosseous muscle is in the fourth layer. It arises from the facing sides of the first and second metatarsal shafts, forming a bipennate muscle whose tendon crosses dorsal to the deep transverse metatarsal ligament on its way to insert in the second toe. It bulges into the dorsum, although a membrane keeps the two compartments distinct. In the third layer, the lateral head of flexor hallucis brevis and the oblique head of adductor hallucis are in the interspace. The first lumbrical, in the second layer, lies plantar to the oblique head. It crosses inferior to the deep transverse metatarsal ligament.

Nerves. The first common plantar digital nerve travels between the first and second metatarsals. The space also includes muscular and articular twigs.

15. Which blood vessels are found in the first intermetatarsal space?

Although the first dorsal metatarsal artery is a dorsal structure, it often penetrates the first dorsal interosseous to run within the muscle. The plantar arch, a continuation of the lateral plantar artery, runs across the foot at the proximal ends of the intermetatarsal spaces. At the first space, it gives off the first plantar metatarsal artery, which for most of its path, lies in relation to the first metatarsal shaft. However, its distal part lies in the intermetatarsal space. The plantar arch anastomoses with the deep plantar branch, often a rather large vessel derived from the arteria dorsalis pedis. Farther anteriorly, there is an anterior perforating artery between the dorsal and plantar metatarsals. Near the distal ends of the spaces, the metatarsal arteries divide into digital arteries. The arteries are, of course, accompanied by venae comitantes.

16. Which nerves innervate the intrinsic muscles of the foot?

Nerve Branch	Muscle
Deep peroneal nerve, lateral terminal branch	Extensor digitorum brevis Extensor hallucis brevis
Medial plantar nerve, trunk	Abductor hallucis Flexor digitorum brevis
Medial plantar nerve, proper digital branch to the hallux	Flexor hallucis brevis
Medial plantar nerve, first common digital branch	First lumbrical
Lateral plantar nerve, trunk	Quadratus plantae Abductor digiti minimi
Lateral plantar nerve, superficial branch	Flexor digiti minimi brevis Third plantar interosseous Fourth dorsal interosseous
Lateral plantar nerve, deep branch	Second, third, and fourth lumbricals Adductor hallucis, oblique and transverse heads First and second plantar interossei First, second, and third dorsal interossei

The innervation of the muscles in the foot can be considered constant. In addition to the major motor nerves listed here some additional nerve supplies have been reported, although their functions are not clear. The first and second dorsal interosseous muscles may also receive twigs from the interosseous branches of the deep peroneal nerve. A nerve has also been described as branching from the lateral plantar nerve in the region of the calcaneal tuberosity, and entering flexor digitorum brevis.

BIBLIOGRAPHY

1. Mayer DB, Hirsch BE, Simon WH: Foot and Ankle: A Sectional Imaging Atlas. Philadelphia, W.B. Saunders, 1993.
2. Sarrafian SK: Anatomy of the Foot and Ankle, 2nd ed. Philadelphia, J.B. Lippincott, 1993.
3. Williams PL (ed): Gray's Anatomy, 38th ed. New York, Churchill Livingstone, 1995.

2. THE DIAGNOSTIC EVALUATION: LABORATORY WORKUP

Thomas M. DeLauro, D.P.M.

1. What is the lowest hemoglobin level considered safe for elective surgery?
< 10 gm/dl, regardless of sex.

2. In a patient taking exogenous corticosteroids, what tests may be used to evaluate the need for steroid coverage during surgery?
Exogenous corticosteroid dosages of 7.5 mg/day or greater taken for 3–4 weeks can suppress endogenous cortisol production for up to 1 year. Low plasma cortisol and ACTH levels indicate this suppression and demand that steroid coverage be ordered.

3. Which tests effectively screen for thyroid function abnormalities?
The simplest tests are the thyroid-stimulating hormone (TSH) and free thyroxine (FT_4), bearing in mind that they function in a negative feedback loop.

4. What is the relationship between serum calcium and phosphorus in evaluating bone disease?
Serum calcium and phosphorus exist in an inverse relationship—i.e., elevated serum calcium leads to decreased serum phosphorus, and vice versa.

5. Which tests of hemostasis screen for causes of petechial hemorrhage?
Petechial hemorrhages may result from vessel fragility, thrombocytopenia, or abnormalities of platelet function. A bleeding time and platelet count screen for these abnormalities, with the bleeding time often being used to evaluate platelet function.

6. In petechial hemorrhage, how does one interpret an elevated bleeding time with a normal platelet count?
The combination of an elevated bleeding time and normal platelet count identifies abnormalities of platelet *function* (the *number* of platelets is normal), such as von Willebrand's disease. Because aspirin and other NSAIDs can affect platelet function, a careful drug history should be obtained.

7. Which tests are normally included in a rheumatologic profile for patients suspected of having inflammatory joint disease?

CBC with differential
Erythrocyte sedimentation rate (ESR)
Rheumatoid factor
Antinuclear antibodies (ANA)
Serum chemistry

ANA subtypes and C-reactive protein also can be ordered, but these tests are often deferred until abnormalities in the first set of studies are discovered.

8. Explain the significance of eosinophilia on a peripheral blood smear.
Eosinophilia is found in association with parasitic infestations, allergies, drug reactions, dermatologic diseases, and collagen vascular diseases.

9. In patients with a family history of anesthesia death, which enzyme should be measured to assess an individual's susceptibility for malignant hyperthermia?
Preoperative elevation of a patient's **creatine kinase** level occurs in approximately 79% of patients susceptible for developing malignant hyperthermia.

10. What level of hypokalemia is considered a contraindication for elective surgery?
3 meq/l or less.

11. How can a patient's uric acid level be used to distinguish between primary and secondary hyperuricemia?
Normal uric acid levels range between 4–8 mg/dl. Primary (or inherited) hyperuricemia is usually associated with levels < 12 mg/dl, whereas secondary (due to increased cellular breakdown) hyperuricemia is 12 mg/dl and above.

12. What is the lowest platelet count considered safe for elective surgery?
Usually 100,000 cells/mm^3, with platelet transfusions considered only if the count reaches 50,000 cells/mm^3 or less. Platelet counts normally range between 150,000–400,000 cells/mm^3. In the absence of a history of bleeding, a normal prothrombin time (PT) and partial thromboplastin time (PTT) in patients with preoperative platelet counts > 50,000 but < 100,000 cells/mm^3 usually indicate that the patient may undergo elective surgery safely.

13. Explain the significance of a reversed albumin-globulin ratio.
The liver manufactures all of the body's albumin and most globulins. Reversal of the normal 2:1 ratio may indicate either hepatocellular disease (especially in the case of hypoalbuminemia) or abnormal production of globulins (as in myeloma).

14. Is the erythrocyte count the only true measure of anemia? At what levels is a further workup necessary?
No. Because the **hemoglobin concentration** truly measures the body's ability to deliver oxygen to the tissues, it is the most significant measure of anemia. A patient does not require further workup for anemia unless he or she is symptomatic and the hemoglobin is < 13 gm/dl in a male, < 12 gm/dl in a nonpregnant female, and < 11 gm/dl in a pregnant female.

15. Name two simple tests recommended for evaluating the progression or remission of osteomyelitis.
The erythrocyte sedimentation rate (ESR) and complete blood count (CBC).

16. Is there a certain level of leukocytosis that is considered indicative of a left shift even though band cells are not apparent?
Yes. Leukocytosis > 75% is considered the equivalent of a left shift, even though band cells are not apparent.

17. What finding on a peripheral blood smear can help distinguish between the different types of macrocytic anemia?
Macrocytic anemias can be divided into two types, megaloblastic and nonmegaloblastic. One of the most sensitive and specific signs of megaloblastic anemia is the presence of **hypersegmented neutrophils** on a peripheral blood smear.

18. What is the significance of a positive test for fluorescent treponemal antibody (FTA) in a patient previously treated for syphilis?
While the VDRL and rapid plasma reagin (RPR) tests in such patients revert to normal after successful treatment of syphilis, the FTA remains positive for the patient's lifetime.

19. Which tests of hemostasis are used to monitor heparin and warfarin (Coumadin) effectiveness?
Warfarin (Coumadin) interferes with the extrinsic and common coagulation pathways, specifically the vitamin K-dependent factors II, VII, IX, and X. The **prothrombin time** (PT) is used to monitor warfarin therapy, aiming for an international normalized ration (INR) of 2.0–3.0.

Heparin blocks the intrinsic and common pathways and is considered therapeutically effective when the **partial thromboplastin time** (PTT) is 1.5–2.0 times normal.

20. In the examination of synovial fluid under a polarizing microscope with a red-plate compensator, how can diagnosis be facilitated by the orientation of mixed yellow and blue crystals?

The red-plate compensator has a black line etched in it that is visible through the microscope eyepiece when you are looking at a slide. If yellow crystals are arranged parallel to that line and blue crystals are perpendicular to that line, then the crystals are negatively birefringent and consistent with monosodium urate (i.e., gout). On the other hand, if parallel crystals are blue and perpendicular ones are yellow, then positive birefringence exists, which is consistent with calcium pyrophosphate (i.e., pseudogout).

21. Prior to an in-office surgical procedure, a dipstick urinalysis demonstrates bilirubinuria. Should this finding alter your decision to perform the surgery?

Bilirubin is found in the urine only when the level of serum conjugated bilirubin is high, indicating hepatobiliary disease. Unconjugated (indirect) bilirubin is lipid-soluble, and so unconjugated hyperbilirubinemia does not spill over into the urine. Because amide local anesthetics, which are metabolized in the liver, are commonly employed in podiatric surgery, the possibility of hepatobiliary disease would definitely influence how and when the surgery would be performed.

22. Preoperatively, an elevated alkaline phosphatase is discovered in an adolescent female about to undergo juvenile hallux abductovalgus correction. Is this finding significant?

Alkaline phosphatase can be used as a marker of osteoblastic activity. In an adolescent still undergoing bony growth, one would normally expect to find an elevated alkaline phosphatase level. In the absence of any other abnormality, this finding would be considered insignificant.

23. Can other tests be ordered to distinguish between liver and bone as the source of an elevated alkaline phosphatase?

Either 5'-nucleotidase or gamma-glutamyl transpeptidase (GGT) can be ordered to confirm a hepatic origin for the elevated alkaline phosphatase, since neither 5'-nucleotidase nor GGT is found in bone.

Even mild associated elevations of alanine aminotransferase (ALT, or SGPT) or aspartate aminotransferase (AST, or SGOT) confirm a hepatic source. Bone disease does not cause elevations of AST or ALT.

24. How can the level and ratio of AST and ALT elevation be used diagnostically?

Enzyme levels > 500 U/L usually indicate acute viral hepatitis, whereas lower elevations (< 300 U/L) are more consistent with alcoholic liver disease, autoimmune hepatitis, and several other diseases. In alcoholic liver disease, the AST:ALT ratio is often > 2:1, but the level is still < 300 U/L.

25. Is it possible to use the alkaline phosphatase elevation versus aminotransferase elevation to divide patients into two groups for workup?

If the alkaline phosphatase elevation is more marked than that of AST and ALT, think of cholestatic or infiltrative (e.g., sarcoidosis, tuberculosis) disease. If the reverse is true, consider hepatocellular injury (e.g., viral hepatitis, autoimmune disease, drug-induced injury).

26. What is the diagnostic value of glycosylated hemoglobin (HbA$_{1c}$)?

Glycosylated hemoglobin provides an indication of the "average" blood glucose level during the preceding 120-day period (the average lifespan of an erythrocyte). High levels are generally associated with poor blood glucose control and vice versa.

27. In an elderly man complaining of leg cramps and weakness, what electrolyte deficiency may be causative, especially if he is taking a diuretic?

Probably one of the most common electrolyte deficiencies in this setting involves **potassium**. It becomes especially prominent when elderly patients eat poorly, because obligatory renal loss of potassium (in exchange for sodium reabsorption) that occurs daily is not compensated for in the diet.

28. When hypokalemia is discovered, an etiologic classification is possible if what other blood value is considered?

Potassium balance is intimately associated with acid-base homeostasis, and therefore an examination of the **serum bicarbonate** level is important as a first step toward recognizing an associated acid-base disturbance. Abnormalities of the serum bicarbonate (either elevated or decreased) warrant blood gas determinations.

29. Following a long podiatric surgery under tourniquet control, hyperkalemia is discovered during a routine blood chemistry panel. The patient is asymptomatic, and systemic etiologies have been excluded. What possible explanation remains?

Pseudo- or **spurious hyperkalemia** is the term applied to this situation, in which platelets in static blood (from the tourniquet) release their intracellular potassium into the serum. This is an in vitro phenomenon that does not occur in vivo. The same phenomenon occurs in blood that has been allowed to stand (and therefore coagulate) for 30–60 minutes before being analyzed.

30. A patient complaining of leg muscle fatigue is found to be hypocalcemic and have a low level of parathormone. Hypothalamic and parathyroid disease have been excluded, and the patient does not respond to exogenous calcium. Should another mineral abnormality be evaluated?

Patients with magnesium deficiency present with the described clinical picture. Magnesium is the second greatest intracellular cation (potassium is first). As intracellular magnesium is depleted (most commonly via gastrointestinal or renal loss, since oral intake is more than adequate in normal patients), parathormone release is decreased leading to hypocalcemia. The administration of parathormone or calcium will not correct the situation, and magnesium repletion is mandatory.

31. What is the RDW? What is its significance?

RDW stands for **red blood cell distribution width**, and it is used to distinguish between anemias that share similar mean corpuscular volumes (MCV). For example, both thalassemia and iron-deficiency anemia are microcytic; however, only iron-deficiency anemia has an abnormal RDW.

32. In the assessment of cardiac risk for patients undergoing noncardiac surgery (Goldman's criteria), a number of abnormal laboratory values indicate poor general health. Name these.

$PaO_2 < 60$ mmHg	BUN > 50 mg/dl
$PaCO_2 > 50$ mmHg	Creatinine > 3.0 mg/dl
$K^+ < 3.0$ meq/l	Abnormal AST (SGOT)
$HCO_3 < 20$ meq/l	

33. Explain the significance of a patient testing positive for HBsAg.

HBsAg, or hepatitis B virus surface antigen, is found on the surface of the viral particles, and its presence indicates that the patient has been infected with the hepatitis B virus. He or she now may remain asymptomatic, become an asymptomatic carrier, or progress to hepatitis (as evidenced by elevated aminotransferase levels). In any case, it is a sign that the patient may transmit the disease to others.

34. What is the significance of a patient testing positive for HBsAb?

HBsAb, or antibody to hepatitis B surface antigen, indicates that the body defenses have produced an immunoglobulin (or the patient has received a vaccine) against the surface antigen. The appearance of HBsAb coincides with the disappearance of HBsAg from the serum and signifies that the patient is now immune from the disease and noninfectious.

35. HIV positivity is established by what testing sequence?

The initial screen is an enzyme-linked immunosorbent assay (ELISA). Positive results are submitted to Western blot testing for confirmation.

36. Why are leukocyte esterase and nitrite tests performed during urinalysis?

Each of these tests is meant to be an indirect measure of bacteriuria, since they detect bodily responses to urinary tract infection or bacterial byproducts, respectively. They do not replace bacterial culture or quantitative analysis, which would be appropriate followup investigations.

37. An order for electrolytes testing returns a value for serum chloride but not bicarbonate. Can this value be useful?

Chloride is the most abundant extracellular anion, followed by bicarbonate. Because dietary salt is abundant, the body has no shortage of chloride. Chloride is passively absorbed from the intestine and renal tubule with sodium but is "exchanged" for bicarbonate (in the same organs) to maintain electroneutrality.

As a result of these regulations, chloride measurement per se is of little value; instead, its measurement is of great value from what one can infer as an indicator of acid-base and water balance. In metabolic alkalosis, serum chloride is low because bicarbonate is high; the reverse is true in metabolic acidosis. In aldosteronism, chloride is carried along with the increase in serum sodium, leading to water retention.

38. Is a measurement of CO_2 content in serum the same as that found in an arterial blood gas?

No. In serum, 95% of CO_2 comes from bicarbonate (which is regulated by the kidneys), and only 5% is dissolved CO_2 gas (controlled by the lungs). Whereas CO_2 determined by arterial blood gas is a measure of pulmonary ventilation, serum CO_2 content is a measure of bicarbonate and therefore a general estimate of alkalinity or acidity.

39. Why are absolute white blood cell counts preferred over differential white cell counts?

Differential counts merely indicate the relative percentage of one cell type over another in a count of 100 random leukocytes. The differential does not distinguish between true elevations or decreases in a cell type versus apparent changes because a different cell type actually changed. For example, it is unclear if an increase in the percentage of neutrophils is the result of an *increase* in the actual number of neutrophils or the result of a *decrease* in the actual number of non-neutrophil leukocytes. Absolute cell counts can be calculated for each type of WBC.

40. How can an absolute lymphocyte count be used as a measure of immunodeficiency?

Lymphocytes are important in maintaining immunocompetence. The absolute lymphocyte count is determined by multiplying the percentage of cells (in a differential count) that are lymphocytes by the total number of leukocytes. For example, if 25% of cells in a different count were lymphocytes and the WBCs measured 8000/mm^3, then the absolute lymphocyte count is 0.25 × 8000, or 2000 lymphocytes/mm^3. Any patient with an absolute lymphocyte count of < 1000 lymphocytes/mm^3 should be considered immunocompromised.

41. Is a single ASO titer sufficient in following a patient with a streptococcal infection?

Single measurements are inadequate because they do not indicate whether the titer is rising (which would indicate an exacerbation) or decreasing (signifying cure or remission). Serial ASO titers are therefore required if the diagnosis has been confirmed or is the primary working diagnosis awaiting corroborating laboratory evidence.

42. Should patients who are hyponatremic automatically be given exogenous salt?

No, since hyponatremia can occur in patients with elevated, decreased, or normal plasma osmolarity. Exogenous salt would worsen a hyperosmolar patient and is not indicated in patients with normal plasma osmolarity.

43. The lab reports several bacteria on Gram stain but only one organism on culture and sensitivity testing. How do you interpret this finding?

This combination of findings could indicate the presence of anaerobes that appear on the Gram stain but are not recovered when the typical aerobic culture (without consideration of the need for anaerobic cultures) is performed.

44. How do you determine a patient's LDL cholesterol fraction from the values for total cholesterol, HDL cholesterol, and triglycerides (the values normally given on SMAC testing)?

$$LDL = \text{total cholesterol} - HDL - \left(\frac{\text{triglycerides}}{5}\right)$$

The value of triglycerides divided by 5 represents the very low density lipoprotein (VLDL) fraction.

45. In a patient with mildly elevated levels of serum AST, ALT, and gamma-glutamyl transpeptidase, what follow-up tests are immediately in order?

Mild elevations of these substances indicate some degree of hepatocellular injury. In view of the widespread nature of the hepatitis viruses, these diseases should be excluded as the cause of the enzyme elevations. Hepatitis viruses A and E are transmitted by the fecal-oral route, while types B, C, and D are blood-borne. In terms of frequency and potential complications, it would probably be wise to order HBsAg and HCV studies for hepatitis B and C, respectively.

46. In the workup for a patient for anemia, can a few simple tests distinguish among hemolysis, hypoproliferation, and defective erythropoiesis?

- High reticulocyte counts (> 3 after correction for changes in hematocrit) indicate hemolysis.
- The combination of an elevated indirect bilirubin and lactate dehydrogenase (LDH) is indicative of defective erythropoiesis.
- If all of these tests are normal, a low transferrin saturation level (calculated by dividing the serum iron by the total iron-binding capacity and expressed as a percent) is a warning of hypoproliferative disease.

47. In patients with a low transferrin saturation level, what additional test can separate individuals with iron-deficiency anemia from those with anemia of chronic disease?

The **serum ferritin** level: if low, iron-deficiency anemia is suggested; if normal, anemia of chronic disease.

48. Aspiration of an inflamed first metatarsophalangeal joint reveals a yellow, opaque fluid with numerous polymorphonuclear leukocytes on microscopic examination. What is your interpretation?

This finding is consistent with a class III joint aspirate (septic arthritis). If the fluid was cellular but more transparent, an inflammatory or class II aspirate would be diagnosed (as in acute gouty arthritis). Lastly, a clear fluid with few cells is termed class I and is found in normal joints.

CONTROVERSIES

49. After an individual has been confirmed as HIV-positive, is elective foot surgery considered "safe" for the patient?

The danger posed by invasive procedures to HIV-positive patients is related to that patient's ability to avoid and fight infection. The best measure to determine a person's immunocompetence is the number of T lymphocytes with the CD4 surface marker (HIV selectively destroys these lymphocytes).

The normal CD4 lymphocyte count in non–HIV-infected individuals is 600–1500 cells/mm^3. One may safely presume that persons with a CD4 count < 500 cells/mm^3 may be HIV-positive. As these cells further decrease in number, so does a patient's ability to avoid and defend against bacterial (including acid-fast types), fungal, or viral colonization. HIV-positive patients should have their CD4 lymphocytes recounted every 2–6 months: every 6 months for counts that are near-normal, but more frequently as the counts drop lower.

The generally accepted cutoff for **elective** surgery is 200 CD4 lymphocytes/mm^3. Lower counts are believed to put the patient at great risk for infection, making elective foot surgery contraindicated. Obviously, in the case of limb or life-saving procedures (i.e., diabetic foot infections), this risk becomes a moot point since preservation of the patient's limb or life is paramount. The **date** of the last CD4 count is always important in HIV-positive patients, because the value may have increased, stabilized, or decreased since it was last checked.

50. Should HLA-B27 assays be ordered in a patient suspected of having spondyloarthropathy-associated heel pain?

The seronegative spondyloarthropathies include psoriatic arthritis, Reiter's disease, ankylosing spondylitis, and the enteroarthropathies (ulcerative colitis, regional enteritis). The HLA-B27 marker has proved to be a sensitive marker for each of these diseases. The utility of this test, however, is diminished by the following factors:

1. As high as 10% of the normal population will test positive for HLA-B27.

2. Despite the test's high sensitivity and specificity for the listed diseases, only a fraction of individuals with positive results actually go on to develop a spondyloarthropathy.

The first discovery leads to a high number of false-positives, while the second finding limits the predictive value of an affirmative test. HLA-B27 testing, therefore, should probably be reserved as a last resort. Reliance on clinical and radiographic findings, as well as serologic markers of inflammation and autoimmune disease, are probably the wiser choice.

BIBLIOGRAPHY

1. Bhopale S, Gundling K: Superficial thrombophlebitis and DVT: When to suspect the latter when you see the former. Consultant 36(1):140–143, 1996.
2. Davenport J: Macrocytic anemia. Am Fam Phys 53(1):155–162, 1996.
3. Ginsberg AL: Liver enzyme abnormalities: How to interpret the diagnostic implications. Consultant 36(3):575–578, 1996.
4. Lipshitz DA, Wheby MS: How far to go in the anemia workup. Patient Care August 15, 1993, pp 76–94.
5. Nadler JL, Rude RK: Disorders of magnesium metabolism. Endocrinol Metab Clin North Am 24:623–641, 1995.
6. Noskin GA, AMA Advisory Group: Prevention, diagnosis, and management of viral hepatitis. Arch Fam Med 4:923–934, 1995.
7. O'Duffy JD: Acute monarthritis: Managing the swollen, painful joint. Consultant 36(3):431–438, 1996.
8. Riegel RT, Neushwander-Tetri BR: Liver function tests. Hosp Phys 32(4):13–16, 19, 58, 1996.
9. Rutecki GW, Whittier FC: Hypokalemia: Clinical implications, consequences, and corrective measures. Consultant 36(1):124–139, 1996.
10. Rutecki GW, Whittier FC: Hyperkalemia: How to identify—and correct—the underlying cause. Consultant 36(3):564–573, 1996.
11. Woodley M, Whelan A (eds): Manual of Medical Therapeutics, 27th ed. Boston, Little, Brown and Co., 1992.
12. Zier B: Essentials of Internal Medicine in Clinical Podiatry. Philadelphia, W. B. Saunders, 1990.

3. DIAGNOSTIC RADIOLOGY

Kim Felder-Johnson, D.P.M.

1. What conditions could be associated with a radiographic finding of a well-marginated spur present at the insertion of the plantar aponeurosis?
- Rheumatoid arthritis
- Normal variation
- Reiter's syndrome
- Acromegaly
- Diffuse idiopathic skeletal hyperostosis

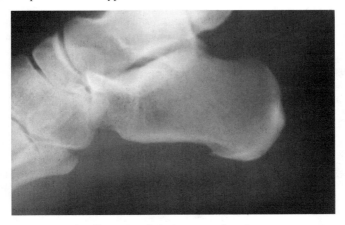

A well-marginated plantar spur on the calcaneus.

2. What conditions could be associated with a radiographic finding of an ill-defined erosive alteration present along the posteroanterior aspect of the calcaneus?
- Psoriatic arthritis
- Hyperparathyroidism
- Rheumatoid arthritis
- Reiter's syndrome
- Ankylosing spondylitis

3. The density of anatomic structures varies on computed tomography. List anatomic structures from highest to lowest density.
Cortical bone, cancellous bone, muscle, nerve, tendon, ligament, subcutaneous fat, air.

4. What is the difference between T1- and T2-weighted images on MRIs?
T1 and T2 are tissue-specific constants which are different for each tissue. T1-weighted images demonstrate differences in T1 between tissues and are obtained with a short TR (repetition time) and short TE (echo time). T2-weighted images demonstrate differences in T2 between tissues and are obtained with a long TR and a long TE. T1 values for tissue generally are dependent on the fat content of the tissue, while T2 values for tissue are dependent on the water content of the tissue. Thus on T1-weighted images, body tissues or structures containing greater amounts of fat will be most intense or bright. On T2-weighted images, body tissues or structures containing greater amounts of water will be most intense or bright.

5. Which radiographic views are used in evaluating ankle injuries and which of these views is most useful?

The most useful radiographic view of the ankle joint for evaluating injury is the anterior-posterior view. Most avulsion, malleolar, and distal fibular fractures can be identified and evaluated. The anterior tibial tubercle overlaps the fibula more than the posterior tibial tubercle. The joint spaces between the tibia, talus, and fibula should be uniform and clearly defined in a normal study. The lateral view is most helpful in evaluating posterior tibial fractures. The lateral also allows the joint space and contour to be evaluated. The distal aspect of the fibula is superimposed on the tibia and talus; however, the distal aspect of the tibia can be observed beyond the posterior aspect of the fibula. The mortise view, which is taken with the leg approximately 20–30 degrees internally rotated, is used in conjunction with the other two views to evaluate ankle injuries. The mortise view allows the medial and lateral malleoli to be in the same plane, reducing the amount of overlap. This view allows for evaluation of the congruity of the talus, which in the normal view should have a smooth fit of the talar dome with the lateral tibia malleolus, the tibial plafond, and the medial fibula malleolus. This view also allows for the determination of associated soft tissue injuries.

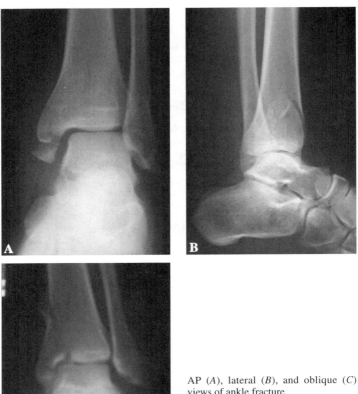

AP (*A*), lateral (*B*), and oblique (*C*) views of ankle fracture.

6. What is Hawkin's sign?

Hawkin's sign is the radioluceny present in the subchondral area of the talar dome seen 6 to 8 weeks post-talar neck fracture-dislocation on an anteroposterior radiograph of the ankle. This rules out the diagnosis of talar body avascular necrosis.

7. What is avascular necrosis?

Avascular necrosis, also known as osteonecrosis, is bone death resulting from a vascular insult. The vessels may be damaged directly as in trauma or occluded by emboli or elevated marrow pressure. The most common sites include the hips, shoulders, medial femoral condyle, and talus.

8. What is the earliest radiographic sign of avascular necrosis?

The radiographic appearance of avascular necrosis can vary but the earliest sign is often a "crescent" sign, which represents a subchondral fracture through the insertion of the individual trabeculae, which are infarcted, and the subchondral bone, which receives some of its nutrients from the synovial fluid and overlapping cartilage. Areas of dead bone appear normal radiographically and do not change density except when the bone impacts or when reactive new bone is laid down alongside the dead trabeculae.

9. What are some common causes of avascular necrosis?

Avascular necrosis can be caused by post-traumatic, non-traumatic, or idiopathic conditions. Post-traumatic causes include fractures, dislocations, and microfractures. Non-traumatic conditions include emboli (which can be seen with hemoglobinopathies-sickle-cell disease, caisson disease, alcoholism, pancreatitis), small vessel disease (such as in systemic lupus erythematosus and giant cell arteritis) and abnormal deposition of cell (such as in Cushing's disease and Gaucher's disease). Some idiopathic presentations may be seen with degenerative arthritis, gout, prolonged immobilization, cytotoxic therapy, associated hyperparathyroidism, metastases, lymphoma, and pregnancy.

10. What are some differential diagnoses for calcaneal erosions?

A list of differential diagnoses for calcaneal erosions can include rheumatoid arthritis, ankylosing spondylitis, Reiter's syndrome, psoriatic arthritis, lipoid dermatoarthritis, and hyperparathyroidism.

11. What is the hallmark radiographic sign of a peroneal subluxation/dislocation?

Peroneal tendon dislocations involve avulsion of the osteocartilaginous attachment of the peroneal tendon sheath to the fibula. The result is a small avulsion fracture that is best seen on the posterolateral corner of the distal fibula. This fracture is the hallmark radiographic sign of the peroneal subluxation/dislocation.

12. What are the guidelines for evaluating ankle fractures radiographically?

1. The fibula and then the medial malleolus and posterior lip of the tibia are examined for a fracture.

2. The width of the medial clear space (joint) and the width of the syndesmosis are determined.

3. If a fracture is present on one side of the joint, the opposite side of the joint should be examined closely for evidence of fracture or ligament avulsion.

4. If no fracture is seen in the distal fibula but there is an isolated transverse fracture of the medial malleolus, isolated widening of the medial clear (joint) space or syndesmosis, or isolated fracture of the posterior tibial lip, a radiograph of the entire tibia and fibula is required to rule out fracture of the proximal fibula. Inspection of the medial and lateral malleoli and the posterior lip of the distal tibia for fractures after an ankle injury is elementary, since fractures are present in these areas in as many as 90 percent of ankle injuries with fractures.

13. What is Boehler's angle and what is its significance?

Boehler's angle is evaluated on a lateral radiograph and formed by a line drawn from the superior posterior margin of the tuberosity through the superior tip of the posterior facet. A second line is drawn from the superior tip of the posterior facet through the superior margin of the anterior process of the calcaneus. Normal Boehler's angle measures 20–40 degrees and is decreased in calcaneal fractures. In severe fractures the angle may even be negative. Bilateral lateral films should always be compared to determine if Boehler's angle has changed following an injury involving the calcaneus.

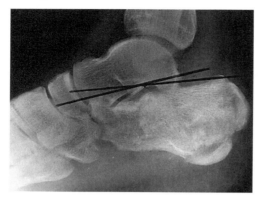

The Boehler's angle is decreased in this calcaneal fracture. (From Katz D, Math K, Groskin S: Radiology Secrets. Philadelphia, Hanley & Belfus, 1998.)

14. What is a true Jones fracture?

A Jones fracture is a transverse fracture of the fifth metatarsal base. The fracture is located 1.5 to 2 cm from the tip of the metatarsal tuberosity or styloid process. The original description of this fracture was made in 1902 by Sir Robert Jones, who reported a fracture that he had sustained while dancing and had diagnosed by radiographic examination. Thus this fracture is sometimes known as dancer's fracture. It is the result of the plantarflexion and inversion of the foot. It is

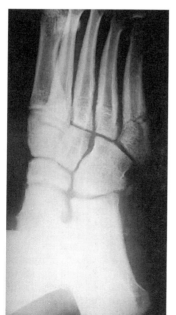

Jones fracture. (From Katz D, Math K, Groskin S: Radiology Secrets. Philadelphia, Hanley & Belfus, 1998.)

actually an avulsion injury mediated through the peroneous brevis tendon. It is differentiated from a styloid fracture, which occurs in the metaphysis and can be observed on an oblique view of the foot.

15. What are some considerations when evaluating and classifying a bone tumor?
Points of value when evaluating and classifying a bone tumor include:
- The origin of growth (medullary, cortical or periosteal, epiphyseal, diaphyseal or metaphyseal)
- The presence of new bone and its character
- The presence of any bone destruction
- The presence of any soft tissue invasion
- Whether the lesion is expansile or extends up or down the shaft of the bone
- Whether there is a sharp line of demarcation or irregular, ill-defined border
- Whether the cortex has been disrupted
- Whether the lesion is single or multiple
- The rapidity of the growth of the lesion

16. What are the radiographic features of a benign or slow-growing bone tumor?
Characteristics of benign or slow-growing bone lesions include: small, well-demarcated lesions that have little or no soft tissue mass; preserved cortical margins that appear sclerotic; solid, uninterrupted periosteal reaction with a narrow zone of transition; the overall appearance is geographic and there is usually trabeculation.

17. What are the radiographic features of a malignant bone lesion?
Characteristics of malignant bone lesions include large lesions with ill-defined or absent margins, usually there is cortical erosion or destruction, periosteal reaction is common and may be irregular, onion peeling or Codman's triangle presentations, the boundaries are usually indistinct, there is a wide zone of transition with permeation into the surrounding soft tissue and bone, there is no sclerosis of the margins, and the overall appearance is moth-eaten or permeative.

18. What is Codman's triangle?
Codman's triangle is a characteristic periosteal elevation and spicule formation that represents tumor extension into the periosteum with calcification.

19. The location of a bone lesion is of diagnostic significance with respect to the portion of the bone that is involved. List the preferential site of origin or the portion of bone the following lesions are most likely to originate from: (a) Ewing's tumor, (b) chondroblastoma, (c) myeloma, (d) giant cell tumor, after fusion of the growth plate, (e) osteogenic sarcoma, (f) fibrosarcoma, (g) unicameral bone cyst, (h) nonossifying fibroma, (i) giant cell tumor, prior to fusion of the growth plate, (j) reticulum cell sarcoma, (k) chondrosarcoma.
Those tumors that preferentially originate in the epiphysis are the chondroblastoma and the giant cell tumor after fusion of the growth plate. The metaphysis is usually the site of origin for the osteogenic sarcoma, fibrosarcoma, unicameral bone cyst, nonossifying fibroma, and the giant cell tumor prior to fusion of the growth plate. The myeloma, Ewing's tumor, and reticulum cell sarcoma are located in the diaphysis.

20. What is the difference between an enthesophyte and osteophyte?
Osteophytes are the result of new bone formation following cartilage degeneration due to any cause. Osteophytes typically form around joints. Osteophyte formation occurs mostly with degenerative arthritis, osteoarthropathy such as with Charcot foot, acromegaly, and trauma. Enthesophytes occur at the site of insertion of tendons, ligaments, or articular capsule into bone. Enthesopathies appear radiographically as calcification of a tendon, capsule, or ligament at or near the site of insertion. Enthesopathy can be seen with inflammatory arthropathies, arthrosis, and metabolic and endocrine disorders.

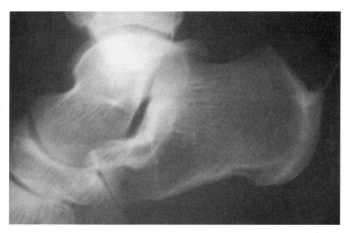

Enthesophyte.

21. Three months following effective hallux abducto valgus corrective surgery, a 30-year-old woman is experiencing chronic pain and swelling in the surgical foot. The surgery was uneventful except for problems with the tourniquet compression. The patient after six weeks began experiencing vasomotor changes and hair loss to the affected foot. Early radiograph demonstrated good alignment and well-approximated osteotomy of the metatarsal head. Both three and four month x-ray demonstrated loss of joint space and patchy areas of osteoporosis with clean cut margins. Clinically, the patient is hypersensitive to touch around the incision site and to motion of the joint, soft tissue swelling, and edema. There are no clinical signs of infection and the patient has completed six weeks of physical therapy with minimal improvement. What is the most likely diagnosis?

Reflex sympathetic dystrophy. The radiographic appearance shows patchy areas of osteoporosis that appear to have clean cut margins. This process is characteristically painful and associated with soft-tissue swelling. It usually presents clinically about three to six months following the insult, which may be trauma, surgery, or anything resulting in a neurocirculatory disturbance. It is also suggested that there may be an imbalance between the sympathetic and parasympathetic nervous system.

22. What is the classification system used to define epiphyseal injuries in children and what are the types?

The Salter-Harris classification system is used to assess epiphyseal fractures in children. The classification consists of five types of fractures.

Type I consists of a fracture that runs completely through the cartilaginous plate with no fracture of the actual osseous fracture. This type is sometimes referred to as a pure epiphyseal separation and radiographically presents as a separation of the epiphyseal ossification center. This injury is common under the age of five and represents approximately six percent of all epiphyseal injuries.

Type II is the most common injury and presents as a fracture that extends partially through the plate and also breaks off a portion of the metaphysis of the bone. This is usually due to shearing or avulsive forces and occurs most frequently in the 10–16 year age group. The hallmark of this injury is an associated triangular metaphyseal fragment, referred to as a "corner sign."

Type III is a fracture that runs partially through the plate and then extends distally through the joint. Radiographically, the epiphysis is detached and there is no associated fracture of the metaphysis. This fracture is the result of an intra-articular shearing force and is frequently seen in the 10–15 year age group.

Type IV is a fracture that starts proximal to the epiphysis and runs through the epiphysis and into the joint. The fracture is usually vertically oriented, resulting from a splitting force that extends across the epiphysis, growth plate, and metaphysis. Radiographically, the fragment consisting of a portion of both the metaphysis and epiphysis is evident.

Type V is a crushing injury to the epiphysis. This type is rare and usually there is no immediate radiographic evidence. The effects of this injury usually appear later and are observed as bone shortening and joint deformation. Sport and auto accidents account for the majority of these injuries.

23. Due to excellent soft tissue contrast and good spatial resolution, magnetic resonance imaging is useful in evaluating osteomyelitis. How would osteomyelitis present on MRI and how can this be differentiated from neuroarthropathy?

The sensitivity of MRI in detecting the presence of osteomyelitis is 94–100 percent. The specificity has had variable reports, ranging from 69–96 percent. With MRI, osteomyelitis appears as decreased signal intensity on T1-weighted images and increased signal intensity on T2-weighted images within the intramedullary space. Neuroarthropathy may present with low signal intensity within the bone marrow on both T1- and T2-weighted images, with ill-defined joint spaces in contrast to the low signal intensity on T1-weighted images and high signal intensity on T2-weighted images. It has been reported, however, that although chronic Charcot joints can be of low signal intensity on all pulse sequences, acute, rapidly progressive neuroarthropathy creates high signal intensity on T2-weighted images. In such cases, osteomyelitis may be indistinguishable from non-infected, rapidly progressing neuroarthropathic disease.

24. How will an abscess present on MRI and how can an abscess be distinguished from soft tissue edema?

Abscesses can be detected as well-defined regions of strikingly high signal intensity on T2-weighted or STIR images, indicating fluid. Abscess can be distinguished from soft tissue edema or cellulitis by a smooth margin and higher signal intensity than that of the surrounding edema. This differentiates abscess from cellulitis, in which the margins are ill-defined. The differentiation between an abscess and cellulitis may be difficult in some patients due to decreased contrast between the abscess and surrounding abnormal signal in the soft tissues.

25. What is the classic appearance of a stress fracture on MRI?

A linear zone of decreased signal intensity on T1-weighted sequences that is surrounded by a broad and more poorly defined area that is of lower signal intensity than the linear component. Typically, the linear component remains dark on T2-weighted sequences, but the surrounding zone of presumed hemorrhagic and nonhemorrhagic edema becomes inhomogeneously brighter. The linear components may be short and straight or long and serpiginous and are typically perpendicular to the adjacent cortex.

26. What is the hallmark of osteonecrosis due to an uncomplicated infarction of medullary bone on MRI?

The appearance of a reactive interface. The reactive interface represents a distinctive layer of inflammatory fibromesenchymal tissue that develops at the margin between viable and infarcted medullary bone in osteonecrosis. On MRI the reactive interface is represented as a well-defined low signal intensity line or arc demarcating the margin of the necrotic segment from viable bone on T1-weighted images. This line represents replacement of fat by granulation tissue.

27. In an abnormal arthrogram of the ankle, the contrast medium always extravasates in a predictable manner, which allows for diagnosis of ligamentous injuries about the ankle. What is the arthrographic pattern in disruption of the posterior talofibular ligament and in the disruption of the calcaneofibular ligament?

There is no distinctive pattern associated with a rupture of the posterior talofibular ligament because this type of rupture is associated with tears of other lateral collateral ligaments. The arthrographic pattern of a calcaneofibular ligament is extravasation of the dye into the peroneal sheath. A rupture of the calcaneofibular ligament is always associated with a tear of the anterior talofibular ligament, which results in the dye flowing anterior and lateral to the lateral malleolus. The dye may overlie the syndesmosis, but on the lateral view there will remain a clear space between the dye and the syndesmosis.

28. Describe the phases of a three-phase bone scan.

The first is the early or immediate phase, which can be seen the first few seconds after the IV injection. The distribution of the radionuclide is in the arterial tree. The presentation of this phase would be an arteriogram. The second phase is the blood pool phase. This phase can be seen two to five minutes post IV injection. This phase represents the regional blood flow. The third is the delayed or static phase. This phase is seen two to three hours post IV injection of the radionuclide material. This phase represents bone uptake and urinary excretion.

29. What would the bone scan of a person with reflex sympathetic dystrophy look like?

Increased blood flow with increased activity during the blood pool images will be seen in the affected limb. In the third phase or delayed images, the joints of the affected limb will demonstrate increased periarticular activity.

30. What are the best planes to evaluate a suspected middle facet subtalar coalition by computed tomography?

The axial and coronal planes. This is because the facet usually has a slope of 45 degrees and therefore is equidistant from both planes.

BIBLIOGRAPHY

1. Deutsch AL: Traumatic injuries of bone and osteonecrosis. In Deutsch AL, Mink JH, Kerr R (eds): MRI of the Foot and Ankle. New York, Raven Press, 1992.
2. Haller J, Resnick D, Sartoris D, et al: Arthrography, tenography, and bursography of the ankle and foot. Clin Podiatr Med Surg 5(4):893–908, 1988.
3. McGlamry ED (ed): Comprehensive Textbook of Foot Surgery, 2nd ed. Baltimore, Williams & Wilkins, 1992, pp 300–310.
4. Perlman MD, et al: Traumatic classifications of the foot and ankle. J Foot Surg 28(6):551–558, 1989.
5. Rogers LF: Radiology of Skeletal Trauma. New York, Churchill Livingstone, 1982.
6. Sartoris DJ, Resnick D: Test of radiologic interpretation: The calcaneus. J Foot Surg 27(5):484–487, 1988.
7. Solomon MA, Oloff-Solomon J: Computed tomographic scanning of the foot and ankle. Clin Podiatr Med Surg 5(4):931–944, 1988.
8. Spaeth HJ, Dardani M: Magnetic resonance imaging of the diabetic foot. MRI Clin North Am 2(1):123–129, 1994.
9. Weissman SD: Radiology of the Foot, 2nd ed. Baltimore, Williams & Wilkins, 1989.

4. DERMATOLOGY

Richelle Day, D.P.M., and Mardon Day, D.P.M.

1. Name the three most common dermatophytes infecting the skin and nails of the feet.
Trichophyton rubrum
Trichophyton mentagrophytes
Epidermophyton floccosum

2. List the four clinical types of fungal nail infections.
• Distal subungual onychomycosis
• Superficial white onychomycosis
• Proximal subungual onychomycosis
• Candida onychomycosis

3. Name the three types of tinea pedis. Which dermatophyte is most commonly associated with each?
Interdigital infections, moccasin distribution, and vesiculobullous or inflammatory infection. **Interdigital** infections present as scaling, maceration, fissuring, or erythema of the webspaces between the toes. This infection is usually associated with *Trichophyton rubrum* or *T. mentagrophytes*. **Moccasin distribution** presents as generalized scaling and hyperkeratosis of the plantar surface and is frequently associated with nail involvement. Moccasin-type tinea pedis is typically caused by *T. rubrum*. The **inflammatory** or **vesiculobullous** type will cause a vesicular eruption on the arch or side of the foot and is most often caused by *T. mentagrophytes*.

4. What is erythrasma?
Erythrasma is a chronic bacterial infection caused by *Corynebacterium minutissimum* affecting the interdigital spaces. The interspace appears macerated with erythematous, sharply defined borders. A characteristic "coral-red" fluorescence is seen when viewing the lesions under a Wood's lamp.

5. What are the diabetes-related skin disorders?
Diabetic dermopathy, necrobiosis lipoidica diabeticorum, diabetic xanthomatosis, bullosis diabeticorum.

6. Describe the lesions seen with necrobiosis lipoidica diabeticorum.
These lesions are irregularly shaped, depressed, atrophic plaques with a yellow-brown center and red borders and with possible areas of ulceration. They most commonly occur on the anterior lower leg (see figure, top of next page).

7. What are the ABCDE's of melanoma.
The development of a new or changing pigmented lesion is the classic initial presentation of melanoma. A lesion that demonstrates a noticeable increase in size over a period of weeks to months or development of pigment irregularity (black, hues of brown, red, blue, or white) should be evaluated by a physician and biopsied. The **ABCDE's** of melanoma are a helpful guideline for determining which moles could be suspicious for melanoma:
  A—Asymmetrical shape.
  B—Border is irregular.
  C—Color is mottled.
  D—Diameter is usually large (> 6.0 mm).
  E—Elevation is usually present.

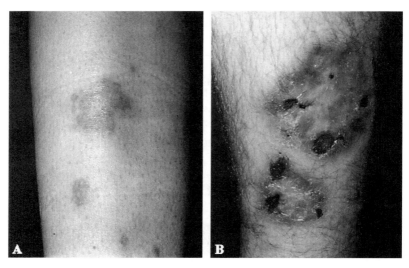

Necrobiosis lipoidica diabeticorum. *A,* Typical yellow-red plaque of an early lesion. *B,* Late lesion, with central atrophy, focal ulceration, and peripheral hyperpigmented rim. (From Fitzpatrick JE, Aeling JL: Dermatologic Secrets. Philadelphia, Hanley and Belfus, 1996, with permission.)

8. Which types of melanoma are seen most frequently?

Superficial spreading is the most common form of melanoma in whites. It is a slowly enlarging brown (usually) or black spot that may have both a macular and papular component. The lesion may show color variegation and irregular borders.

Nodular is a pigmented (usually brown or black) papule that slowly enlarges and frequently ulcerates. Nodular melanomas may ulcerate, presenting as a nonhealing skin ulcer.

Acral lentiginous is the most common form in blacks, Asians, and Hispanics. It usually appears as brown or black macules arising on palms, soles, or nailbeds.

Lentigo maligna usually presents as an irregularly shaped, flat, pigmented lesion on actinically damaged skin. More advanced lesions can develop papules or nodules, indicating the lesion has developed a vertical or downward growth component.

9. List the anatomical components of the toenail unit from distal to proximal.

1. Nail plate	4. Medial and	6. Eponychium
2. Hyponychium	lateral nail fold	7. Cuticle
3. Nail bed	5. Lunula	8. Matrix

10. What are the primary skin lesions?

Primary Skin Lesions

PRIMARY LESION	DEFINITION	MORPHOLOGY	EXAMPLES
Macule	Flat, circumscribed skin discoloration that lacks surface elevation or depression	Macule	Café au lait Vitiligo Freckle Junctional nevi Ink tattoo

Table continued on following page.

Primary Skin Lesions (Continued)

PRIMARY LESION	DEFINITION	MORPHOLOGY	EXAMPLES
Papule	Elevated, solid lesion < 0.5 cm in diameter	Papule	Acrochordon (skin tag) Basal cell carcinoma Molluscum contagiosum Intradermal nevi Lichen planus
Plaque	Elevated, solid "confluence of papules" (> 0.5 cm in diameter) that lacks a deep component	Plaque	Bowen's disease Mycosis fungoides Psoriasis Eczema Tinea corporis
Patch	Flat, circumscribed skin discoloration; a very large macule	Patch	Nevus flammeus Vitiligo
Nodule	Elevated, solid lesion > 0.5 cm in diameter; a larger, deeper papule	Nodule	Rheumatoid nodule Tendon xanthoma Erythema nodosum Lipoma Metastatic carcinoma
Wheal	Firm, edematous plaque that is evanescent and pruritic; a hive	Wheal	Urticaria Dermographism Urticaria pigmentosa
Vesicle	Papule that contains clear fluid; a blister	Vesicle	Herpes simplex Herpes zoster Dyshidrotic eczema Contact dermatitis
Bulla	Localized fluid collection > 0.5 cm in diameter; a large vesicle	Bulla	Pemphigus vulgaris Bullous pemphigoid Bullous impetigo
Pustule	Papule that contains purulent material	Pustule	Folliculitis Impetigo Acne Pustular psoriasis
Cyst	Nodule that contains fluid or semisolid material	Cyst	Acne Epidermoid cyst Pilar cyst

From Fitzpatrick JE, Aeling JL: Dermatology Secrets. Philadelphia, Hanley and Belfus, 1996, with permission.

11. What are the secondary skin lesions?

Secondary Skin Lesions

SECONDARY LESION	DEFINITION	MORPHOLOGY
Crust	A collection of cellular debris, dried serum, and blood; a scab Antecedent primary lesion is usually vesicle, bulla, or pustule	
Erosion	A partial focal loss of epidermis; heals without scarring	
Ulcer	A full-thickness, focal loss of epidermis and dermis; heals with scarring	
Fissure	Vertical loss of epidermis and dermis with sharply defined walls; crack in skin	
Excoriation	Linear erosion induced by scratching	
Scar	A collection of new connective tissue; may be hypertrophic or atrophic Scar implies dermoepidermal damage	
Scale	Thick stratum corneum that results from hyperproliferation or increased cohesion of keratinocytes	

From Fitzpatrick JE, Aeling JL: Dermatology Secrets. Philadelphia, Hanley and Belfus, 1996, with permission.

12. How do the Auspitz sign, Koebner phenomenon, and Nikolsky sign differ?

Auspitz sign—Pinpoint bleeding that occurs when the scale of a psoriatic lesion is removed

Koebner phenomenon—Secondary skin lesion, such as psoriasis or eczema, caused by physical trauma

Nikolsky sign—Epidermal detachment produced by lack of skin cohesion, often seen in blistering skin diseases

13. What causes plantar verrucae? Describe their clinical appearance.

Plantar verrucae are caused by the human papilloma virus, which invades the skin usually by trauma. Verrucae typically have a hyperkeratotic border, without skin lines traversing the lesion, and display pinpoint bleeding on debridement. They occur singly, in groups, or in large numbers in a widespread distribution (mosaic verrucae).

14. Describe the appearance of a typical psoriatic skin lesion.

It consists of sharply defined "salmon pink" papules or plaques covered by silvery scales.

15. What nail changes can occur with psoriasis?

Pitting
Subungual hyperkeratosis
Onycholysis
"Oil spot," a yellow-brown spot under the nail plate (pathognomonic!)

16. Describe the lesions seen with lichen simplex chronicus.

The lesions are puritic red or hyperpigmented solid plaques of thick lichenification (attenuated skin lines) usually seen around the ankle area. They are caused by the predilection of the skin to respond to physical trauma with epidermal hyperplasia, which results in the skin becoming highly sensitive to touch due to the proliferation of nerves in the epidermis.

17. How do the lesions seen with dyshidrotic eczematous dermatitis present clinically?

Early in the disease course, there are small deep-seated vesicles, resembling tapioca, in clusters that may form large bullous lesions. The bullous form is called pompholyx. Late in the disease, scaling, lichenification, painful fissures, and erosions may occur.

18. What are the possible treatment options for dyshidrotic eczema?

Wet-to-dry dressings in the vesicular stage and Burow's soaks.
Topical steroids in the later stage when fissuring, scaling, and lichenification are seen.
Oral antibiotics if signs of bacterial infection are also seen.
Dietary restriction of certain metals (nickel, cobalt, chromium) that may cause a reaction.
PUVA oral or topical as soaks.
Systemic corticosteroids.

19. Define onychocryptosis and the other nail disorders.

Onychocryptosis—chronic pressure on the lateral nail fold by the nail plate
Onychauxis—hypertrophic nail plate
Leukonychia—idiopathic white nail formation
Koilonychia—spoon-shaped nail usually caused by iron deficiency
Onycholysis—distal-to-proximal separation of the nail from the nail bed
Onychomadesis—proximal separation of the nail from the nail bed
Onychogryphosis—hypertrophic nails resembling ram's horns

20. Describe the clinical appearance of basal cell carcinoma.

It presents as a skin-colored lesion with raised borders, and the central area of the lesion may be depressed and crusted. The lesion bleeds easily with friction.

21. How do the lesions of Kaposi's sarcoma present clinically? In which populations are these lesions most commonly found?

The lesions are purple or echymotic in color and consist of raised macules, papules, plaques, nodules, or tumors. They are most commonly seen in patients with AIDS (epidemic Kaposi's sarcoma) and middle-aged males of Jewish or Eastern European heritage.

22. What are the main clinical features of a glomus tumor?
- Slow-growing solitary lesion, extremely painful
- Often located subungually at the end of a digit or completely beneath the nail plate
- Red to purple color, blanches on pressure
- Recurrence common with incomplete excision

23. List the differential diagnosis for a glomus tumor.

Subungual fibroma	Pyogenic granuloma
Kaposi's sarcoma	Malignant melanoma

24. How is a hypertrophic scar differentiated from a keloid formation?
Hypertrophic scar—Results from abnormal collagen proliferation laid down parallel to the skin surface; encapsulated staying within the original scar
Keloid—Fibrous tissue hyperplasia with fibroblasts arranged in randomly oriented parallel strands; nonencapsulated, extending beyond the limits of the original scar

25. How does erythema nodosum present? Who is most commonly affected?
- Lesions present as deep red, tender, circumferential nodules on the anterior aspect of the lower leg.
- They are most commonly seen in females and associated with pregnancy, birth control pills, infections (strep, fungal, tuberculosis), and inflammatory bowel disease
- Treatment consists of aspirin, bed rest, warm compresses, and system steroids.

26. Where is an interdigital corn most often found?
Between adjacent surfaces of the fourth proximal interphalangeal joint and the fifth distal interphalangeal joint.

27. Which disease processes may cause splinter hemorrhages in the nail?
Subacute bacterial endocarditis and trichinosis.

28. What are Beau's lines within the nail? List the proposed etiologies.
Beau's lines are horizontal depressions across the nail plate. They are caused by transient arrest in nail growth due to acute stress, such as high fever, circulatory shock, myocardial infarction, or pulmonary embolism.

29. With which associated disorder is periungual fibroma frequently seen?
A periungual fibroma is a flesh-colored nodule seen usually at the nail fold. When found at the proximal nail fold, a longitudinal groove in the nail plate is seen, which is caused by pressure on the matrix cells. It is very commonly seen with tuberous sclerosis.

30. What is the nail matrix?
These specialized epithelial cells begin 7–8 mm under the proximal nail fold and undergo division to form the nail plate.

31. Describe the clinical presentation of a glomus tumor.
This painful, bluish to red, vascular tumor regulates distal digital blood flow. The associated pain is pulsating and worse at night.

32. How do the lesions of lichen planus present?
Lichen planus in an inflammatory skin disorder which presents as violaceous, polygonal, flat-topped papules. The surface of the lesion possesses fine whitish dots and lines called Wickham's striae.

BIBLIOGRAPHY

1. Albert SF: Disorders of the nail unit. Clin Podiatr Med Surg 13(1):13–27, 1996.
2. Brooks KE, Bender JF: Tinea: Diagnosis and treatments. Clin Podiatr Med Surg 13(1):31–46, 1996.
3. Cobb MW: Human papillomavirus infection. J Am Acad Dermatol 22:547, 1990.
4. Ditre C, Howe N: Surgical anatomy of the nail unit. J Dermatol Surg Oncol 18:665–671, 1992.
5. Dockery GL: Dermatology flow sheet. Clin Podiatr Med Surg 3(3):391–397, 1986.
6. Graff GE: General cutaneous examination of the podiatric patient. Clin Podiatr Med Surg 3(3):385–389, 1986.
7. Hoffman AF, Driver VR: Onychomycosis. Clin Podiatr Med Surg 13(1):13–27, 1996.
8. Hutchinson BL: Malignant melanoma in the lower extremity. Clin Podiatr Med Surg 3(3):533–550, 1986.
9. McCarthy D: Anatomic consideration of the human nail. Clin Podiatr Med Surg 12:164, 1995.
10. McCarthy D: Therapeutic considerations in the treatment of pedal verrucae. Clin Podiatr Med Surg 3(3): 433–448, 1986.

5. NAIL ANATOMY AND PATHOLOGY

L. V. Grant, D.P.M., and Simon Nzuzi, D.P.M.

1. Name two well-defined clinical disorders of nails that are brought on or exacerbated by HIV infection.
Onychomycosis and psoriatic nail.

2. How do you treat leukonychia and longitudinal nail-ridging caused by osteoarthritic changes of the distal interphalangeal joints?
Local steroidal and anti-inflammatory treatment of the osteoarthritic node.

3. How do you diagnose the yellow nail syndrome?
Yellow nail syndrome is usually described as the combination of yellow nails, lymphedema, and respiratory manifestations, such as chronic sinusitis, bronchiectasis, and pleural effusions. The diagnosis is clinical, not requiring any specialized tests, but all the above features need not be present.

4. Separation of the nail plate from the bed is common with which conditions?
Psoriasis
Eczema
Candida or *Pseudomonas* infection

5. Which anatomic structures help form the nail base angle?
The nail base angle is formed by the proximal nail fold and nail plate.

6. The nail and base angle are increased in which four diseases?
1. Glandular disease
2. Hyperthyroidism
3. Hyperparathyroidism
4. Cardiovascular disease

7. The lunula is absent in which local and systemic conditions?
Club nail, acromegaly, hypopituitarism.

8. Define ONYX.
ONYX is a term used to describe onychocryptosis, or an ingrown nail.

9. Moisture and wetness considerably decrease nail discomfort of what nail condition?
Onychophosis, which is a corn in the nail groove. It is softened by moisture, which also makes it easier to reduce.

10. What is Terry's nail?
It is a nail presentation involving an opaque and white nail plate with a 1–3-mm pink band at the free edge of the nail on digits 1, 3, and 4 associated with diabetes mellitus. It was originally described in chronic liver disease (cirrhosis).

11. In which systemic conditions do Beau's lines appear?
Arsenic poisoning, eczema, diabetes mellitus, and malaria cause change of the nail plate, leading to one or more white lines across the nail, which disappear after the condition is corrected.

31

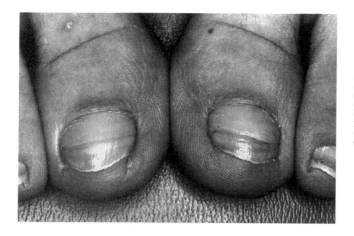

Beau's lines, with an abrupt demarcation across the nail from a systemic insult. (From Fitzpatrick JE, Aeling JL: Dermatology Secrets. Philadelphia, Hanley & Belfus, 1996, with permission.)

12. Muehrcke's lines are present in which systemic conditions?
Muehrcke's lines are white bands with loss of lunula and are present in liver disease, hypoalbuminemia, and nephrotic syndrome.

13. Roseneau's depression of the nail plate is found in which systemic disease?
Diabetes mellitus.

14. Why is tinea unguium (onychomycosis) rarely seen in children?
Children are rarely affected by trichophytosis, which is the cause of 70% of fungal nail infections.

15. Give two other names for Osther's Lori nail.
Osther's Lori nail, an extensive overgrowth of the nail plate caused by neglect, is also known as ram's horn or onychogryphosis.

16. What is the name of the process by which the nail plate may fall off in onychogryphosis, onychauxis, and diabetes mellitus?
Phlogosis. In this process the thickening of the nail plate causes the nail plate to lift off the nail bed.

17. What is the fungal etiology of chronic paronychia in children?
Candida albicans.

18. Describe the differential diagnosis of nail pitting seen in psoriatic nails.
Psoriatic nails are characterized by superficial pits about 1 mm or less in diameter. The same kind of nail pitting (onychia punctata) may be found in other inflammatory diseases, such as:

Eczema	Reiter's syndrome
Alopecia areata	Dermatomyositis
Histiocytosis	

19. What is the term used to describe any disorder that causes dystrophy of all 20 nails?
Twenty-nail dystrophy, which is primarily seen in endocrinopathies.

20. How does the Koebner phenomenon affect the toenails?
The Koebner phenomenon, or isomorphic effect, is instrumental in the development of nail and skin reaction at sites of local injury in psoriasis, lichen planus, lichen nitidus, Darier's

disease, and pityriasis rubra pilaris. In it, lesions typical of these diseases appear on uninvolved skin or nails subjected to pressure.

21. Why is tinea unguium more common in toenails than fingernails?
1. Warm, moist environment of the shoe enhances fungal growth.
2. Trauma caused by the shoe provides a site for infection.
3. Hyperhidrosis, diabetes mellitus, and decreased vascular supply can be contributing co-morbid sites.

22. List the four classifications of onychomycosis in order of frequency.
1. Distal subungual onychomycosis (most common)
2. Superficial white onychomycosis (common)
3. Proximal subungual onychomycosis (uncommon)
4. Chronic mucocutaneous candidiasis

23. What two bacterial organisms are commonly found with *Pseudomonas aeruginosa* as the cause of acute paronychia?
Staphylococcus and *Streptococcus* group A.

24. Splinter hemorrhages can be signs of which severe underlying systemic conditions?
Splinter hemorrhages are due to oozing of blood from damaged, longitudinally oriented vessels of the nail bed or matrix region. Trauma is the most common cause, but splinter hemorrhages assume greater clinical importance in subacute bacterial endocarditis, vasculitis, and adverse drug reactions (tetracycline and phototoxic response), in which they signal the underlying disease.

25. How do the histologic findings of Darier's disease in the nail bed differ from the findings of disease in the skin?
The nail bed findings in Darier's disease differ by the absence of **suprabasilar cells**, the presence of **multinucleated epithelial cells**, and the near-absence of **inflammatory infiltrate**.

26. An increase in growth rate of the nails may be associated with which common conditions?
Pregnancy, psoriasis, and nail biting (injury). Normal nail growth averages 0.5–1.2 mm/week, or 0.1 mm/day, but may accelerate to ≥ 2 mm/week in these conditions. Other conditions causing increased nail growth include onycholysis, periungual inflammation, onychophagia, and the premenstrual state.

27. Name four conditions affecting the nail plates that occur as a result of abnormal differentiation of cells in the matrix and with abnormal keratinization.
1. Psoriasis   3. Leukonychia
2. Fungal infection   4. Onychoschizia

28. Which is the most common complication of the nail overgrowth onychogryphosis?
Pyogenic granuloma. In this condition the nail plate becomes loose and irritates the nail bed, which becomes infected.

29. What nail plate change is found in diseases such as psoriasis, alopecia areata, and onychomycosis but not in post-trauma nail changes?
Pitting.

30. Name six benign tumors or tumor-like growths associated with nail disorders.
Garlic clove fibroma (subungual fibroma)   Pyogenic granuloma
Glomus tumor   Mucous cyst
Keratoacanthoma   Pigmented nevus

31. A 67-year-old woman with diabetes mellitus and chronic liver disease presents with dystrophic mycotic nails. What is the local treatment of choice?

Application of urea 40% after mechanical debridement.

32. A 35-year-old woman presents with diffuse grayish-brown toenails. What do you suspect she has?

Onychauxis secondary to syphilis.

33. A red band on one or more nails suggests that the patient has what systemic disease?

Cardiac failure. Thyrotoxicosis causes congestive heart failure, and the nail can develop a red band.

34. Name five malignant tumors that can affect the nails.

1. Epithelioma
2. Bowen's disease
3. Malignant melanoma
4. Squamous cell carcinoma
5. Basal cell carcinoma

35. A 68-year-old man presenting with nail signs of distal red bank, red lunula, and white proximal nail plate is suspicious for what systemic disease?

Cirrhosis.

36. Name four conditions that can cause onycholysis.

1. Paronychia
2. Eczema
3. *Pseudomonas* infection
4. Allergy

37. Blue lunula is suggestive of what systemic disease?

Normally, the lunula is a white, moon-shaped structure at the proximal aspect of the nail plate, but in Wilson's disease it turns blue.

38. What is the typical depth of soft tissue found between the nail bed epithelium and the bone of the distal phalanx?

1 mm.

39. What is the proper method for obtaining a good specimen for culture from suspicious white onychomycosis?

Material is collected by simply scraping the dorsal surface of the nail plate with scalpel blade.

40. What KOH concentration is suitable for nail analysis?

The usual first step in evaluating suspected onychomycosis in the clinician's office is to perform a direct KOH preparation. There are several different KOH preparations, but 20–40% KOH concentration enhances clearing of many artifacts.

41. What is the action of KOH preparation on fungal cells?

KOH dissolves bonds that hold the keratinized cells together. As a result, the fungal elements present are exposed for identification. Elements that have taken up a fluorescent dye are enhanced in their visibility.

42. How do you judge whether an antifungal is clinically effective in onychomycosis (dermatophytosis) and *Candida albicans* infection?

First, a small wedge of the nail plate is cut from the surface of the normal and abnormal junction of the plate of a patient who is receiving the proper antifungal dose. This wedge establishes a clinical barrier to the proximal invasion of the fungus. The part of the new nail plate proximal to the wedge will be normal on subsequent microscopic examination.

43. What is the nail bed?

The nail bed is the epidermal structure beginning with the distal portion of the lunula and terminating with the hyponychium. It produces very small numbers of cells with no granular layer.

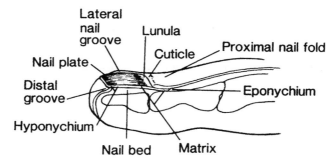

Nail bed and other toenail structures. (From Mellion MB: Office Sports Medicine, 2nd ed. Philadelphia, Hanley & Belfus, 1996, with permission.)

44. What is the hyponychium?

It is the extension of the volar epidermis under the nail plate that ends adjacent to the nail bed.

45. To increase the positive rate for nail specimens sent for fungal culture, which part of the nail should be sent to the laboratory?

Send a portion of the nail over the nail bed, about 3 mm in length, and subungual nail debris.

46. Why don't saprophytes and some yeasts grow in dermatophytic media?

An inhibitor called cycloheximide is present in the media.

47. How long does it take fungal organisms to grow on dermatophytic test cultures for a final identification by the laboratory?

3–6 weeks.

48. One cannot determine and institute a proper treatment for nail fungal infection on the basis of clinical impression alone. Why?

- Many fungal infections are clinically similar to each other.
- Nail infection may be caused by a mixture of dermatophytes, yeasts, and nondermatophyte molds.
- Laboratory identification of the infecting organism is essential for determining a proper treatment.
- Specific fungi respond only to a specific antifungal drug.

49. Most antifungal medications used today are effective primarily against which type of fungi?

Dermatophytic organisms.

50. To ensure a successful clinical management of nail fungal infection, what type of medication should be used?

Broad-spectrum medications specific for yeasts, dermatophytes, or nondermatophytic organisms.

51. Name the drug of choice and oral dosage for tinea unguium.

Itraconazole (Sporanox, Janssen Pharmaceutic Inc.), 200 mg daily orally for 3 months.

52. What is the oral drug of choice and dosage for treatment of *Candida albicans* and *Cryptococcus neoformans* infection in a patient with HIV/AIDS?
Fluconazole (Diflucan, Pfizer), oral "triazone," 150 mg daily for 3 months or 15 mg a month for 12 months.

53. What percentage of patients without joint disease have psoriatic nail abnormalities?
Psoriatic nail involvement in many cases may be the only clue to the diagnosis of psoriatic arthritis, even though nail manifestations are not specific to diagnose psoriasis. Approximately 20% of patients without joint disease have abnormal nails and approximately 20% of the patients with psoriatic nails have joint disease.

54. Name six nail disorders due to nail matrix abnormalities from any source.

Beau's line	Onychorrhexis
Pterygium	Koilonychia
Onychoschizia	Leukonychia

55. List some conditions associated with anonychia.
Anonychia is the complete absence of one or more nails. It is a rare condition and may be due to a congenital ectodermal defect, sequelae of Stevens-Johnson syndrome, frostbite, toxic infection, Raynaud's disease, emotional disorders, Darier's disease, lichen planus, subungual tumors, fungal infection, psoriasis, febral condition, ichthyosis, surgery, or physical, chemical, and mechanical trauma.

56. The presence of green nails with discoloration and discharge suggests what organisms?
Pseudomonas aeruginosa and *Candida albicans*. Onycholysis of the distal portion of the nail is usually present.

57. What are the three types of nail clubbing as described by Stone?
1. Hippocratic fingers
2. Hypertrophic osteoarthropathy
3. Pachydermoperiostosis

Clubbing of the nail was first described by Hippocrates. Friedreich in 1868 described the idiopathic hypertrophic osteoarthropathy, for which Marie coined the term *pulmonary hypertrophic osteoarthropathy*. Finally, Touraine et al. described pachydermoperiostosis.

BIBLIOGRAPHY

1. Beaven DWD, Brooks SE: Fungal infections and onychomycosis. In A Color Atlas of the Nail in Clinical Diagnosis. Weert, Netherlands, Wolfe Medical Publ, 1984, pp 82–89.
2. Burke WA, Jones BE: A simple stain for rapid office diagnosis of fungus infections of the skin. Arch Dermatol 120:1519–1520, 1984.
3. Cutolo M, Cimmino MA, Accardo S: Nail involvement in osteoarthritis. Clin Rheumatol 9(2):242–245, 1990.
4. Daniel CR (ed): The Nail. Dermatol Clin North Am 3:440, 1985.
5. Daniel CR, Lawson LA: Tinea unguium. Cutis 40:326–327, 1987.
6. Elder BL, Roberts GD: Rapid methods for the diagnosis of fungal infections. Lab Med 17:591–596, 1986.
7. Greene RA, Scher RK: Nail changes associated with diabetes mellitus. J Am Acad Dermatol 16:1015–1021, 1987.
8. Kechijian P: Onycholysis of the fingernails: Evaluation and management. J Am Acad Dermatol 12:552–560, 1985.
9. Leahy AL, Timon CI, Craig A, Stephens RB: Ingrowing toenails: Improving treatment. Surgery 107:566–567, 1990.
10. Nzuzi SM: Nail entities: Clin Podiatr Med Surg 6(2):258–259, 1989.
11. Ro B: Granuloma pyogenicum. Int J Dermatol 25:10, 1986.
12. Scher RK, Daniel CR (eds): Nail Therapy. Philadelphia, W.B. Saunders Co. (in press).

6. HALLUX/FIRST RAY: PART I

Richard O. Jones, D.P.M., M.P.H.

ANATOMY

1. Define hallux valgus.

A deformity of the first metatarsophalangeal (MTP) joint involving a lateral and/or rotational deviation of the hallux with or without a medial and/or dorsal prominence of the first metatarsal head.

2. Name the bones of the first ray.

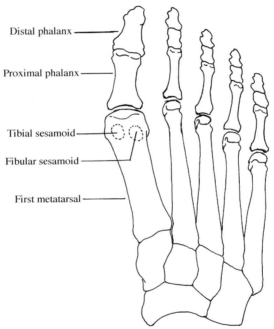

Distal phalanx

Proximal phalanx

Tibial sesamoid

Fibular sesamoid

First metatarsal

Bones of the first ray. (Adapted from Whitney AK: Radiographic Charting Technic, 1978, with permission.)

3. What nerves are anesthetized in a Mayo nerve block?
1. Deep peroneal—terminal branch
2. Terminal saphenous
3. Medial dorsal cutaneous
4. Medial plantar nerve

4. Name the seven muscles that contribute to the sesamoid complex.
1. Extensor hallucis longus
2. Extensor hallucis brevis
3. Abductor hallucis
4. Medial head, flexor hallucis brevis
5. Flexor hallucis longus
6. Lateral head, flexor hallucis brevis
7. Abductor hallucis

5. What first ray structure separates the two sesamoids?
First metatarsal crista.

37

6. List the three types of first metatarsal heads, from least to most stable.
1. Round
2. Square
3. Square with a ridge

7. What is the most likely etiology of a painful callus beneath the distal joint?
Hallux interphalangeal sesamoid (supernumerary sesamoid).

BIOMECHANICS

8. What biomechanical factors influence the rate of hallux valgus progression?
Stage I   Lateral displacement of proximal phalanx to the first metatarsal head
Stage II   Hallux abduction deformity
Stage III   First-ray subluxation
Stage IV   Dislocation or major subluxation

9. Name the biomechanical mechanism of the plantar fascia resulting in first-ray plantarflexion?
The windlass effect of Hicks. As the toes begin to extend, the plantar fascia wraps around the metatarsal heads, which causes the arch to elevate without the use of muscle force.

10. Loss of flexor hallucis brevis stabilization results in what deformity?
Hallux malleus, or cocked-up hallux.

11. Describe the axis of motion of the first-ray joint?
The axis of the first ray parallels the transverse plane, so that there is no motion in that plane. When the first ray plantarflexes, it also everts. When the ground dorsiflexes, first-ray inversion occurs simultaneously.

12. Rupture of what muscle can result in first-ray dorsiflexion, hallux limitus, and/or forefoot supinatus?
Peroneus longus.

13. In evaluation of the first MTP joint, what is considered normal active range of motion of dorsiflexion and plantarflexion?
65–75° dorsiflexion
> 15° plantarflexion

14. What two biomechanical laws result in enlargement of the medial eminence and redundancy of the medial capsule during chronic pronation, lateral first MTP joint deviation, and subluxation?
1. Wolff's law—Law of functional adaptation of bone and traction medial eminence formation. Bone is able to reorient itself by rearranging its lamellae and trabeculae in relation to mechanical tension and stress.
2. Davis' law—Capsular stretch. Soft tissue under constant tension elongates. The adverse is also true.

15. How do structural and functional hallux limitus differ?
Structural—Dorsiflexion of the first MTP joint is decreased when the forefoot is both loaded and unloaded.
Functional—Dorsiflexion of the first MTP joint is decreased only when the forefoot is loaded.

16. How does one determine hallux purchase?
Place a piece of paper under the great toe, ask the patient to stand, and then try to pull the paper out.

RADIOLOGY

17. In a congruent joint, the hallux abductus angle is equal to the sum of what two angles?
Proximal articular set angle (PASA) and distal articular set angle (DASA).

18. What are the normal angles as measured on a weight-bearing anteroposterior radiograph?

1. Hallux abductus angle	0–15°
2. Hallux abductus interphalangeal angle	0–10°
3. Intermetatarsal angles	8–12° in rectus foot
	8–10° in adductus foot
4. PASA and DASA	7.5° each
5. Metatarsus adductus angle	15°

19. What is the normal tibial sesamoid position on a weight-bearing anteroposterior radiograph?
The normal position is 1–3.

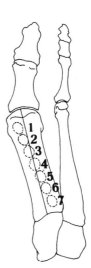

From Whitney AK: Radiographic Charting Technic. 1978, with permission.

20. Describe the radiographic findings in hallux limitus.
1. Joint narrowing
2. Flattening of the first metatarsal head
3. Osteophytes-Geodes-loose bodes in the first MTP joint space
4. Subchondral sclerosis
5. First metatarsal elevatus

21. What is the significance of first metatarsal declination?
It indicates preexisting sagittal plane deformity or elevation. The method for determining its presence is bisecting either the first metatarsal or talus on a weight-bearing radiograph. The normal position is parallel.

22. What are the radiographic findings in performing a hallux interphalangeus arthrodesis?
1. Contracted interphalangeal joint
2. Interphalangeal joint arthritis
3. Abnormal hallux interphalangeal abductus angle
4. Abnormally short or long hallux
5. Adequate bone stock of distal and proximal phalanx

SURGERY

23. In first-ray osteotomies, what three techniques can achieve osseous correction in any plane?
1. Transposition
2. Angulation
3. Derotation

24. List the different fixation and stabilizing methods used in first-ray osteotomies.
1. Casting
2. Kirschner/Steinmann pins (smooth and threaded)
3. Staples
4. Sutures
5. Screw and/or plate fixation
6. External fixators
7. Impaction
8. Non–weight-bearing

25. Describe the function in a nonbiased two-screw fixation position in a closing abductory base wedge osteotomy.
The distal screw perpendicular to the osteotomy gives compression. The proximal screw perpendicular to the shaft prevents translation.

26. Name three soft-tissue correction bunionectomies.
1. Silver
2. McBride
3. Hiss

27. What are the five capital head osteotomies in bunion surgery?
1. Austin
2. Reverdin
3. Reverdin-Green
4. Reverdin-Laird
5. Reverdin-Todd

28. What is the ideal positioning for the frontal, transverse, and sagittal planes in first MTP joint arthrodesis?
1. Frontal   0°
2. Transverse   20–30° valgus
3. Sagittal   15–20° dorsiflexion

29. What nine types of first MTP joint capsulotomies are used in bunion surgery?
1. Mediovertical
2. Medial-U
3. Medial-H
4. Medial-T
5. Inverted-L
6. Dorsolinear
7. Dorsal-T
8. Lenticular
9. Washington Monument

30. In a unicorrectional Austin bunionectomy, what is the angle between the two arms of the V-osteotomy? Why this angle?
60°. Angles greater or less than 60° can result in overcorrection, undercorrection, displacement of capital fragment, or delayed union (see figure).

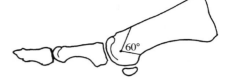

Adapted from Whitney RAK: Radiographic Charting Technic, 1978, with permission.

31. What are the indications for arthrodesis of the first MTP joint?
1. Recurrent hallux valgus
2. Previous infection
3. Traumatic arthritis
4. Hallux rigidus
5. Failed Keller
6. Severe hallux valgus
7. Neuromuscular instability

32. What combination of procedures is performed with the Logracino?
Reverdin, closing abductory wedge base osteotomy, and capsule tendon-balancing procedure.

33. List eight hallux limitus procedures.
1. Arthrodesis
2. Watermann
3. Modified Waterman
4. Kessel-Bonney
5. Implant arthroplasty
6. Regnauld
7. Lambrinudi
8. Green-Watermann

34. What is the advantage of a crescentric base osteotomy compared to a closing base wedge osteotomy?
No wedge of bone is removed in the crescentric procedure, and so there is negligible shortening of the first metatarsal.

35. What are the indications for hallux nail matricectomies?
1. Onychocryptosis (ingrown nail)
2. Onychomycosis (fungal infection)
3. Onychauxis (thickened nail)
4. Onychogryphosis (dystrophic nail)
5. Onycholysis (separated)
6. Incurvation

36. What are the possible complications of performing a tibial sesamoidectomy?
1. May increase a hallux abductus deformity.
2. Loss of range of motion of first MTP joint.
3. If flexor hallucis longus tendon is injured, a hallux extensus or cocked-up hallux may occur.

POSTOPERATIVE CARE

37. Following a closing abductory base wedge osteotomy, how long should a patient avoid weight-bearing?
6–8 weeks.

38. Following an Austin bunionectomy, when should the Steinmann pin(s) be removed?
3–6 weeks.

39. Following bunion surgery, when should the sutures be removed?
10–21 days.

40. Prophylaxis during implant arthroplasty should be performed with which drug? Against what primary organism?

Vancomycin, 1 gm administered over 60–90 minutes, to protect against *Staphylococcus epidermidis*, which is the primary pathogen in infections following implant arthroplasty.

41. Patients requiring tricortical bone grafting for a failed first MTP implant arthroplasty or failed fusion should be kept non–weight-bearing for how long?

12 weeks.

COMPLICATIONS

42. What are the potential disadvantages of performing the traditional Keller resectional arthroplasty?

1. Shortened hallux
2. Cocked-up hallux
3. Loss of function of first MTP joint
4. Metatarsalgia
5. First-ray instability
6. Need for orthosis with Morton's extension
7. Lesser metatarsal stress fractures
8. Painful joint pseudoarthrosis and joint osseous proliferation

43. Which organism causes most postoperative infection in hallux valgus surgery?

Coagulase-positive *Staphylococcus aureus*.

44. What are the contributing etiologies of iatrogenic hallux varus?

1. Staking the first metatarsal head
2. Overcorrection of the intermetatarsal angle
3. Overzealous capsulorrhaphy
4. Overcorrection of the proximal articular set angle
5. Overzealous bandaging
6. Excising fibular sesamoid

CONTROVERSY

45. In performing a first metatarsal closing abductory base wedge osteotomy, do you orient the osteotomy perpendicular to the metatarsal or to the weight-bearing surface?

Before the 1980s, it was generally accepted to orient the osteotomy cut perpendicular to the long axis of the first metatarsal. Today, most surgeons perform the osteotomy to the weight-bearing surface. If the cut is to the shaft, you get frontal plane rotation, which results in a net loss of ground contact. However, Steven Palladino, using a mathematical model, found that the difference in outcomes was statistically insignificant with either method of orientation. Therefore, it might be acceptable to orient the osteotomy according to the surgeon's preference or level of expertise.

BIBLIOGRAPHY

1. Austin DV, Leventen EO: A new osteotomy for hallux valgus: A horizontally directed "V" displacement osteotomy of the metatarsal head for hallux valgus and primus varus. Clin Orthop Rel Res 157:25, 1981.
2. Bonney G, Macnab I: Hallux valgus and hallux rigidus: A critical survey of operative results. J Bone Joint Surg 34B:366, 1952.
3. Clough JG, Marshall HJ: The etiology of hallux abducto valgus: A review of the literature. J Am Podiatr Med Assoc 75:238, 1985.
4. Draves DJ: Anatomy of the Lower Extremity. Baltimore, Williams & Wilkins, 1986.
5. Fortman D, Keating SE, DeVincentis AF: Prophylactic antibiotic usage in podiatric implant surgery of the 1st metatarsophalangeal joint. Foot Surg 27:66, 1988.

6. Gerbert J: Textbook of Bunion Surgery, 2nd ed. Mount Kisco, NY, Futura, 1991.
7. Higgins KR, Lavery LA, Ashy HR, et al: Structural analysis of absorbable pin and screw fixation in first metatarsal osteotomies. JAMA 85:528–532, 1995.
8. Joseph WS (ed): Clin Podiatr 1990.
9. Jules KT (ed): Clin Podiatr 1989.
10. Keller WL: Surgical treatment of bunions and hallux valgus. N Y Med J 80–741, 1904.
11. Mann RA (ed): Surgery of the Foot, 5th ed. St. Louis, C.V. Mosby, 1986.
12. Mann RA, Coughlin MJ: Hallux and valgus and implications of hallux valgus. In Mann RA (ed): Surgery of the Foot. St. Louis, C.V. Mosby, 1986, pp 65–67.
13. McGlamry ED (ed): Comprehensive Textbook of Foot Surgery, 2nd ed. Baltimore, Williams & Wilkins, 1992.
14. Marcus SA, Block BH: American College of Foot Surgeons Complications in Foot Surgery: Prevention and Management, 2nd ed. Baltimore, Williams & Wilkins, 1984.
15. Nelson JP, Fitzgerald RH Jr, Jaspers MT, et al: Prophylactic antimicrobial coverage in arthroplasty patients. J Bone Joint Surg 72A:1, 1990.
16. Palladino SJ: Orientation of the first metatarsal base wedge osteotomy: Perpendicular to the metatarsal wedge versus weight-bearing surface. J Foot Surg 27:294–298, 1988.
17. Root ML, Orien WP, Weed JH: Normal and Abnormal Function of the Foot. Los Angeles, Clinical Biomechanics Corporation, 1977.
18. Schuberth JL, et al: Hallux Valgus in the Healthy Adult: Preferred Practice Guidelines. The American College of Foot Surgeons, 1992.
19. Sgarlato TE: A Compendium of Podiatric Biomechanics. San Francisco, California College of Podiatric Medicine, 1971.
20. Swanson AB: Implant arthroplasty of the great toes. Clin Orthop 85:75, 1972.
21. Williams DN, Gustillo RB: The use of preventative antibiotics in orthopaedic surgery. Clin Orthop 190:83, 1984.
22. Yu GV, Nagle CJ: Hallux interphalangeal joint sesamoidectomy. J Am Podiatr Med Assoc 86:105–111, 1986.

7. HALLUX/FIRST RAY: PART II

Richard A. Bellacosa, D.P.M.

1. What makes up the first ray?

The first ray consists of the first or medial cuneiform, first metatarsal, and hallux toe, consisting of a proximal and distal phalanx. It includes the metatarsocuneiform joint, a plane joint demonstrating relatively minimal range of motion in the sagittal plane, and the first metatarsophalangeal (MTP) joint, which is best described as a ginglymoarthrodial joint. The first ray also includes the interphalangeal (IP) joint, which is a ginglymus or hinge joint.

2. What ligaments are associated with the first MTP joint?

1. Medial and lateral collateral ligaments
2. Medial and lateral sesamoid ligaments
3. Medial and lateral plantar sesamoidal ligaments
4. Intersesamoidal ligament
5. Deep transverse ligament

3. Which tendons are associated with the first MTP joint?

Six tendons are incorporated about the first MTP joint: three intrinsic and three extrinsic:

Intrinsic	**Extrinsic**
Flexor hallucis brevis	Extensor hallucis longus
Abductor hallucis	Extensor hallucis brevis
Adductor hallucis	Flexor hallucis longus

4. How much dorsiflexion is necessary for normal function of the first MTP joint?

Approximately 50–60° of dorsiflexion are necessary for normal function in gait.

5. What is the incidence of bipartite hallucal sesamoids?

Dobas and Silvers reviewed 1000 adult foot radiographs and found the incidence of bipartite sesamoids to be 19.3%. There was equal occurrence in males and females, with the ratio of bipartite tibial:fibular sesamoids being 7:1.

6. How frequent are interphalangeal sesamoids?

Yanklowitz and Jaworek reviewed 690 adult foot radiographs and found a 43.5% incidence of IP joint sesamoid. The male:female ratio was 2.5:1. Only 6% of those patients with positive findings had unilateral involvement.

7. Describe the blood supply to the first metatarsal.

Vogler describes the blood supply to the first metatarsal as coming essentially from three sources: the periosteal supply, metaphyseal supply, and nutrient artery. The periosteal supply contributes to the outer third of the cortex, and the medullary supply contributes to the inner two-thirds. The primary nutrient foramen is located laterally at the middle of the shaft. Metaphyseal arteries penetrate both proximally and distally (see figure at top of next page).

8. Describe the blood supply to the sesamoids.

Sobel et al. found that the blood supply to the hallucal sesamoids comes from three sources. The major blood supply comes from proximal and plantar branches from off the first plantar metatarsal artery. Proximal supply is located within the sesamoid attachment to the flexor hallucis brevis muscle. A less significant distal supply originates from the distal capsular attachment to the sesamoid (see figures A and B on next page).

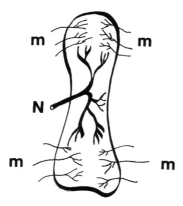

Blood supply to the first metatarsal. *N* = nutrient artery entering through the lateral cortex; *m* = metaphyseal arteries.

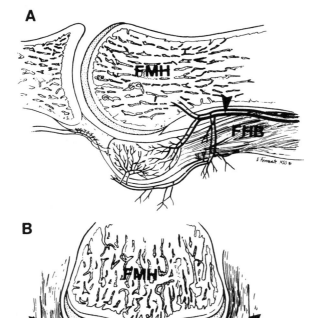

A, Sagittal section through the tibial sesamoid demonstrating the typical blood supply of the sesamoid complex. The proximal and plantar supply arises from branches of the first plantar metatarsal artery (*arrow*). The distal supply is minimal and enters through the capsular attachment. *B,* Coronal section through the sesamoid complex demonstrating the rich plantar blood supply and absence of vascularity from the capsule (*small arrows*) and intersesamoid ligament (*large arrow*). FMH = first metatarsal head; FHB = flexor hallucis brevis. (From Sobel M, et al: The microvasculature of the sesamoid complex: Its clinical significance. Foot Ankle 13(6):359–363, 1992; with permission.)

9. What is the best approach for removing the tibial sesamoid without bunionectomy?

The tibial sesamoid is easily exposed through a medial linear incision made at the junction of the plantar and medial skin at the level of the first metatarsal head. A linear capsulotomy in line with the skin incision is made just superior to the sesamoid, dropping it away from the first metatarsal head.

10. What is the best approach for removing a fibular sesamoid without bunionectomy?

The most direct approach is to use a plantar linear incision placed lateral to the fibular sesamoid in the relatively non–weight-bearing area between the first and second metatarsal heads. A fibular sesamoidectomy can also be carried out as an isolated procedure through a dorsal approach over the first interspace, using a small lamina spreader for exposure and a sesamoid clamp. The more direct plantar approach is preferred.

11. How is a hallux valgus deformity clinically evaluated preoperatively?

The severity of the deformity is noted visually in both non–weight-bearing and stance positions. The hallux is manually placed through range of motion, and quality and quantity are noted. Additionally, hypermobility of the first ray is evaluated, along with reducibility of the hallux abductus and metatarsus primus varus. Being able to place your index finger between the first and second metatarsal heads indicates an increase in the IMA, suggesting the need for a basal osteotomy for correction. Tracking, suggestive of articular adaptation, is evaluated by placing the hallux toe through a range of motion in both the deviated and corrected positions. Decreased motion or motion that deviates from the sagittal plane while the toe is held in a corrected position indicates a tract-bound joint with articular adaptation, suggesting the need to realign the articular surface with a metatarsal head osteotomy.

12. What radiographic angles are used to evaluate hallux valgus?

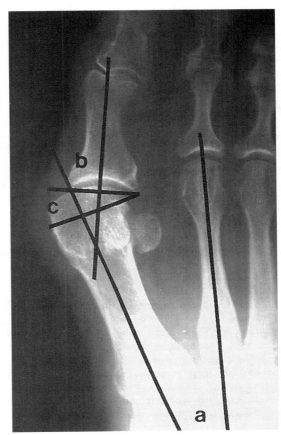

Radiographic Angles Evaluated in Hallux Valgus

ANGLE	NORMAL VALUE
Intermetatarsal angle (IMA, *a* in figure)	8°
Hallux abductus angle (HAA, *b* in figure)	Up to 15°
Proximal articular set angle (PASA,* *c* in figure)	Up to 8°
Distal articular set angle (DASA)	Up to 6°
Hallux interphalangeal angle	Up to 10°

* Also known as distal metatarsal articular angle (DMAA).

Tibial sesamoid position is also evaluated along with whether the first MTP joint articulation is congruous, deviated, or subluxed. Concomitant metatarsus adductus is also identified (normal value up to 14°).

13. What role does metatarsus adductus play in the planning of hallux valgus surgery?

Metatarsus adductus present with hallux valgus can make a bunion deformity more significant than it appears on x-ray. In these cases, x-rays may demonstrate a relatively normal intermetatarsal angle (IMA), while clinically the first metatarsal protrudes medially. Trepal suggests that the true IMA in these cases is actually:

$$\text{Measured IMA} + (\text{MAA} - 15°)$$

where MAA is the metatarsus adductus angle. As a rule of thumb in these cases, this author adds 3° to the measured IMA for the sake of surgical planning.

14. Categorize the procedures for hallux valgus repair and list the indications for each.

Procedures for Repair of Hallux Valgus

PROCEDURES	EXAMPLES	INDICATIONS
Capsule tendon balance	McBride bunionectomy	Positional deformities demonstrating low to normal IMAs
Head osteotomy	Chevron, distal-L, Z, Mitchell	Structural deformities with IMA up to 15–16°
Proximal osteotomies	Closing abductory wedge, crescentic, proximal chevron	Structural deformities with IMA > 15–16°
Arthrodesis	First MTP joint, first MTC joint	Deformities with marked hypermobility of first MTC joint; severe hallux valgus with MTP joint pain
Arthroplasty with or without prosthetic implant	Keller bunionectomy	Pain or crepitus on range of motion

MTC = metatarsocuneiform.

15. What is the recommended hallux position in first MTP joint arthrodesis?

The recommended position of the hallux in a fused great toe joint is 20° dorsiflexed from the supporting surface and 15° abducted.

16. What are the advantages of a lenticular capsulotomy of the first MTP joint?

A lenticular capsulotomy of the first MTP joint is used primarily in hallux valgus repair and provides several advantages:

1. It allows for the greatest amount of exposure and is helpful especially in cases in which joint replacement is considered.

2. Capsulorrhaphy following lenticular capsulotomy allows for correction of the soft-tissue component of hallux valgus.

3. Derotation of the of the sesamoids is possible, especially if sutures are placed from distal medial to proximal lateral and capsular closure is performed from distal to proximal. An occasional "pulley" suture (thrown twice through the capsule before being tied down) can facilitate the derotation effect.

17. How is an adductor transfer done?

The adductor transfer technique is employed in the repair of the positional deformity of hallux valgus. The adductor hallucis tendon and oblique head of the adductor hallucis muscle are freed and tagged and then passed medially over the dorsal aspect of the first MTP joint capsule and inferior to the extensor hallucis longus tendon. The adductor is then secured to the medial capsule, derotating the sesamoids and capsular sleeve in the process.

18. Describe the proper method of removing the medial eminence in hallux valgus repair.

The proper method for removing the medial eminence of bone at the head of the first metatarsal depends on the procedure being performed. In a metatarsal head osteotomy, the medial eminence is removed in a line parallel with the second metatarsal shaft and "straight up and down" or parallel to the sagittal plane (see figure on next page). This allows for slight shortening of the metatarsal and slackening of the joint after osteotomy, resulting in better postoperative range of motion.

In capsule tendon balance procedures, particularly the McBride bunionectomy, the medial eminence is removed in line with the medial aspect of the shaft of the first metatarsal and angled slightly from dorsal-lateral to plantar-medial in the frontal plane (see figure). This approach allows for preservation of the plantar articular surface of the first metatarsal head to prevent tibial sesamoid peeking, which can lead to the unfortunate complication of iatrogenic hallux varus.

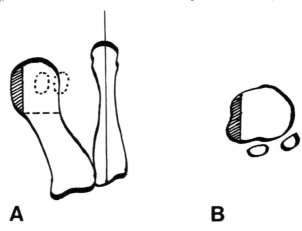

Removing medial eminence via head osteotomy bunionectomy. *A,* Bone removed parallel to second metatarsal shaft. *B,* Bone removed parallel to sagittal plane.

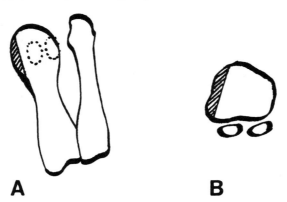

Removing medial eminence via capsule tendon balance procedure. *A,* Bone removed in line with medial metatarsal shaft. *B,* Bone removed from dorsal-lateral to plantar-medial to keep tibial sesamoid covered.

19. What factors predispose to iatrogenic hallux varus?

Factors that contribute to the formation of hallux varus following hallux valgus repair include:
1. Fibular sesamoidectomy
2. Overcorrection of the IMA
3. Improper removal of medial eminence
4. Overly aggressive reefing of the medial joint capsule
5. Malposition of a first metatarsal osteotomy
6. Long first metatarsal

Bandaging in a varus position has often been implicated as a cause for hallux varus. In this author's experience, bandaging alone without one of the other factors present rarely results in hallux varus. At present, we rarely perform fibular sesamoidectomy with hallux valgus repair, but if it is done, it *never* is used with the presence of a long first metatarsal. Hallux varus is most commonly seen following McBride bunionectomy.

20. What is "reverse buckling"?

Buckling refers to the retrograde force placed on the first metatarsal head by the proximal phalangeal base when the pathomechanics of hallux valgus cause the hallux toe to abduct and the first metatarsal to adduct, resulting in pathologic metatarsus primus varus deformity.

Reverse buckling then refers to those techniques used to adduct and derotate the hallux toe, resulting in abduction of the first metatarsal and a decrease in the IMA. This phenomenon can also be explained as reciprocal motion: abduction of the hallux results in adduction of the first metatarsal, while adduction of the hallux results in abduction of the first metatarsal.

21. How does first-ray insufficiency present clinically? How is it treated?

In first-ray insufficiency, the first ray fails to bear its share of body weight during stance and propulsion. It can be the result of a short or elevated first metatarsal, present from birth or iatrogenically induced following first metatarsal osteotomy or failed first metatarsocuneiform arthrodesis. Clinically, patients often complain of lateral forefoot pain, usually manifested by second MTP joint capsulitis/synovitis (with or without hammer toe formation) or intermetatarsal neuroma of the second or, more commonly, third interspace.

Treatment is directed toward symptomatic relief of forefoot symptoms, which can be controlled with a functional orthotic with metatarsal raise. Morton's extension built into the orthotic device is sometimes helpful. Surgical intervention is also directed toward specific forefoot symptoms, along with restoring the weight-bearing capability of the first ray. The latter can be accomplished with plantarflexory arthrodesis of the first metatarsocuneiform joint with or without bone graft.

22. How is hallux rigidus or limitus classified?

The American College of Foot and Ankle Surgeons Preferred Practice Guidelines classify hallux limitus/rigidus into four stages:

Stage I	Functional hallux limitus with pronatory foot type, elevation of the first ray, and hyperextension of the hallux IP joint.
Stage II	Joint adaptation, flattening of the metatarsal head, limitation of passive motion, and beginning of dorsal exostoses.
Stage III	Pain on range of motion, spurring about the joint becomes pronounced, and crepitus with motion.
Stage IV	Ankylosis of the joint.

23. Which capsulotomy is favored in hallux rigidus/limitus surgery?

A **long linear capsulotomy** provides adequate exposure without reducing the amount of capsule available for closure. Capsulorrhaphy is usually carried out with simple interrupted 3–0 absorbable suture, allowing for "slack" in the capsule after removal of hypertrophic bone, which allows for greater postoperative range of motion.

24. Which nerve can be entrapped in medial and dorsomedial approaches to the first MTP joint?

The proper digital branch along the medial aspect of the great toe emerging from the terminal portion of the medial dorsal cutaneous nerve can be entrapped in this area.

25. Which nerve can be entrapped following first interspace release?

The first common digital nerve, which emerges from the medial plantar nerve, can be entrapped in scar tissue following aggressive dissection in adductor tendon release, transection of the deep intermetatarsal ligament, lateral capsulotomy, and fibular sesamoid release during hallux valgus repair.

26. What is Joplin's neuroma?

Joplin described a traumatic lesion of the plantar proper digital nerve, arising as a terminal branch of the medial plantar nerve and coursing plantar and medially across the first MTP joint and hallux toe. Treatment consists of excision, although this author has treated some cases with corticosteroid injection and biomechanical control with an orthotic.

27. Name four methods for fixating a hallux interphalangeal joint arthrodesis.

1. Single 2.7-mm cortical bone screw placed obliquely across the fusion site
2. Crossed 0.045 or 0.062 Kirschner wires
3. Two 0.045 or 0.062 Kirschner wires placed parallel to the long axis of the digit
4. Single 4.0 cancellous screw placed parallel to long axis of the digit

Single Kirschner wire and monofilament wire fixation are not recommended. Staples provide a viable alternative means of fixation.

28. When is hallux interphalangeal joint arthroplasty indicated?

Rosenblum et al. describe hallux IP joint arthroplasty as a salvage procedure in the treatment of chronic neuropathic plantar ulcerations of the hallux in patients without significant structural deformity at the first MTP joint. The procedure is used in an effort to avoid hallux amputation.

29. How is turf toe treated?

Turf toe is a sprain of the first MTP joint caused by hyperflexion and, more commonly, hyperextension. It is usually a sports-related injury, sustained by football players on artificial playing surfaces. Clinically, it must be differentiated from sesamoid fracture, avulsion fracture of the hallux or first metatarsal, tendon rupture, and dislocation. Treatment is conservative and consists of various degrees of immobilization, depending on severity of injury (see figure on p. 112).

30. How does first MTP joint dislocation occur?

Forced hyperextension, such as that sustained in a motorcycle accident, is the mechanism for this relatively rare dislocation.

31. How are first MTP joint dislocations classified? How does this classification affect treatment?

Type I	Sesamoids and intersesamoid ligament remain intact.
Type IIA	Sesamoids are not fractured, but the intersesamoid ligament is disrupted.
Type IIB	Transverse fracture of one of the sesamoids is sustained.

Closed reduction is usually possible in type II injuries, whereas type I injuries usually require open reduction.

CONTROVERSIES

32. Does head osteotomy with lateral release in hallux valgus lead to avascular necrosis?

Avascular necrosis (AVN) of the first metatarsal head can be seen following first metatarsal osteotomy. Lateral release of the fibular sesamoid, conjoined adductor tendon, deep intermetatarsal ligament and joint capsule, and excessive dissection, especially of the periosteal tissues, can compromise the vascular supply to the first metatarsal. Wilkinson et al. using MRI found a 50% incidence of AVN following Austin or chevron bunionectomy, with 10% of plain films in this study showing signs of AVN. Wallace et al., using a mailed survey to 45 podiatric surgeons, reported an incidence of only 0.11% in 13,000 head osteotomy bunionectomies.

Although AVN is a recognized complication of first metatarsal head osteotomy and may occur at a higher incidence than first recognized, clinical signs and symptoms are relatively rare.

The use of rigid internal screw fixation, minimal dissection, and minimal lateral release performed through the first MTP joint help minimize the possibility of clinically significant AVN.

33. Discuss the current philosophy regarding the use of first MTP joint implants.

Implants available for use in the first MTP joint currently include the silicone plastic polymer single-stem or **hemi-implant**, the silicone plastic polymer double-stem or **total implant**, and **component implants** made of titanium, cobalt, or chromium and polyethylene. Titanium grommets are available for use with the silicone plastic polymer implants.

Currently, there is a trend away from the use of joint implants in the foot, following less than ideal long-term results with silicone polymer implants, including the occurrence of detritus synovitis and implant breakage. The two-part component implants are reminiscent of implants tried and failed prior to the accepted use of silicone polymer implants. The present-day component implants are not time-tested, and long-term results are unknown. For these reasons, reconstructive techniques consisting primarily of cheilectomy, shortening or plantarflexory osteotomy of the first metatarsal, and arthrodesis of the first MTP joint are preferred, depending on the symptoms and severity of joint disease.

BIBLIOGRAPHY

1. American College of Foot and Ankle Surgeons: Hallux Rigidus in the Healthy Adult: Preferred Practice Guideline. Park Ridge, IL, American College of Foot and Ankle Surgeons, 1994.
2. Cavaliere RG: New concepts in metatarsal head osteotomies: Reverse buckling techniques. Clin Podiatr Med Surg 6:161–178, 1989.
3. Dobas DC, Silvers MD: The frequency of partite sesamoids of the first metatarsophalangeal joint. J Am Podiatry Assoc 67:880–882, 1977.
4. Dykyj D: Pathologic anatomy of hallux abducto valgus. Clin Podiatr Med Surg 6:1–15, 1989.
5. Hanft JR, Merrill T, Marcinko DE, et al: First metatarsophalangeal joint replacement [grand rounds]. J Foot Ankle Surg 35:78–85, 1996.
6. Jahss MH: Traumatic dislocations of the first metatarsophalangeal joint. Foot Ankle 1:15–21, 1980.
7. Jaworek TE: The intrinsic vascular supply to the first metatarsal: Surgical considerations. J Am Podiatry Assoc 63:555–562, 1973.
8. Joplin RJ: The proper digital nerve, vitalium stem arthroplasty, and some thoughts about foot surgery in general. Clin Orthop 76:199–207, 1971.
9. Rosenblum BI, Giurini JM, Chrzan JS, et al: Preventing loss of the great toe with the hallux interphalangeal joint arthroplasty. J Foot Ankle Surg 33:557–560, 1994.
10. Ruch JA, Banks AS: Anatomical dissection of the first metatarsophalangel joint. In McGlamry ED (ed): Comprehensive Textbook of Foot Surgery, vol 1, 2nd ed. Baltimore, Williams & Wilkins, 1992, pp 469–492.
11. Sobel M, Hashimoto J, Arnoczky SP, et al: The microvasculature of the sesamoid complex: Its clinical significance. Foot Ankle 13:359–363, 1992.
12. Trepal MJ: Hallux valgus and metatarsus adductus: The surgical dilemma. Clin Podiatr Med Surg 6:103–113, 1989.
13. Vittetoe DA, Saltzman CL, Krieg JC, et al: Validity and reliability of the first distal metatarsal articular angle. Foot Ankle 15:541–547, 1994.
14. Vogler HW: Shaft osteotomies in hallux valgus reduction. Clin Podiatr Med Surg 6:47–69, 1989.
15. Wallace GF, Bellacosa RA, Mancuso JE: Avascular necrosis following distal first metatarsal osteotomies: A survey. J Foot Ankle Surg 33:167–171, 1994.
16. Weissmann SD: Biomechanically acquired foot types. In Weissmann SD (ed): Radiology of the Foot, 2nd ed. Baltimore, Williams & Wilkins, 1989, pp 66–90.
17. Wernick J, Volpe RG: Lower extremity function and normal mechanics. In Valmassy RL (ed): Clinical Biomechanics of the Lower Extremities. St. Louis, Mosby, 1996, pp 1–57.
18. Wilkinson SV, Jones RO, Sisk LE, et al: Austin bunionectomy: Postoperative MRI evaluation for avascular necrosis. J Foot Surg 31:469–477, 1992.
19. Yanklowitz B, Jaworek TA: The frequency of the interphalangeal sesamoid of the hallux: A retrospective roentgenographic study. J Am Podiatry Assoc 65:1058–1062, 1975.

8. LESSER DIGITS

Thomas B. Leecost, D.P.M., F.A.C.F.A.S.

MALLET TOE

1. What are the positions of the DIP, PIP, and MTP joints in mallet-toe deformity?

Distal interphalangeal (DIP)   Flexed
Proximal interphalangeal (PIP)   Unaffected
Metatarsophalangeal (MTP)   Unaffected

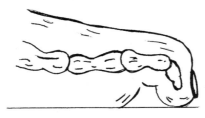

Mallet-toe deformity.

2. Why does the digit lose length in the surgical correction of a rigid mallet toe?

Resection of the head of the middle phalanx is usually required to reduce the mallet-toe's deformity, thus causing the digit to shorten.

3. How are elongated digits which produce mallet toes treated surgically?

The middle phalanx or the proximal phalanx is longer than normal in an elongated digit; therefore, in correcting an elongated digit with a mallet toe deformity, decreasing the length of the digit is very important. A DIPJ arthroplasty will reduce the length of the digit as well as correct the mallet toe deformity.

4. Which is the procedure of choice for a flexible mallet toe of normal length?

DIP joint arthroplasty is reduced by use of a capsulotomy and flexor tenotomy at the DIP joint for this condition.

5. In which plane(s) does the mallet-toe deformity occur?

Primarily in the sagittal plane.

FLEXIBLE HAMMER-TOE DEFORMITY

6. Which procedure is used most often in the correction of flexible hammer toe?

PIP joint resection (arthroplasty). This procedure may be used alone or in conjunction with soft-tissue releases to correct the flexible hammer toe.

7. What force in the hammer-toe condition affects the MTP joint to cause a plantar prominence of the metatarsal head on the plantar surface?

A retrograde force from the hammer toe contributes directly to plantar prominence of the metatarsal head.

8. Describe the positions of the DIP, PIP, and MTP joints in the flexible hammer toe.

PIP   Plantarflexed
DIP   Neutral or hyperextended
MTP   Dorsiflexed

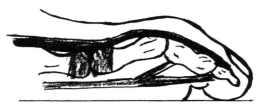

Hammer-toe deformity.

9. Why is flexor tendon transfer sometimes used in the correction of a flexible hammer toe?

This procedure, first described by Girdlestone in 1947 and later reintroduced by Taylor in 1951 and Parish in 1973, is used to assist the intrinsics by plantarflexing the MTP and extending the PIP joint.

10. How are the interphalangeal joints viewed on anteroposterior (AP) x-ray to locate the flexible hammer-toe deformity?

The normal lesser-digit AP view should show phalanges aligned directly over each other, with joints parallel and equally spaced. Viewing the film for digits that are "out of line" assists in locating the hammer-toe deformity.

SEMIRIGID OR RIGID HAMMER TOE

11. How are K-wires usually used for hammer-toe correction?

K-wires are used to maintain reduction of the hammer-toe deformity. They are placed within the medullary canals through all phalanges and across the MTP joint. The distal end of the K-wire is bent at 90° and capped to prevent migration of the wire.

12. Why does the PIP joint arthrodesis have validity in the correction of the semirigid and rigid hammer toe?

Lambrinudi fused the interphalangeal joint to compensate for the ineffectiveness of the intrinsic muscles. In cases in which greater stability of the PIP joint is required in the reduction of the hammer toe, the arthrodesis is the procedure of choice.

13. In which plane(s) does the hammer-toe deformity occur?

Primarily in the sagittal plane.

14. Describe the joint positions in the boutonnière deformity as part of the hammer-toe complex.

MTP   Dorsiflexed
PIP   Plantarflexed
DIP   Hyperextended

15. Which corrective procedure for hammer-toe deformity causes destabilization of the MTP joint, transfer lesions, and flail toes?

The important stabilizing structures of the MTPJ are the collateral ligaments and capsule along with the extensor apparatus; these structures have attachments to the base of the proximal phalanx. When the base is removed in a surgical procedure, it will destabilize the MTPJ.

CLAW TOES

16. Describe the positions of the PIP, DIP, and MTP joints in a claw toe.
MTP   Dorsiflexed
PIP   Plantarflexed
DIP   Plantarflexed

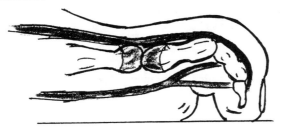

Claw toe deformity.

17. Why does the correction of claw toe require a combination of osseous and soft-tissue procedures?
The MTP joint is very unstable in the claw-toe deformity, the interphalangeal joints have varied degrees of flexibility, and all joint capsules are contracted, which therefore requires osseous as well as soft tissue corrections.

18. In which plane does the claw-toe deformity occur?
Primarily in the sagittal plane.

19. How do the flexor digitorum brevis (FDB) and the flexor digitorum longus (FDL) contribute to the claw-toe deformity?
The flexors create a strong plantarflexor force by retrograding the digit proximally. The FDB's primary force flexes the PIP joint. The FDL's primary force flexes the DIP and PIP joints, retrograding the digit and causing dorsiflexion of the MTP joint.

20. Which foot type most often develops claw-toe deformity?
The cavus foot. Often, this foot type is induced by a neuromuscular disorder, which contributes to the foot's becoming cavus.

DIGITI QUINTI VARUS

21. Which procedure is usually used with a skinplasty to correct digiti quinti varus?
Reducing digiti quinti varus correction requires an osseous procedure as well as a skinplasty. This deformity reduction is best achieved by using a head resection of the proximal phalanx (arthroplasty).

22. In which plane(s) does digiti quinti varus occur?
The transverse and frontal planes are usually involved.

23. Describe the skinplasty used to assist in realigning of the fifth digit.
The elliptical incision running distal medial to proximal lateral corrects the varus direction of the digit when closed because it is perpendicular to the axis of rotation of the varus toe.

24. How are the fifth digits seen clinically in digiti quinti varus deformity?
The fifth digit underriding the fourth digit, with the PIP joints in a varus attitude.

25. Why does the abductor digiti quinti muscle elongate and become weaker in digiti quinti varus deformity?

The flexor digitorum longus muscle causes stabilization late in the stance phase of gait, creating digiti quinti varus but also aiding the third plantar interossei to become stronger and contracted.

CLINODACTYLY

26. Describe the positions of the DIP, PIP, and MTP joints in clinodactyly.

Clinodactyly is usually observed in the DIP joint, at times with the PIP showing a possible varus rotation. The MTP usually is unaffected.

27. How are x-rays used to determine the location or levels of deformity in clinodactyly?

The interphalangeal joints are involved in clinodactyly (curly toe); they are best viewed on AP and oblique views of the foot. Joint deviation as well as flexion is easily observed.

28. Which skinplasty is useful in the correction of clinodactyly?

Clinodactyly often has a varus rotation of the digit, which will require a derotational skinplasty in conjunction with the osseous correction required.

29. Why does the elliptical incision have to be placed carefully to correct clinodactyly?

When the derotational skinplasty is carefully placed so that it is perpendicular to the axis of rotation of that deformed digit, it properly aligns or corrects the rotational deformity.

30. In which plane does clinodactyly occur?

The transverse plane.

OVERLAPPING FIFTH TOE

31. Which component of the overlapping fifth toe is reduced by a skinplasty, extensor digitorum longus (EDL) lengthening, EDL tenotomy, and/or MTP capsulotomy?

The **dorsal contracture** may be reduced using a combination of these procedures.

32. In which plane(s) does the overlapping fifth toe deformity occur?

In the sagittal, frontal, and transverse planes.

33. Describe the Lapidus procedure used for correction of overlapping fifth toes.

A hockey incision is made over the dorsum of the fifth toe. A second incision is made over the middle of the shaft of the fifth metatarsal, through which the EDL is tenotomized. The tendon then is brought through the first incision and freed to its distal attachment of the distal phalanx. A hole is drilled through the proximal third of the shaft of the proximal phalanx. The EDL is fed through the drilled hole from medial to lateral and attached to the lateral side of the capsule of the MTP joint. The tendon is then sutured to the abductor digiti quinti tendon to help stabilize the lateral side of the fifth MTP joint.

34. When does syndactylization of the fourth and fifth digit have application in an overlapping digit?

In resistant or recalcitrant deformities of overlapping fifth digits or in iatrogenic instability of the fifth digit resulting from correction of an overlapping fifth digit, syndactylization of the fourth and fifth toes may be necessary.

35. How are moderate deformities of overlapping fifth toes treated using DuVries technique?

DuVries technique requires an EDL tenotomy, MTP capsulotomy, and skinplasty performed distal and dorsal to the fourth and fifth metatarsal interspace.

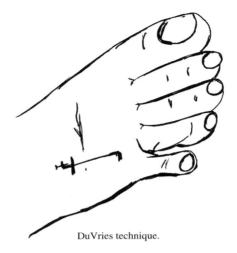

DuVries technique.

HYPEROSTOSIS/EXOSTOSIS

36. Describe the accepted procedure to correct hyperostosis/exostosis.
Excision of exostosis, or bone reduction, is the acceptable procedure used to reduce the offending bone.

37. Why does the interdigital heloma occur?
Opposing bony prominences create pressures on the skin.

38. Which x-ray views are useful in identifying hyperostosis or exostosis?
The AP and oblique x-ray views are used to confirm the location of hyperostosis or exostosis.

39. Where is hyperostosis of the condyles in digits most often found?
The fourth interdigital webspace is the most frequent location for hyperostosis, usually involving the lateral base of the fourth proximal phalanx and the medial head of the fifth proximal phalanx.

40. What procedure is used most often when hyperostosis/exostosis is found on the head of the MTP and PIP?
Joint resection arthroplasty.

41. Which radiologic finding is seen commonly with heloma durum located at the PIP joint?
Widening of the proximal phalangeal head.

42. What is the procedure of choice to prevent recurrence of interdigital heloma of the fourth interspace?
Syndactylization of the fourth and fifth digits may be used. It also stabilizes the fifth digit.

43. Describe the radiologic appearance of diaphyseal allosis.
On radiographs, multiple hereditary exostoses (osteochondromas) are seen arising at the ends of tubular bones.

44. Why does the surgeon create a concavity in bone when removing the exostosis?
A small concavity is created in the area where the exostosis is removed to prevent recurrence of lesions.

45. How are enchondromas (Ollier's disease) differentiated from exostosis on normal x-ray views?

Enchondromas may present clinically as exostosis, but on x-rays, these solitary lesions show a circumscribed lucent area that affects both the ends of the phalanx as well as the adjacent shaft. Exostosis affects only the ends of bone and does not resemble a lesion.

DIGITAL PEARLS

46. What is the most common etiology of a digital deformity?

Unlike genetic conditions, which cause structural deformities or neuromuscular disorders resulting in muscle imbalances, the most common etiology of digital deformities is **biomechanical dysfunction**.

47. Why does the extensor complex become important in evaluating digital deformities of the PIP and DIP joints?

The extensor digitorum brevis and longus combine to form the extensor complex. The middle slip attaches to the base of the MTP to extend the PIP, and the medial and lateral slips attach to the base of the DIP to extend the DIP.

48. Which muscles control function and must be considered when correcting a digital deformity?

Extensor digitorum longus (EDL)	Interossei
Extensor digitorum brevis (EDB)	First dorsal interosseous (FDOB)
Flexor digitorum longus (FDL)	Lumbricals
Flexor digitorum brevis (FDB)	Quadratus plantae

49. What three considerations determine whether surgical corrections of multiple digital deformities can be completed at the same surgical session?

• The patient's ability and willingness to follow postoperative instructions.
• The complexity of the procedure.
• The rehabilitative process will not compromise the patient.

These indicators should have priority in considering correction of multiple digital deformities at the same surgical session.

50. What are the two most common complications following a lesser metatarsal neck osteotomy?

• Transfer lesion
• Lack of toe purchase

51. What is the etiology of lack of toe purchase following a lesser metatarsal neck osteotomy?

The collateral ligaments insert into the metatarsal head and base of the proximal phalanx. When the metatarsal head is dorsiflexed, the toe follows the metatarsal, leading to lack of purchase, or floating toe.

52. How do you determine the exact location in which to inject a painful lesser MTP joint?

Measure on x-ray with a centimeter ruler the exact distance from the tip of the toe to the joint and mark this area.

53. How does this facilitate injecting the joint?

The toe is hyperextended, and the pucker indicates the location of the joint. However, if edema is present, this may not be visible or may be difficult to locate. Measuring with a centimeter ruler corrects for this problem.

BIBLIOGRAPHY

1. Barbari SC, Brevig K: Correction of clawtoes by the Girdlestone-Taylor flexor-extensor transfer. Foot Ankle 5(2):67–73, 1984.
2. Coughlin J: Lesser toe deformities. Orthopedics 10(2):63–75, 1987.
3. Gillett HG: Incident of interdigital clavus. J Bone Joint Surg 56B:(4):752, 1974.
4. Girdlestone GR: Physiotherapy for hand and foot. J Chart Soc Physiol 32:167, 1947.
5. Jimenez AL, McGlamry ED, Green DR: Lesser ray deformities. In McGlamry ED (eds): Comprehensive Textbook of Foot Surgery. Baltimore, Williams & Wilkins, 1987, pp 71–73.
6. Kelikian H: Deformities of the lesser toes. In Hallux Valgus, Allied Deformities of the Forefoot, and Metatarsalgia. Philadelphia, W.B. Saunders, 1965, pp 282–336.
7. Mann RA: Conservative treatment and office procedures. In Inman V (ed): DuVries Surgery of the Foot, 5th ed. St. Louis, Mosby, 1973, pp 425–434, 1973.
8. Parrish TF: Dynamic correction of clawtoes. Orthop Clin North Am 4(1):97–102, 1973.
9. Reginald B: Congenital Malformations: The Foot. Berlin, Springer-Verlag, 1986, pp 424–461.
10. Selig S: Hammer toe: A new procedure for its correction. Surg Gynecol Obstet 72(1):101–105, 1941.
11. Shaw AH: The use of digital implants for the correction of hammer toe deformity and their potential complications and management. J Foot Surg 31:63–74, 1992.
12. Sorto LA: Surgical correction of hammer toes. J Am Podiatr Assoc 64:930–940, 1974.
13. Turain J: Deformities of the smaller toes and surgical treatment. J Foot Surg 29:176–178, 1990.
14. Weissman SD: Radiology of the Foot. Baltimore, Williams & Wilkins, 1983.
15. Yale I: Congenital and acquired deformities of the foot. In Podiatric Medicine, 2nd ed. Baltimore, Williams & Wilkins, 1980, pp 278–300.
16. Zeringue G, Harkless LB: Evaluation and management of the web corn involving the fourth interdigital space. J Am Podiatr Med Assoc 76:210–213, 1986.

9. METATARSALS

Kevin R. Higgins, D.P.M.

1. The condyles of which metatarsal interfaces least directly with the supporting surface?
The first metatarsal, because its weight-bearing surface articulates with the sesamoid apparatus.

2. The anatomic neck of the metatarsals is distal to the surgical neck. True or false?
False.

3. What shape is the base of the second metatarsal at its cuneiform articulation?
Triangular with the apex plantar.

4. Osteophytic lipping and limited first metatarsophalangeal (MTP) joint range of motion correlate with what underlying anatomic cause?
Long or dorsiflexed metatarsal.

5. Which is normally the longest metatarsal?
The second.

6. Finding a short contracted toe, usually the fourth, suggests what cause?
Brachymetatarsia. This suspicion will be supported by transverse creasing of the dorsal skin, relative dorsal position of this toe in comparison to adjacent toes, and definitively by radiographic evaluation.

7. Which angle is of primary concern in the treatment of bunion deformity?
The first intermetatarsal angle. Evaluation of this angle will determine the primary corrective osteotomy or procedure. Obliquity of the first metatarsal cuneiform articulation coupled with a marked increase in first intermetatarsal angle or first ray hypermobility may validate a Lapidus-type first metatarsal cuneiform articulation fusion. For higher first intermetatarsal angles, basilar osteotomies are indicated, while moderate increases are usually addressed with metatarsal head osteotomies.

8. In the tailor's bunion deformity, what two measurements guide surgical decision-making?
The fourth intermetatarsal angle and lateral bowing angle of the distal aspect of the fifth metatarsal. Usually one or the other will be significantly elevated. Correction for lateral bowing is amenable to distal osteotomies, while increase in the proximal angle may warrant a proximal osteotomy.

9. What treatments are available for tailor's bunion deformity?

Shoewear adjustment	Distal osteotomy
Accommodative padding	Proximal osteotomy
Orthotics	Metatarsal head resection
Exostectomy	

10. A high school athlete complains of stiffness in the second toe joint, which he bruised a year earlier while jumping hurdles. He has bony fullness about the joint. What is your diagnosis?
Freiberg's infraction, which is osteochondrosis at the second metatarsal head.

11. What is osteochondrosis?
Epiphyseal injury with related vascular insult and subsequent degenerative changes about the affected MTP joint.

12. How are these treated surgically?

Cheilectomy	Shortening osteotomy
Soft-tissue interposition	Implant arthroplasty
Resection arthroplasty	Interpositional arthroplasty

These represent patient or problem-specific choices and are not exclusive. If soft tissue interposition is considered, it should be part of the preoperative plan and incorporated into the capsulotomy approach. I prefer an aggressive cheilectomy or reshaping of the joint surfaces, which might be considered an arthroplasty. I commonly find soft tissue interposition unnecessary and would not usually advocate implant placement in this pathologic bone stock. Temporary Kirschner wire stabilization of the entire segment can be helpful.

13. Name the one aspect always missing from the diagnosis of stress fracture.
Abrupt trauma. By definition, it is an insidious process.

14. Which clinical indicator is usually found with stress fractures?
Point tenderness along the metatarsal shaft.

15. Outline the treatment choices for stress fractures.

Metatarsal padding	Ankle–foot orthoses
Surgical shoe	Bone stimulation
Cast immobilization	Orthotics

16. What are the common fifth metatarsal fractures?
Styloid process (e.g., avulsion fracture) and the Jones' fracture.

17. When a patient sustains an inversion ankle sprain, what metatarsal should be examined for fracture?
The fifth metatarsal. Avulsion of the base is commonly seen, which results when tension on the peroneus brevis pulls off the bony attachment.

18. Is this the injury sustained by Sir Robert Jones?
No. He describes a fracture 1.5 cm from the fifth metatarsal base.

19. Why are Jones' fractures such notorious injuries?
Repetitive trauma and migration of the fracture fragments contribute to a high rate of delayed union. Additionally, the union process can be worsened by compromised nutrient arterial flow associated with the injury.

20. How are Jones' fractures commonly fixated?
Intramedullary screw.

21. How do osteochondromas occur?
Osteochondromas (shown in the radiograph at top of next page) are the most common benign metatarsal tumors. They develop following a spontaneous accident in cartilage development, usually arising at growth plate closure (metaphyseal-epiphyseal junction). Hereditary forms also occur.

22. Are osteochondromas usually symptomatic?
Only when they impinge on adjacent soft tissues.

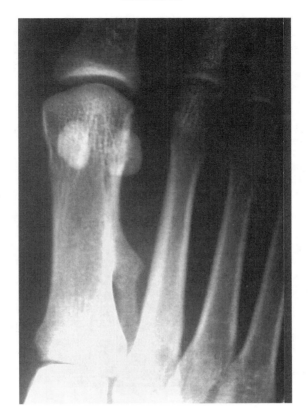

23. What can be gleaned from additional imaging studies in osteochondroma?

A **CT scan** (below) shows that the lesion is bony and well-delineated from the surrounding soft tissues without an inflammatory response. It is benign.

A triphasic **technetium-99** image (at top of next page) confirms the fracture of the lesion base, which is the cause of the patient's symptoms.

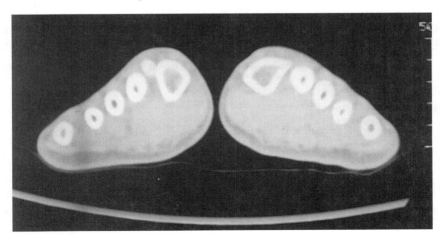

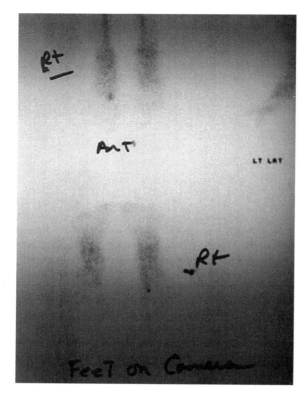

24. What exactly does a technetium-99 late-phase scan indicate?
Osteoblastic activity.

25. Which pathologic processes provide similar uptake on Tc-99 scans?
Fracture, tumor, and infection. The patient's history will provide important clues as to the underlying process. Events contributing to fractures can usually be better defined than the insidious course of tumor evolution. Likewise, tumor symptoms, especially in the event of malignancy, are not consistently precipitated by weight bearing alone, as is often the case with fractures. Foot infections rarely evolve, particularly in adults, without a portal of entry. Clinicians should beware of fractures which present in the pathologic setting, such as in the presence of tumors when either diagnosis may be missed.

26. What features on a CT scan (see top of next page) might suggest a malignant process?
Marked edema
Soft-tissue extension
Demineralization of adjacent bones

27. Can osteomyelitis present with similar findings on CT scan?
No. Osteomyelitis is most likely to involve a single bone and migrate longitudinally rather than transversely.

28. Discuss the changes seen radiographically with rheumatoid arthritis.
Juxta-articular osteoporosis with decreased bone density at the metatarsal heads are found symmetrically. This finding is often coupled with erosive changes in more than one metatarsal and bilateral involvement.

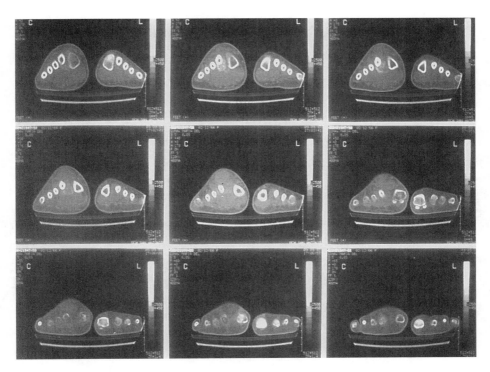

BIBLIOGRAPHY

1. Dameron TB Jr: Fractures and anatomic variations of the proximal portion of the fifth metatarsal. J Bone Joint Surg 57A:788, 1975.
2. Fallat LM, Buckholz J: An analysis of the tailor's bunion by radiographic and anatomical display. J Am Podiatr Assoc 70:597, 1980.
3. Jimenez AL: Brachymetatarsia: A study in surgical planning. J Am Med Podiatr Assoc 69:245–251, 1979.
4. Jones R: Fracture of the base of the first metatarsal by indirect violence. Ann Surg 35:697, 1902.
5. Kavanaugh JH, Brower TD, Mann RV: The Jones' fracture revisited. J Bone Joint Surg 60A:776, 1978.
6. Kinnard P, Lirette R: Dorsiflexion osteotomy in Freiberg's disease. Foot Ankle 9:226, 1989.
7. McKeever DC: Excision of the fifth metatarsal head. Clin Orthop 13:321, 1959.
8. Siffert RS: Classification of the osteochondroses. Clin Orthop 158:10, 1981.
9. Taylor PM: A review of changes of the hands and feet in rheumatoid arthritis. J Am Podiatr Assoc 68:817, 1978.

10. SUBTALAR COMPLEX

George F. Wallace, D.P.M.

1. Define the subtalar complex.
The subtalar complex consists of the entire talocalcaneal joint and related structures. Jahss includes the midtarsal joints (Chopart's joint) as well. The talocalcaneal joint comprises the anterior, middle, and posterior facets of the talus and calcaneus. The anterior facets may be hypoplastic. The middle facet of the calcaneus is on the sustentaculum tali.

2. What is the difference between the functional and anatomic subtalar joints?
The functional subtalar joint contains all facets on both the talus and calcaneus. The anatomic subtalar joint only contains the posterior facets of each bone. The posterior facets are found in their own capsule, while the anterior and middle facets along with the midtarsal joint are in another capsule.

3. Where is the axis of the subtalar complex located?
The axis is directed 42° from the transverse plane and 16° from the sagittal plane. The axis passes obliquely from the posteroinferolateral border of the calcaneus to the anterosuperomedial border of the talar neck.

4. Describe the motion of the subtalar complex.
Triplane motion exists around the two axes: pronation and supination. Total motion is two parts supination to one part pronation. Because one axis is only 16° from the sagittal plane, the amount of dorsiflexion and plantarflexion is relatively low. Supination produces obliquity of the midtarsal joint.

5. In closed kinetic chain motion, what happens to each bone in pronation and supination?

Pronation	Calcaneus everts
	Talus adducts and plantarflexes
Supination	Calcaneus inverts
	Talus abducts and dorsiflexes

6. Define the sinus tarsi.
The sinus tarsi is an anatomic landmark formed when the talus and calcaneus articulate. It is just like a tunnel, formed by the sulcus calcanei as the floor and the sulcus tali as the roof. It is found distal to the posterior facets. The sinus tarsi is wider laterally.

7. What is the tarsal canal?
The tarsal canal is another name for the sinus tarsi.

8. What are the contents of the sinus tarsi?
1. Artery of the sinus tarsi
2. Artery of the tarsal canal
3. Deltoid artery
4. Unnamed nerves
5. Interosseous talocalcaneal ligament
6. Fibroadipose tissue
7. Medial root of the inferior extensor retinaculum

9. Where is Hoke's tonsil?
The fibroadipose tissue, sometimes described as a plug, contained in the sinus tarsi is Hoke's tonsil. When performing sinus tarsi decompression surgery, this tissue is excised.

10. Describe the interosseous talocalcaneal ligament.

This ligament is found within the sinus tarsi. The fibers are somewhat transverse and run plantar and lateral from the talus to the calcaneus. During inversion, it is taut.

11. Describe the cervical ligament.

The cervical ligament can be found just lateral to the sinus tarsi. The fibers are directed dorsal and medial from the calcaneus to the talus. During inversion, it is taut. When performing a STA-peg procedure, the cervical ligament may have to be incised.

12. Where is the sinus tarsi on the surface of the foot?

The sinus tarsi can be palpated by measuring approximately one fingerbreadth inferior and one fingerbreadth anterior to the lateral malleolus. When located, a dell can be created in the skin while pressing into the sinus tarsi.

13. How does the sinus tarsi appear on radiographs?

On lateral views, the sinus tarsi appears as an oval of decreased density just anterior to the lateral process of the talus and superior to the sustentaculum tali. In a supinated foot, the oval appears larger. When there is a high degree of pronation, such as a flatfoot, the oval decreases and may disappear.

14. What is sinus tarsi syndrome?

Sinus tarsi syndrome usually occurs after an inversion injury to either the ankle or subtalar joint. The interosseus talocalcaneal ligament is primarily affected. The patient presents with sub-acute or chronic pain on the lateral aspect of the foot. The sinus tarsi is palpated and pain is elicited. Also, pain occurs when the subtalar joint is put through its range of motion. In some instances, treatment consists of a steroid injection into the sinus tarsi. Failure of this and other conservative measures may necessitate excising the contents of the sinus tarsi. Pathology can be reported as "chronic inflammation" when the talocalcaneal ligament is analyzed.

15. Are there other causes of pain within the sinus tarsi?

Degenerative joint disease (osteoarthritis) from a traumatic episode, usually a fracture of the calcaneus, and rheumatoid arthritis may lead to pain within the sinus tarsi. Another cause may be a coalition of the subtalar joint.

16. What is the most common subtalar joint dislocation?

The medial subtalar joint dislocation. The foot is medial to the talus, which remains in the mortise, and both the subtalar and talonavicular joints are dislocated. After relocation of the joints, the patient is immobilized for approximately 6 weeks.

17. What are the other types of subtalar dislocations?

Lateral subtalar dislocations are the second most common type. They are caused by forceful eversion. Both anterior and posterior dislocations have been described but are rare.

18. Can degenerative joint disease develop following a subtalar dislocation?

Degenerative arthritis may develop, but for an isolated subtalar dislocation, it is of low frequency. However, if a concomitant intra-articular fracture occurs, then the likelihood for developing degenerative joint disease is great. If a fracture is suspected along with the dislocation, a CT scan is appropriate.

19. How is subtalar instability related to lateral ankle instability?

One can have subtalar instability in conjunction with lateral ankle instability, or it can exist separately. Both can follow inversion injuries. Primarily, the calcaneofibular ligament is torn in subtalar-unstable patients. The cervical and interosseous talocalcaneal ligaments may also be affected.

Stress radiographs, stress tomograms, and subtalar arthrograms aid in the diagnosis. Surgical procedures that reconstruct any of the ruptured ligaments may be used if conservative measures fail. Suspicion is heightened when there is no objective ankle instability but the patient has a feeling of instability and pain.

20. Arthroscopy of the subtalar joint uses which portals?
The anterior, middle, and posterior portals laterally are used for observation of the subtalar joint, but due to the interosseous talocalcaneal and cervical ligaments, only the posterior portal provides ready access to the posterior facet. A 2.5-mm arthroscope is commonly employed.

21. Why do peroneal spasms occur when there is a coalition of the subtalar joint?
When the subtalar joint is everted, there is less stress on the various facets. The peroneal spasms try to keep the foot everted, thereby decreasing stress and hopefully lessening subtalar pain. Also, after prolonged spasms, the peroneals become painful and have to be treated to "break the spasms."

22. What is the number-one coalition found in the foot?
A talocalcaneal coalition, specifically of the middle facet. Some argue that it is the calcaneonavicular joint. Semantically, a **coalition** is between two bones within an anatomic joint, whereas a **bar** is between bones not within an anatomic joint.

23. Name the types of coalitions or bars.
Synchondrosis (cartilaginous), synostosis (osseous), and syndesmosis (fibrous) are the various types of coalitions or bars, depending on their tissue characteristics.

24. How does one assess movement of the subtalar joint?
With the patient prone (although sitting may give a general idea), the heel is grabbed and then inverted and everted. Bisection of the heel and the lower leg and measuring of the angles between the two after inversion and eversion will provide numerical values.

BIBLIOGRAPHY

1. Bohay DR, Manoli A: Occult fractures following subtalar joint injuries. Foot Ankle Int 17:164–169, 1996.
2. Clanton TO: Instability of the subtalar joint. Orthop Clin North Am 20:583–592, 1989.
3. Frey CC, Gasser S, Feder KS: Arthroscopy of the subtalar joint. Foot Ankle Int 15:424–428, 1994.
4. Jahss MH (ed): Disorders of the Foot and Ankle, 2nd ed. Philadelphia, W.B. Saunders, 1991.
5. Marcinko DE (ed): Medical and Surgical Therapeutics of the Foot and Ankle. Baltimore, Williams & Wilkins, 1992.
6. O-Connor D: Sinus tarsi syndrome: A clinical entity. J Bone Joint Surg 40A:720, 1958.
7. Root ML, Orien WP, Weed JH: Normal and Abnormal Function of the Foot. Los Angeles, Clinical Biomechanics Corp., 1977.
8. Roukis TS, Hurless JS, Page JC: Functional significance of torsion of the tendon of tibialis posterior. J Am Podiatr Med Assoc 86:156–163, 1996.
9. Zimmer TJ, Johnson KA: Subtalar dislocations. Clin Orthop 238:190–194, 1989.

11. ANKLE PATHOLOGY

Thomas J. Chang, D.P.M.

1. What are the classifications for ankle fractures?

In the adult, the most common fracture classifications are the Lauge-Hansen and the Danis-Weber. The **Lauge-Hansen** classification is based on a two-word description. The first word describes the position of the foot at the time of injury, and the second word describes the motion of the talus within the ankle mortise. The **Danis-Weber** classification focuses on the importance of the fibular injury and describes the level of the fibular fracture with respect to the ankle joint line.

In the pediatric ankle, Salter-Harris and Dias-Tachdjian are the two classifications. **Salter-Harris** describes the fracture according to anatomic location of the fracture, whereas **Dias-Tachdjian** describes the foot position and mechanism similar to the Lauge-Hansen adult classification.

2. Which fractures are possible with an inversion ankle injury?

Lateral malleolar—Avulsion or push-off
Medial malleolar—Avulsion or push-off
Posterior tibial malleolus—Volkmann fracture
Wagstaffe fracture—Avulsion of the anterior inferior tibiofibular ligament from the fibula
Tillaux-Chaput fracture—Avulsion of the anterior inferior tibiofibular ligament from the tibia
Talar dome fracture (Berndt-Harty)
Shepard's fracture—Fracture of the os trigonum
Fracture of the anterior calcaneal beak—Avulsion of the bifurcate ligament
Styloid fracture—Avulsion of the peroneus brevis
High fibular fracture—Maisonneuve fracture

3. What is the status of the anterior talofibular (ATF) ligament in a SER-II ankle injury?

In a SER-II, the anterior inferior tibiofibular (AITF) ligament has been involved along with a spiral oblique fracture of the fibula. In this external rotation mechanism, the talus is externally rotating against the fibula, causing the fibula to fracture in a spiral-oblique fashion. The ATF ligament is slack during this process and is therefore intact.

4. How many ankle fracture mechanisms does Lauge-Hansen describe?

In 1960, Lauge-Hansen described five ankle fracture mechanisms:
1. Supination-adduction (2 stages)
2. Pronation-abduction (3 stages)
3. Supination-external rotation (4 stages)
4. Pronation-external rotation (4 stages)
5. Pronation-dorsiflexion (4 stages)

5. What are the most common portals for ankle arthroscopy?

Anterior medial—Medial to the anterior tibial tendon
Anterior lateral—Lateral to the peroneal tertius tendon
Anterior central—Dangerous due to the proximity of the anterior neurovascular bundle
Posterior lateral—Potential for sural nerve injury
Posterior medial—Most dangerous portal

71

6. What are some potential complications of ankle arthroscopy?
- Nerve injury/neuropraxia
- Vascular injury
- Iatrogenic damage to the chondral surfaces
- Hemarthrosis
- Foreign body/instrumentation left within the joint

7. How is the "squeeze test" done?

This test helps to diagnose syndesmotic ruptures. If a compressive force is applied to the tibia and fibula at mid-leg, pain will be elicited in cases in which the syndesmosis has been injured. This test will apply a direct force to the injured syndesmotic region.

8. What is Hawkin's sign?

Hawkin's sign is used to describe the radiographic appearance of the talus on the anteroposterior (AP) view of the ankle after a talar injury. Because the talus has a tenuous blood supply, the potential for avascular necrosis is present in talar neck fractures. At roughly 6–8 weeks after injury, the talus may appear sclerotic on the AP view. This is due to the dead bone in the talus surrounded by the relatively radiolucent tibia and fibula with intact circulation. As the circulation returns, the talus will once again appear relatively radiolucent. This is termed Hawkin's sign and is an indication of vascular healing. Sometimes, it may take several years for healing to occur, but healing almost always does occur with time.

9. What are the common areas of talar dome injuries?

Berndt and Harty described the anterior-lateral and posterior-medial areas as the classic regions of talar dome fractures. A helpful mnemonic to describe both the anatomic location and mechanism of these fractures is **DIAL-A-PIMP** (Dorsiflexion Inversion Anterior Lateral—Plantarflexion Inversion Medial Posterior). However, transchondral fractures are reported to occur in other areas of the talar dome, and these also need to be treated in the same fashion.

10. Why is the transfixation screw used?

The transfixation screw is used to anatomically approximate the fibula back to the tibia in situations of syndesmotic ruptures and, subsequently, ruptures of the interosseous membrane. This is seen commonly in PER ankle fracture mechanisms. The fibula is placed back into the fibular notch, and then the transfixation screw is placed in a noncompressive manner from the fibula anteriorly into the tibia. Common practice is to catch three cortices with two screws or all four cortices with one screw.

11. Describe a triplane fracture.

Triplane fractures occur in pediatric patients with open epiphyseal plates. Due to the variable ossification of the distal tibial growth plates during ages 12–18 years, unique fractures can occur. Fracture forces will usually find areas of least resistance, so the fracture lines will be variable depending on the areas of ossification in the patient. Although the fracture line appears to change planes as it travels, the triplane fracture is a Salter-Harris IV fracture because the fracture line starts at the ankle joint, passes through the growth plate, and then progresses proximally to exit in the tibial metaphysis. Interestingly, this fracture resembles a Salter-Harris II on the lateral view and a Salter-Harris III on the AP ankle view.

12. What is the Thurston-Holland sign?

This sign describes the fracture fragment found radiographically in a Salter-Harris II ankle injury. This fragment is seen extending from the growth plate and traveling proximally to exit the posterior surface of the tibia.

13. What is the classic radiographic sign of a peroneal dislocation?

Peroneal dislocation injuries can often involve avulsion of the peroneal retinaculum from the posterior fibula. When this occurs, it is possible to observe a ridge of periosteum or bone parallel to the lateral aspect of the distal fibula on the AP view of the ankle.

14. Which tendon is intimately associated with the posterior processes of the talus?

The tendon of the **flexor hallucis longus** courses through the two posterior tubercles of the talus. This tendon then courses underneath the sustentaculum tali of the calcaneus to insert in the distal phalanx of the hallux. It has been described that a fracture of the posterior lateral tubercle of the talus (Shepard's fracture) can be diagnosed clinically by pain on dorsiflexion of the hallux, which is caused by irritation of the fracture fragment by the tendon. Clinically, this may be present only in an acutely diagnosed fracture.

15. Name the six nerves around the ankle.

The six nerves at the level of the ankle can be separated into superficial and deep nerves. The superficial nerves all lie above the deep fascia and are the saphenous, medial dorsal cutaneous, intermediate dorsal cutaneous, and sural nerves. The deeper nerves lie deep to the deep fascia and are the posterior tibial and deep peroneal nerves.

16. Describe the classifications of equinus.

Equinus can be broken down into several different classifications. One differentiation concerns spastic versus nonspastic forms of equinus. The nonspastic forms are by far the more common and are generally separated into either soft-tissue equinus, osseous equinus, or pseudo-equinus. The soft-tissue types are described as either a gastrocnemius or gastrosoleal equinus. Pseudoequinus is seen in patients with cavus feet.

Types of Equinus

TYPE	KNEE JOINT	DORSIFLEXION AT THE ANKLE JOINT
Gastrocnemius	Knee extended	< 10°
	Knee flexed	> 10°
Gastrosoleus	Knee extended	< 10°
	Knee flexed	< 10°
Ankle	Knee extended	< 10°
	Knee flexed	< 10°
Spastic	Observe gait Calf muscle contraction leads to early heel-off	
Acquired	Calf muscle adapts to shortened position leading to early heel-off	

From Birrer RB, DellaCorte MP, Grisafi PJ: Common Foot Problems in Primary Care. Philadelphia, Hanley & Belfus, 1996, with permission.

17. What are the components of the deltoid ligament?

There is controversy about whether there are four or five general bands of the deltoid ligament. The commonly accepted scheme (see figure, next page) divides the ligament into superficial and deep components.

The superficial division is generally comprised of three bands: anterior tibionavicular, tibiocalcaneal, and posterior tibiotalar.

The deep division has either one main tibiotalar band or two separate tibiotalar bands, one anterior and one posterior.

Medial View

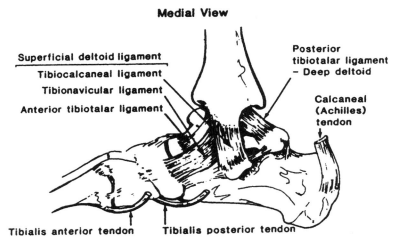

Medial ankle ligaments. (From Mellion MB (ed): Office Sports Medicine, Philadelphia, Hanley & Belfus, 1996, with permission.)

18. What is the order of ossification in the distal tibial growth plate?

From central to lateral to medial. This ossification usually occurs from age 12–16 in females and age 14–18 in males. Ankle trauma during this period of ossification may lead to unique fractures, such as the triplane and juvenile tillaux fractures.

19. Which tests are used to indicate lateral ankle instability?

The classic tests for documenting ankle instability are the stress tests: the anterior drawer and talar tilt. They can be performed either manually or with a calibrated Telos device.

The **anterior drawer** test is used to test the integrity of the anterior talo-fibular ligament (see figure). The talus is brought out anteriorly of the ankle joint by pushing backward on the distal tibia while pulling forward on the posterior calcaneus. A lateral radiograph is taken to assess the amount of shift in the position of the talus out of the ankle joint.

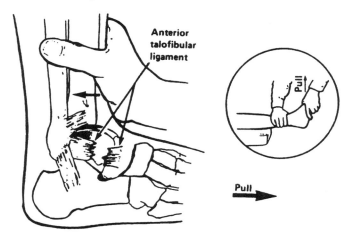

Anterior drawer test. (From Mellion MB (ed): Office Sports Medicine, 2nd ed. Philadelphia, Hanley and Belfus, 1996, with permission.)

The **talar tilt** test is used to test the integrity of the calcaneal-fibular ligament (see figure). this test is done by pushing laterally on the medial distal tibia while inverting the talus from the lateral side. An AP radiograph is taken to assess the degree of angulation between the dorsal cortex of the talar dome and the distal plafond of the tibia. Care should be taken to minimize inversion of the subtalar joint.

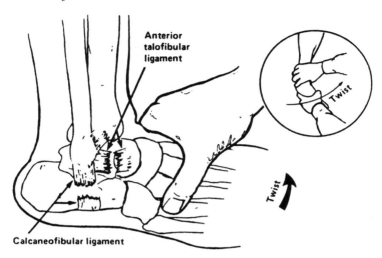

Talar tilt test. (From Mellion MB (ed): Office Sports Medicine, 2nd ed. Philadelphia, Hanley & Belfus, 1996, with permission.)

20. What values are considered abnormal for the talar tilt and anterior drawer tests?

Stress testing for lateral ankle injuries should always be performed bilaterally. This allows one to assess ligamentous laxity and prior trauma in evaluating the unstable ankle.

Abnormal values for the anterior drawer test are described as a > 2-mm excursion of the talus out of the ankle mortise. This is determined by using concentric circles and measuring the amount of anterior displacement of the center points.

An abnormal value for talar tilt is > 4° of inversion. Some authors have described different levels of lateral ligament disruption depending on the degree of angulation.

21. What is the Silfverskiold test?

The Silfverskiold test is used to differentiate between a gastrocnemius and gastrosoleal equinus. The amount of ankle dorsiflexion is assessed with the knee extended, and it is checked again with the knee flexed. Because the gastrocnemius muscle originates from above the knee, any limitation in ankle dorsiflexion with the knee extended should decrease with the knee flexed. If there is limitation of dorsiflexion seen with the knee both extended and flexed, then a tight soleus is also involved in the equinus deformity.

22. What is the recommended position of an ankle fusion?

The optimum position of ankle fusion is described in three planes. In the sagittal plane, the fusion should be in the neutral position. The frontal plane position should be 0–5° of valgus, and the transverse plane position should be abducted with the angle and base of gait.

23. What is a Volkmann fracture?

A posterior malleolar fracture of the distal tibia. This injury is classically seen in both SER and PER ankle fracture mechanisms, and can also be seen in pronation-abduction injuries. It is caused by avulsion by the posterior–inferior tibular–fibular ligament. This fragment usually aligns well after anatomic reduction of the fibula due to the "vassal" principle. If the fragment involves greater than roughly 25% of the joint, then internal fixation is usually recommended.

24. What is a pilon fracture?

This describes a comminuted fracture of the distal tibial metaphysis which extends into the ankle joint. The fibula is commonly involved, but not always. These are most commonly high-velocity/impaction injuries in which the talar body forcibly impacts the tibial surface.

25. How should an osseous equinus be examined radiographically?

The best radiographic exam is a "stress dorsiflexion lateral." This is a lateral radiograph taken with the foot flat on the ground and the leg and knee brought forward maximally on the ankle. This view provides visualization of osseous contact between the distal tibia and talus.

26. List the four steps for sequential reduction of a pilon fracture.

1. Anatomic reduction of the fibula
2. Anatomic reconstruction of the distal tibial articular surface
3. Bone grafting of the tibial deficit
4. Plate fixation to the distal/anterior tibia.

BIBLIOGRAPHY

1. Berndt A, Harty M: Transchondral fractures of the talus. J Bone Joint Surg 41A:988–1020, 1959.
2. Dias LS, Tachdjian MO: Physeal injuries of the ankle in children. Clin Orthop 136:230–233, 1978.
3. Hawkins L: Fractures of the neck of the talus. J Bone Joint Surg 52A:991–1002, 1970.
4. Lauge-Hansen N: Fractures of the ankle. II. Arch Surg 60:957–985, 1950.
5. McGlamry ED, Banks AS, Downey MS (eds): Comprehensive Textbook of Foot Surgery, 2nd ed. Baltimore, Williams & Wilkins, 1992.
6. Salter RB, Harris WB: Injuries involving the epiphyseal plate. J Bone Joint Surg 45A:587–622, 1963.
7. Sarrafian SK: Anatomy of the Foot and Ankle, 2nd ed. Philadelphia, J.B. Lippincott, 1993.
8. Scurran BL (ed): Foot and Ankle Trauma. New York, Churchill Livingstone, 1989.

12. ANKLE ARTHROSCOPY AND ENDOSCOPY

Richard O. Lundeen, D.P.M.

1. Who coined the term arthroscope?

In 1918, Kenji Takagi used a Charriere no. 22 pediatric cystoscope to inspect a knee. Soon after, he developed his own instrument, which was 7.3 mm in diameter, and termed it an "arthroscope."

2. How do arthroscopy and endoscopy differ?

Arthroscopy refers to visualizing the interior of a joint. **Endoscopy** means "to see within," referring to a body cavity.

3. Which joints or body cavities have been reported to be arthroscoped or endoscoped in the lower extremity?

Arthroscopy

Hip	Talonavicular
Knee	First metatarsophalangeal
Ankle	Lesser metatarsophalangeal
Subtalar	Hallux interphalangeal
Calcaneocuboid	

Endoscopy

Tendo Achilles (primary repair)
Laciniate ligament (posterior tibial nerve release)
Plantar fascia (endoscopic plantar fasciotomy)
Intermetatarsal ligament (endoscopic decompression of intermetatarsal neuroma)
Os trigonum/Stieda's process
Haglund's deformity/retrocalcaneal bursa

4. What is a portal?

Portals are small cut-down incisions, placed to access specific anatomic areas and avoid vital structures.

5. What is arthroscope obliquity?

All arthroscopes have a "tip cut," which refers to how the end of the optical tube of the arthroscope is cut. Seldom are they cut blunt, perpendicular to the axis of the tube, but usually they are angled 25–30°. This angle alters the field of view by that many degrees from the axis of the optical tube, allowing the visual field to be deflected in that direction. Thus, the oblique scope allows visualization around bony contours that could not be seen with an arthroscope looking only straight ahead (see figure).

How the angle of the tip cut affects the direction of the field of view.

6. Which portals are used to arthroscope the ankle?

Anterior   1. Two portals (anterolateral, anteromedial)
            2. Three portals (anteromedial, anterolateral, anterocentral)
Posterior   1. Two portals (posterolateral, posteromedial)
            2. From the anterior aspect of the joint through an anterocentral portal, passing through the sagittal groove of the talus, into the posterior aspect of the ankle
            3. Trans-tendo Achilles

7. Describe the four functions of an arthroscope.

1. **Sweeping.** Side-to-side or up-and-down movement to see objects or anatomic areas.

2. **Pistoning.** Moving the tip of the arthroscope closer to an object to magnify it and decrease the field of vision, or moving away from an object to decrease the magnification but increase the field of vision.

3. **Rotation.** Turning the arthroscope about a 360° arc. Because the tip of the arthroscope is usually angled, this rotation increases the field of view due to the obliquity of the tip cut.

4. **Triangulation.** Using sweeping, pistoning, and rotation to place an object in the direct field of vision of the arthroscope through an adjacent portal.

8. What is accomplished with an endoscopic plantar fasciotomy?

The medial band of the plantar fascia is released under direct arthroscopic visualization. This releases the tension within the structure as produced from its "windlass effect," as described by Hicks in 1851, that results from its being tethered between the metatarsal heads and calcaneus in pronatory motions of the subtalar and midtarsal joints.

9. Are infracalcaneal spurs (heel spurs) located in the insertion of the plantar fascia into the calcaneus?

No. They are actually above the plantar fascia in the muscular insertion of the flexor digitorum brevis muscle into the superior surface of the plantar fascia and medial tubercle of the calcaneus.

10. Why is lactated Ringer's solution a better irrigant for arthroscopy than saline?

It is less harmful to chondrocyte metabolism, producing less potential damage during arthroscopic procedures.

11. How many layers can cartilage be divided into?

Three: horizontal, tangential, and vertical layers. The upper layer is thinned and horizontally oriented. The other two layers are formed by deeper, vertical portions of collagen fiber arches that intermingle above the tangential layer and under which is the deeper vertical layer (see figure).

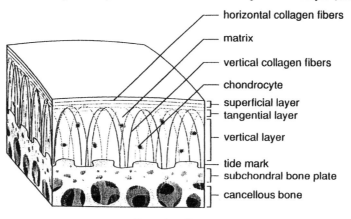

Normal cartilage.

12. What is the matrix of cartilage? What is its significance?

Cartilage is a mixture of substances, consisting primarily of collagen fibrils in a glycoprotein gel which is termed *matrix*. The collagen fibrils form arches that resist tension, to which are attached glycoproteins that resist compression. Any alterations of these two elements result in the start of the breakdown of cartilage.

13. Where is the lamina splendins located?

It is a thin superficial membrane overlying the horizontal layer of cartilage that is firmly attached to the articular margins as it blends with the periosteum. It serves to shield the matrix of cartilage.

14. What is the tidemark?

The tidemark is the eosinophilic-staining area between the zone of calcified and noncalcified cartilage. It represents the location at which the vascular supply to cartilage ends and thus is also the location at which the vascular supply needed to repair cartilage starts when treating cartilaginous defects.

15. Name the two types of degeneration of cartilage.

Superficial and basal. **Superficial** degeneration refers to the breakdown of cartilage that starts in the superficial layer of cartilage. **Basal** degeneration starts under the superficial layer, in the tangential or vertical layers of cartilage.

16. Define chondromalacia.

Literally, it is "softening" of the cartilage. Arthroscopically, it involves various stages of superficial and basal degeneration of cartilage.

17. How do chondral and osteochondral lesions differ?

Articular pathology is divided into chondral and osteochondral lesions. **Chondral** lesions involve only the cartilage, whereas **osteochondral** lesions also involve the underlying subchondral bone.

18. How many types of medial impingement lesions are there?

Medial impingement lesions are of three types and are located at the medial bend of the tibia and the anterior aspect of the ankle joint. They form by traumatic injury from inversion stress, resulting in the impingement of the medial talar shoulder onto the tibial plafond and the inferior portion of the anterior tibial lip at the medial bend (see figure).

- Type A lesions—Chondral
- Type B lesions—Osteochondral
- Type C lesions—Osteochondral with involvement of the underlying cancellous bone of the tibial plafond.

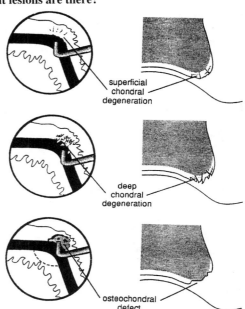

19. What is synovitis?

Inflammation of the synovial lining. The synovium lines everything within a diarthrodial joint, except the surface of the cartilage. Normal synovium is barely visible to the naked eye, yet microscopically it consists of fingerlike projections termed *synovial villi.* Inflammatory processes initiate an almost immediate response in the villous projections, inducing their enlargement and making them visible within the joint when viewed arthroscopically.

20. How can acute and chronic synovitis be differentiated on arthroscopy?

By appearance of the synovial villi. In acute synovitis, the villi are long, fingerlike, and transparent, with a single central vessel that becomes enlarged (injected). With time, the villi become opaque, and the ends fray and break off, which can give the joint a cloudy appearance on initial arthroscopic entrance. The synovium accumulates and "piles up" in the various joint recesses, becoming a source of reinflammation.

21. What is a meniscoid lesion?

This term was developed by Irwin Wolin, an orthopedist, who first described the lesion as hyalinized (compressed and thickened) fibrous tissue between the talus and fibula under the anterior talofibular ligament resulting from a sprain. Meniscoid lesions can occur in other joint recesses and are often termed meniscoid bodies. These also result from the hyalinization of synovium that has piled up in the joint recesses and become compressed between the capsule and articular surfaces.

22. How are meniscoid bodies (lesions) differentiated from osteochondral bodies?

Meniscoid bodies are directly connected to synovium.

23. What mediates the pain resulting from intra-articular pathology?

Cartilage has no nerves, and there are few nerve endings in synovium or subchondral bone. Therefore, it is the capsule, which arises from the periosteum, that is responsible for mediating pain production.

24. How is inflammation within a joint responsible for the breakdown of cartilage?

With inflammation, synovitis always occurs, as synovium is the primary filter of noxious substances out of a joint. Synovium cannot differentiate whether the inflammation is caused by trauma, bacteria, sodium urate, etc., and so it hypertrophies to increase its efficiency. Simultaneously, it produces enzymes that are released into the joint which also cannot differentiate a particular cause for the inflammation. As a result, enzymatic degradation of the lamina selenoins and superficial layer of the cartilage can occur, resulting in a loss of cartilage matrix and initiating the breakdown of the articular surface.

25. How does synovial pile-up cause chondral and osteochondral erosions (lesions) at the articular margins?

By reducing the washing of cartilage by synovial fluid, thereby decreasing chondrocyte nourishment, and through enzymatic degradation.

26. Which ligaments about the ankle are intra-articular?
1. Anterior talofibular ligament
2. Anterior inferior tibiofibular ligament
3. Deltoid ligament (specifically the anterior tibiotalar ligament)
4. Posterior talofibular ligament
5. Posterior tibiofibular ligament
Not the calcaneofibular ligament.

27. Can the hallucal sesamoids be seen in arthroscopy of the first MTP joint?

No. The tight association between the sesamoidal and collateral ligaments and the contour of the inferior surface of the plantar condyles of the first metatarsal head prevents this visualization.

28. Which six structures make up the lateral gutter in the ankle?
1. Lateral trochlear surface of the talus
2. Medial surface of the fibula
3. Anterior border of the fibula
4. Tip of the lateral malleolus
5. Anterior inferior talofibular ligament
6. Joint recess between the talus and fibula

29. What structures make up the lateral interval of the ankle?
1. Lateral talar shoulder
2. Anterior inferior tibiofibular ligament
3. Anterior tibial tubercle
4. Tibiofibular synovial recess
5. Tibiofibular synovial fringe
6. Anterior border of the fibula
7. Medial surface of the fibula

30. Does the anterior inferior tibiofibular ligament impinge on the lateral talar shoulder?
Not always, but often it does. Rarely is this impingement pathologic, and only when there is distinct degenerative changes under it on the lateral talar shoulder should portions of the ligament be resected.

31. When entering the ankle with the arthroscope, should you first visualize the joint medially or laterally?
The medial aspect of the ankle should be approached first, as it is a larger pouch and contains no ligaments. Also, most pathology occurs laterally, and so there are usually less synovitis and fewer degenerative changes medially.

32. List 10 locations where intra-articular avulsion fractures occur in the ankle.
Anterior inferior tibiofibular ligament
    1. Anterior tibial tubercle (Chaput)
    2. Anterior border of the fibula (Tilleaux)
Anterior talofibular ligament
    3. Anterior border of the fibula
    4. Lateral trochlear surface of the talus
Deltoid ligament
    5. Tip of the medial malleolus
    6. Medial trochlear surface of the talus
Posterior tibiofibular ligament
    7. Posterior tibial tubercle
    8. Medial border of the fibula
No ligament involved
    9. Anterior tibial lip
    10. Posterior tibial lip

33. What is the fracture classification described by Berndt and Harty in 1959?

Four Stages of Transchondral Fractures of the Talus

Stage I	Compression injury with secondary cystic formation of a talar shoulder
Stage 2	Incomplete fracture
Stage 3	Complete fracture
Stage 4	Complete fracture with an avulsed central fragment, leaving a crater or defect in the talus

34. In which two areas of the talus do transchondral fractures usually appear?
Anterolateral shoulder
Posteromedial shoulder

35. When is continuous passive motion (CPM) useful in ankle arthroscopy?
CPM is not intended to increase the postoperative range of motion of the ankle, but rather to promote neochondrogenesis following resection of a chondral or osteochondral lesion. CPM increases healing through the regeneration of cartilage, forming a more mature tissue and filling the defect with a higher number of chondrocytes.

36. Why is abrasion arthroplasty used?
Abrasion arthroplasty is a method whereby a small burr is used to resect a chondral or osteochondral defect approximately 1.5 mm below the chondral surface, the level at which vascularity exists in the cartilage. Histologically, this is the tidemark zone. By vascularizing the defect, the lesion then has a means to heal by filling with a covering of "pseudo" cartilage.

37. How is a posteromedial transchondral fracture approached arthroscopically?
From the anterior aspect of the joint. In most cases, an impingement lesion is identified at the medial bend of the anterior tibial lip. When resected posteriorly on the tibial plafond, this lesion forms a triangular defect. At its apex, the obliquity of the arthroscope is turned toward the medial talar shoulder, which is then probed, and the posteromedial transchondral fracture is found. The bone is then curetted and/or abraded until fully resected.

38. What is the best method to make a lateral portal in the anterior aspect of the ankle?
By transillumination, with the arthroscope placed through an adjacent, more medial portal.

39. Which two joints have been reported to be fused arthroscopically?
Ankle joint
Subtalar joint

40. Which nerve is most at risk during arthroscopy of the anterior aspect of the ankle?
Intermediate dorsal cutaneous nerve.

41. What three nerves are most at risk in endoscopic plantar fasciotomy?
Lateral plantar branch of the posterior tibial nerve
Muscular branch to the digiti quinti brevis muscle
Medial calcaneal branch of the posterior tibial nerve

42. Which nerve is most at risk when a leg holder is used?
The common peroneal nerve at the fibular head, caused when the leg holder is placed too caudally.

43. Where are the portals placed in the arthroscopic resection of the os trigonum?
Two stacked portals are placed over the lateral aspect of the ankle, just behind the peroneal tendons, 1 and 3 cm above the superior surface of the calcaneus.

44. Where are the portals placed in the arthroscopic fusion of the subtalar joint?
Two stacked portals over the sinus tarsi, 1 and 3 cm above the calcaneal sulcus, just in front of the lateral talar process.

45. What is the most common complication of endoscopic decompression of an intermetatarsal neuroma (EDIN)? Of endoscopic plantar fasciotomy (EPF)?
  EDIN: Entrapment neuropathy of the second or third plantar intermetatarsal nerve, secondary to inadvertent resection or secondary entrapment.

EPF: Lateral and midtarsal joint instability with secondary pain from jamming, due to the resection of more than only the medial band of the plantar fascia.

46. Which structure visibly separates the central from the medial band of the plantar fascia?
An intermuscular septum and its associated fat pad.

47. During resection of an os trigonum or Stieda's process arthroscopically, which tendon is at most risk for injury?
The flexor hallucis longus tendon as it passes just lateral to the posterior lateral process of the talus.

CONTROVERSIES

48. Should the anterior inferior tibiofibular ligament be resected in the lateral impingement syndrome in the ankle?
Lateral impingement syndrome in the ankle has been defined as hypertrophic synovial tissue in the lateral interval and a hypertrophic anterior inferior tibiofibular ligament. Actually, the tibiofibular synovial fringe is normal, but it often appears as being hypertrophic. It is a normal anatomic structure and does *not* need to be resected. The anterior inferior tibiofibular ligament often hoods the lateral interval and is usually observed in close association with the lateral talar shoulder. Think of the posterior tibiofibular ligaments as it forms a labrium to deepen the posterior articular surface of the ankle. Only if secondary degenerative changes are present on the talus with associated degenerative changes of the anterior inferior tibiofibular ligament should any portions of the ligament be resected.

49. Is an endoscopic or modified-open approach more successful for plantar fasciotomy?
The controversy over endoscopic plantar fasciotomy versus modified open plantar fasciotomy rests on issues of expense, overutilization, complication rate, lack of research, and so on. In the late 1970s, there was a similar controversy between the "minimal incision" surgeons versus surgeons who performed traditional open surgeries. The bottom line is:
  1. Surgery for "heel spur surgery" should be performed only when conservative care has failed to achieve a realistic resolution of the patient's heel pain.
  2. The surgeon is adequately trained to perform either surgery.
  3. The patient has been informed of realistic outcomes and potential postoperative problems.
  4. The procedures have been performed properly.
  5. The surgeon uses the procedure which works best in his or her hands.
The controversy over how to surgically approach infracalcaneal heel pain appears to be favoring a selective medial band fasciotomy without spur resection by any appropriate method in the case of failed conservative care.

BIBLIOGRAPHY

1. Amendola A, Petrik J, Webster-Bogaert S: Ankle arthroscopy: Outcome in 79 consecutive patients. Arthroscopy 12:565–573, 1996.
2. Ferkel RD, Heath DD, Guhl JF: Neurologic complications of ankle arthroscopy. Arthroscopy 12:200–208, 1996.
3. Lundeen RO: Manual of Ankle and Foot Arthroscopy. New York, Churchill Livingstone, 1992.
4. Menche DS, Frenkel SR, Blair B, et al: A comparison of abrasion burr arthroplasty and subchondral drilling in the treatment of full-thickness cartilage lesions in the rabbit. Arthroscopy 12:280–286, 1996.
5. Ogilvie-Harris DJ, Sekyi-Otu A: Arthroscopic debridement for the osteoarthritic ankle. Arthroscopy 11:433–436, 1995.

13. PEDIATRICS: PART I

Richard Martin Jay, D.P.M., F.A.C.F.A.S.

SUBTALAR JOINT DEFORMITIES

1. What diagnostic characteristic of congenital vertical talus can be seen radiographically?
The dorsal dislocation of the navicular off the head of the talus and onto the neck of the talus.

2. Describe the clinical findings seen on examination of the congenital vertical talus foot.
The foot shows a break in the area of the midtarsal joint. The forefoot is abducted and dorsiflexed, while the rearfoot is plantarflexed due to the equinus. The talar head is noted plantarly and medially.

3. What other pathologic changes are noted in the congenital vertical talus?
The talar head and neck rotate downward and medially due to the loss of the sustentaculum tali and the spring ligament. The navicular rides dorsally onto the talar neck and head. The posterior tibial tendon slides upward along with the flexor digitorum longus and now acts anteriorly as a dorsiflexor of the forepart of the foot.

4. How is congenital vertical talus treated?
Conservative treatment is usually unsuccessful. The operative procedures needed to reduce the deformity are intended to relocate the dislocated midfoot plantarly and reduce the equinus of the rearfoot. This is usually accomplished through a staged procedure. In older children, an extraarticular subtalar arthrodesis is indicated.

5. In determining the clinical and differential diagnosis between calcaneovalgus and congenital vertical talus, which radiographs are helpful?
A lateral view of the actively plantarflexed foot.

6. How does this radiograph differentiate congenital vertical talus from calcaneovalgus?
When the foot is plantarflexed in the lateral view, in a flexible calcaneovalgus foot, the bisection of the talus approximately bisects the first ray. In a rigid vertical talus, the bisection of the talus is plantarly displaced in relation to the bisection of the first ray.

CAVUS FOOT

7. When presented with a cavus foot deformity, what consideration is paramount?
Most cases of cavus foot deformity are of neurologic origin. Neuromuscular deficits should be ruled out immediately.

8. Outline the possible pathogenesis of a cavus foot deformity.
A cavus foot type is a cyclical deformity. Depending on the level of neurologic involvement within the foot, different changes can be expected. For example, with a strong peroneus longus tendon as it is inserting into the first ray, the first ray will plantarflex. With this mechanism, the anterior groove is weakened, and the foot loses its dorsiflexory power but gains the clawing or dorsiflexion component of the digits. In turn, this creates the windlass effect. The plantar fascia starts to contract, the first ray is further plantarflexed, and the calcaneal inclination is increased. With a young child, this soft-tissue change will result in osseous changes if left untreated.

9. How does a cavus foot of different planes present on lateral radiographs?
  • The sagittal-plane cavus foot yields a high calcaneal inclination, with a plantarflexed first metatarsal.
  • A frontal-plane cavus foot results in inversion of the calcaneus, yielding a calcaneovarus or heel varus.
  • A transverse cavus results in a cavovarus, in which the forefoot is adducted.

10. Describe the different types of cavus foot as seen radiographically.
  • Posterior cavus yields an increase in the calcaneal inclination.
  • Anterior cavus yields an increase in the plantarflexion of the first ray.
  • Anterior local cavus has a first-ray plantarflexion only.
  • Global anterior cavus is plantarflexion of all five metatarsals.
  • A combined deformity consists of an anterior and posterior cavus.

11. What surgical options are available for the treatment of a rigid cavus foot deformity?
    If the first ray is plantarflexed, a dorsiflexory wedge osteotomy can be performed. If it is a rearfoot component with an increase in the calcaneal inclination, a Dwyer osteotomy can be performed to lower the calcaneal inclination and reduce the varus rearfoot.

12. What surgical options are available for the severely deformed cavus foot after osseous development is complete?
    Midfoot osteotomies and triple arthrodeses.

13. Which conservative measures can be used in treating a cavus foot deformity?
    Orthotic devices with valgus forefoot posting. Depending on the flexibility of the first ray, the first ray can be cut out and allowed to float to an acceptable height, or the forefoot can be posted in valgus, first metatarsal through fifth metatarsal, if there is a complete forefoot valgus. If the first ray is only plantarflexed and metatarsals 2–5 are inverted, then a 1–5 valgus forefoot posting and an intrinsic 2–5 varus posting are used.
    Rearfoot posting can be used with the cavus foot type, but care must be taken to prevent lateral ankle instability. When posting the forefoot and rearfoot with varus rearfoot and forefoot valgus, a stabilizing effect will occur and prevent the supinatory rock in the rigid foot and thereby lateral ankle instability.

CLUBFOOT (TALIPES EQUINOVARUS)

14. What clinical findings are seen on physical examination of a clubfoot?
    The medial malleolus abuts against the navicular medially. The head of the talus is noted to be prominent on the dorsolateral side of the foot. The forefoot is in adduction, and the rearfoot is maximally inverted.

15. What is the range of motion of the ankle joint in a clubfoot?
    The ankle joint has a limitation of dorsiflexion and is usually in a fixed, plantarflexed position due to the equinus deformity.

16. Describe the anatomic relationship between the calcaneus and talus in talipes equinovarus.
    The calcaneus is inverted and in equinus with respect to the talus.

17. In a clubfoot deformity, as compared to metatarsus adductus, the navicular lies in which position in reference to the talar head?
    The navicular is displaced medially on the talar head. In metatarsus adductus, the reverse is noted, and the navicular lies laterally.

18. On a lateral x-ray of a clubfoot, how do the bisection of the calcaneus and the talus relate to each other?

The calcaneus and talus are in an equinus position. When the foot is maximally dorsiflexed, there is no change in the relationship between the bisection of the calcaneus and the talus, and this bisection remains parallel.

19. On anteroposterior x-rays of clubfoot, what is the relationship between the talus and calcaneus? What is the name of this angle?

This angle is known as the talocalcaneal angle, or kite angle. The angle is narrow, and the talus and calcaneus are often parallel to one another.

20. On the first day of treatment of a clubfoot deformity, what should be a primary consideration?

The subtalar joint should be maximally abducted, thus pronating and increasing the talocalcaneal angle, *before* any other manipulative procedures.

21. Forcible dorsiflexion during the initial treatment may result in what deformity?

A flat top talus or rocker-bottom flatfoot may be iatrogenically induced.

22. After an unsuccessful soft-tissue release, what osseous procedures might be considered to reduce a resistant clubfoot?

Cuboid osteotomy with decancellation
Evans procedure removing an anterior wedge from the calcaneus
Evans calcaneocuboid joint resection

METATARSUS ADDUCTUS

23. What is the difference between a total metatarsus adductus and a compensated metatarsus adductus?

Total metaductus involves only the forefoot, distal from the Lisfranc articulation. These metatarsals are adducted 1 through 5. The **compensated** metaductus, also known as a skew foot or serpentine "Z" foot, results in an adduction of the forefoot and hyperpronation out of the midfoot. The result leaves the subtalar joint completely unlocked, giving an impression of a valgus deformity increasing the cuboid and midfoot abduction.

24. By what age should serial casting treatment be started for the reduction of metatarsus adduction?

Cast reduction should be attempted before the child is ambulatory.

25. Describe the position that is held during the manipulative procedure in casting a child for metatarsus adductus.

The rearfoot is held in neutral to an inverted position. The cuboid and fifth metatarsal base are stabilized, and counterpressure is maintained to abduct the metatarsals 1 through 5. Care must be taken not to abduct the foot from the digital area, as this may induce a hallux valgus deformity.

26. How can metatarsus adductus be reduced surgically?

Soft-tissue release of the abductor hallucis tendon
Release of the intermetatarsal ligaments at the Lisfranc articulations (Heyman-Herndon-Strong procedure)
Osteotomies of the bases of the metatarsals
Osteotomies of the cuneiforms

27. What surgical procedure would be recommended for a child who presents with a compensated metatarsus adductus with severe flatfoot deformity?

Metatarsal osteotomies 1–5 with an arthrodesis of the subtalar joint by a Grice-Green procedure or extra-articular arthrodesis. Secondary equinus may be present, and tendo-Achilles or gastrocnemius resection may be indicated.

COALITIONS

28. What are the most common tarsal coalitions?

Talocalcaneal and calcaneonavicular coalitions.

29. What radiographic findings are seen in a subtalar coalition?

Halo sign, talonavicular beaking, anteater nose sign (seen on the elongation of the anterior calcaneus)

30. Which radiographic views of the foot should be taken first to rule out subtalar coalitions?

Anteroposterior and lateral oblique views.

31. When should a Harris-Beath radiograph be performed to rule out coalition?

If the halo sign and broadening of the talus are noted. In the Harris-Beath procedure, on the lateral view, an angle is taken from the weight-bearing surface through the apparent sustentaculum tali and posterior facet. The angle is approximately 30–40°. An axial view is then taken, positioning the central ray at 5° above and 5° below this angle.

32. What other studies can be performed to rule out coalition?

CT and standard radiographic tomography. MRI has been helpful in determining soft-tissue fibrous unions.

33. Describe a treatment plan for a 12-year-old child with a painful subtalar coalition.

The child should be placed into a non–weight-bearing cast in physiologic rest, and nonsteroidal anti-inflammatory drugs are given. This should be followed with orthotic devices.

34. What tendon can enter into spasm during a subtalar coalition?

The peroneus brevis may enter into spasm, creating a peroneal spastic flatfoot.

35. What conservative treatment can be given for this peroneal spastic flatfoot?

A common peroneal block with or without a sinus tarsi block of 2% plain lidocaine. The child is kept immobilized for approximately 3 weeks in a psychologically positioned cast. Nonsteroidal anti-inflammatories are given, followed with a course of physical therapy and orthotics.

36. If a calcaneonavicular coalition is present, what surgical approaches can be recommended?

Resection of the CN bar should be presented first if the child is below age 16 years. A Bagley procedure can be performed by interposing fat or silicone sheathing.

INFECTIONS AND SYSTEMIC CONDITIONS

37. Which organisms are usually prevalent in osteomyelitis in young children below age 5?

Staphylococcus aureus	Group B streptococci
Haemophilus influenzae	Group A streptococci

38. Which organism is usually seen in osteomyelitis in children above the age of 5?

Staphylococcus aureus.

39. What are the causes of rickets?
Vitamin D deficiency, malabsorption syndromes, chronic renal insufficiency, and hypophosphatasia.

40. What is the pathologic basis underlying rickets?
Failure of mineralization of the osteoid tissue.

41. Describe the radiologic signs with rickets.
Trumpeting or lipping of the metaphysis and epiphysis
Bowing of the long bone
Thickening of the medial cortex
Thinning of the lateral cortex

42. How is rickets treated?
Vitamin D replenishment. Usually, exposure to sunlight and the normal intake of milk containing 1500–5000 units daily of vitamin D are sufficient.

43. What is Ehlers-Danlos syndrome?
This is an autosomal dominant genetic disorder that presents with variances of hyperlaxity of the skin and joints as well as capillary fragility that leads to easy bruising. Often seen are lax ligaments of all joints, causing severe flattening of the foot.

44. Describe the recommended course of treatment for the child with Ehlers-Danlos syndrome.
A child presenting with Ehlers-Danlos syndrome who has severe laxity in all ligaments, especially the knee, ankle, and foot, should have these joints held in a neutral-position, deep-seated orthoses.

45. What are the surgical options for a child with Ehlers-Danlos?
In a child presenting with ligament laxity of the ankle and foot, one may consider arthrodesis: either a subtalar extra-articular arthrodesis or, if the child is old enough, total subtalar triple arthrodesis.

BIBLIOGRAPHY

1. Carrel JM: Complications in foot and ankle surgery. In: American College of Foot and Ankle Surgeons. Baltimore, Williams & Wilkins, 1984, pp 190–234.
2. Coleman SS: Complex Foot Deformities in Children. Philadelphia, Lea & Febiger, 1983.
3. DeValentine SJ: Foot and Ankle Disorders in Children. New York, Churchill Livingstone, 1992.
4. Jay RM: Current Therapy in Podiatric Surgery. Philadelphia, B.C. Decker, 1989.
5. Loth TS: Orthopedic Boards Review. St. Louis, Mosby, 1993.
6. Oloff LM: Musculoskeletal Disorders of the Lower Extremity. Philadelphia, W.B. Saunders, 1994, pp 652–672.
7. Tachdjian MO: The Child's Foot. Philadelphia, W.B. Saunders, 1984.
8. Turco VJ: Clubfoot. New York, Churchill Livingstone, 1981.

14. PEDIATRICS: PART II

Edwin Harris, D.P.M.

1. A 6-year-old girl with Rett's syndrome has developed severe ankle equinus contractures and is scheduled for bilateral percutaneous tendo-Achilles lengthenings. What routine preoperative laboratory studies are indicated?

It is inappropriate to order "routine" laboratory tests before surgery, as studies show that randomized preoperative lab tests do little for patient management. They have a low yield for identifying latent disease. Although many tests will be abnormal, identifying these abnormalities usually does not improve care or affect surgical outcome, and frequently the patient receives additional work-up for false-positive tests. This does not mean that there should be no preoperative testing. Testing should be based on the findings from the patient history and physical examination, as well as on the needs unique to the planned procedure.

2. In the case of Rett's syndrome, which specific preoperative tests might be considered?

Rett's syndrome is a neurodegenerative disease of childhood that affects only females. Its etiology, method of inheritance, and biochemical pathophysiology are not known, and there are no laboratory markers. Consequently, there is no role for lab tests in monitoring the progression of the disease. The patient's history and physical examination would suggest any need for lab testing.

In this patient, preoperative lab testing can be limited to hemoglobin and hematocrit and, because she is being treated with the anticonvulsant valproic acid, determination of serum drug level. Urinalysis is not likely to be helpful, because she has no signs of urinary tract disease. If the patient were genetically prone, a screen for sickle cell disease would be indicated. At age 6, she is premenarchal and cannot possibly be pregnant. In a menarchal female, a pregnancy test would be in order.

3. What are acceptable postoperative analgesics for children? How are safe doses determined?

Safe dosages are best calculated using the child's weight in kilograms and the recommended amount per kilogram for the drug in question. This approach is more reliable than calculating the dosage according to a complicated formula using age as the chief variable.

A word of caution about the nonsteroidals (other than acetaminophen) as analgesics: they should be used only when the cause of pain is very clear. When the cause is obscure, their anti-inflammatory action may mask signs of serious infection.

Postoperative Analgesics and Dosages for Children

ANALGESIC	DOSAGE	COMMENTS
Narcotics		
Morphine	0.05–0.1 mg/kg q 2–4 hr	Excellent for pain at any age; must be given IM, IV, or SC.
Fentanyl	1–2 µg/kg/dose	Usually limited to OR or recovery room use.
Meperidine	1–1.5 mg/kg q 3–4 hr	Tablets (50 mg) impractical for children; syrup, given orally, is preferred.
Codeine	0.5–1.0 mg/kg q 4–6 hr	Oral form adequate for less severe pain; often combined with acetaminophen.

Table continued on following page.

Postoperative Analgesics and Dosages for Children (Continued)

ANALGESIC	DOSAGE	COMMENTS
Non-narcotics		
Acetaminophen	10–15 mg/kg q 4 hr	May be given orally or rectally; often combined with codeine or hydrocodone
Aspirin	10–15 mg/kg q 4 hr	Associated with Reye's syndrome in children.
Ibuprofen	20 mg/kg/day, given in divided doses tid	—
Naproxen	10 mg/kg bid	This dosage is double that used for anti-inflammatory purposes.

4. What are the narcotic and benzodiazepine antagonists? What are the pediatric doses?

Naloxone, a narcotic antagonist, is given to infants and children in doses of 0.005–0.01 mg/kg/dose every 2–3 min up to 3 times. Intravenous naloxone has a duration of 30–45 min. Elimination half-time is 60 min. It is possible for the child to become re-narcotized after this time, so it is necessary to observe the child for a sufficient period to ensure narcotic-related symptoms do not return.

Flumenazil is a benzodiazepine-specific antagonist that is ineffective against all other CNS depressants. It is titrated in increments of 0.2 mg up to a maximum dose of 1.0 mg. Reversal of the depressant effects may not be complete. The elimination half-time is 1 hour, which is shorter than the half-life of many commonly used benzodiazepines. Discharge should not be premature.

5. How do you calculate the hourly IV fluid replacement for infants and young children?

The amount is calculated from the child's weight (kg) according to the following schedule:

Calculation of Hourly IV Fluid Replacement for Infants and Young Children

For the first 10 kg	4 ml/kg/hr
For weight between 10–20 kg	40 ml + 2 ml/kg/hr for each kg over 10 kg
For weight between 20–30 kg	60 ml + 1 ml/kg/hr for each kg over 20 kg

6. When should the Heyman-Herndon-Strong procedure be considered for salvage of metatarsus adductus? How is it done?

The Heyman-Herndon-Strong procedure was described in 1958 and has a very specific indication: It is a salvage procedure for failed closed reduction and for children who are too old for successful closed reduction at the time of their diagnosis of metatarsus adductus. It is not a substitute for closed reduction. The principle for its success is based on remodeling of the cartilage that makes up the metatarsal bases and the adjacent tarsals. It is not simply a release of tight structures. There must be adequate remodeling potential remaining, or the procedure will not succeed. Chronologic age is not as important as developmental (bone) age.

The dorsal, medial, and plantar capsule and ligaments of each of the five tarsometatarsal joints are sectioned. Care is taken to protect the insertions of tibialis anterior, tibialis posterior, and peroneus longus when the first metatarso-cuneiform joint is released. The peroneus brevis is protected when the fifth tarsometatarsal structures are released. Because of the anatomy of the second metatarsal base and its relationship to the cuneiforms and the adjacent metatarsals, sectioning the capsule and ligaments does not allow much transverse motion. A second metatarsal osteotomy with abduction and fixation produces correction in this ray. It is appropriate to apply repeat corrective casting for 6 weeks after the procedure, followed by an additional 6 weeks of maintenance casts.

7. How is talipes equinovarus classified?

Classification of Talipes Equinovarus (Clubfoot) in Children

Idiopathic	Small talus
	Abnormal position of the talar neck
	Equinus of the ankle
	Fixed subtalar supination
	Abnormal forefoot-to-rearfoot positioning
	Major joints congruous in abnormal positions
	Calf muscles small, with abnormal fiber size and type disproportion
	Anterior tibial vascular anomalies common
Postural (positional)	Size and shape of talus and calcaneus normal
	Joint surfaces normal, but subluxed
Teratologic (teratogenic)	Includes foot deformities, but other bone and joint lesions predominate, e.g., irreducible bilateral hip dislocation, knee dislocations and subluxations, upper limb pathology, arthrogryposis multiplex congenita
	Associated neuropathies and congenital myopathies
Syndromic	Similar to teratologic form, with non-skeletal abnormalities added
	Includes severe visceral abnormalities, e.g., VATER sequence, congenital constriction band syndrome, glycogen storage diseases, caudal regression sequence

8. How does the prognosis differ among the various types of clubfoot?

Idiopathic: This severe hereditary clubfoot is the most common of the four types. Prognosis is fair, but most of these infants require major release to achieve full reduction of the deformity.

Postural: Not as common as the idiopathic form. Prognosis depends on the cause. Those caused by intrauterine malpositioning have an excellent prognosis, with most going to full lasting reduction after manipulation and casting. In those caused by muscle imbalance, the prognosis then depends on the underlying etiology.

Teratologic: This is an extremely severe form with a very poor prognosis.

Syndromic: Because of its extraskeletal manifestations, even with major reconstructive surgery, the prognosis remains very poor.

9. What are the current principles in treating idiopathic talipes equinovarus?

1. *Early recognition is critical.* The best prognosis is for infants recognized and initially treated within the first 24 hours of life.

2. *Comorbidities must be identified and managed.* Specifically, developmental hip dysplasia and dislocation must be recognized and treated.

3. *Start serial casting and manipulation as soon as possible.* The forefoot deformity and heel varus deformity are managed as a unit. Once these combined deformities are corrected, ankle equinus is corrected.

4. *If the infant's deformity does not fully correct, closed reduction should be stopped* before a secondary deformity is created.

5. *When attempts at closed reduction fail to completely correct the deformity, aggressive surgical release should be performed.* The ideal age is between 6–9 months. The release should be comprehensive. The most common error made by surgeons who infrequently treat this problem is to underestimate the amount of persisting deformity. This results in selecting procedures inadequate for the amount of residual pathology.

10. An 18-month-old girl presents for evaluation of tibia varum. How should you work up this child?

Some amount of tibia varum is physiologic for this age group, so you must determine if this is normal or pathologic bowing. Differential diagnosis is extremely important.

The patient history provides the first clues. If the parents note that the deformity is improving with time, the infant probably is developing normally. Any history of renal, hepatic, or intestinal disease suggests metabolic involvement. Obesity, early standing, and walking before the ninth month in a female are parts of the stereotype for Blount's disease. The outcome in siblings with a similar complaint is also useful.

Examination for symmetry and degree of deformity is critical. Some infants' bowing is so severe that it cannot be accepted as developmentally normal. Unilateral forms are always pathological until proven otherwise.

X-rays for children under age 2 may be helpful if there is osteopenia or abnormality at the growth plates. Lacking these specific changes, the only additional information is the angle formed between the tibial metaphysis and the distal tibial shaft (tibiometaphyseal angle, or Drennan's angle). If this angle is 11° or less, the likelihood of Blount's disease is very low. Above 12°, the probability is very high.

11. A 3-year-old toe-walking boy was examined by a resident who felt that this was a part of normal development. Later, the pediatrician mentions that the child has cerebral palsy. How could this diagnostic error have been avoided?

1. Toe-walking at this age is unlikely to be normal. A **high index of suspicion** for underlying neuromuscular disease is the best tool.

2. A **careful history** will usually uncover risk factors and other clues. Complications of pregnancy are very common. Vaginal spotting during the first two trimesters, treated premature labor, preterm delivery, low birth weight, cesarean section, low Apgar scores, meconium aspiration, need for resuscitation, neonatal apnea, admission to the pediatric intensive care unit, failure to suck, hypotonia at birth, and delayed acquisition of major motor landmarks and cognitive skills are a few of the clues suggesting perinatal CNS insult.

3. **Gait evaluation** often will show adduction of the limbs across midline, abnormal knee extension, equinovarus or equinovalgus feet, and abnormal hand position. There may be balance difficulty suggesting ataxia. Athetosis may also be observed.

4. **Neurologic exam** may show hypertonia in the upper and lower extremities. Deep tendon reflexes may be particularly brisk. There may be an upgoing plantar reflex (Babinsky's sign). Sustained ankle clonus may be present.

12. An 8-year-old girl has as 2-week history of right heel pain. Onset was sudden, with no history of trauma. The remainder of her medical history is unremarkable. Her pediatrician has diagnosed calcaneal apophysitis on clinical findings. How should she be worked up?

The **physical examination** is probably the most important part of the work-up. Pain on side-to-side compression of the calcaneus is characteristic of apophysitis. Absence of edema, erythema, or ecchymosis is also typical. Pain limited to the plantar aspect of the calcaneus is more consistent with plantar fasciitis. Pain on palpating the superior surface of the calcaneus just anterior to the tendo-Achilles suggests stress fracture. Constitutional findings plus edema and erythema suggest infection or one of the juvenile arthropathies.

A very careful **general physical exam** should also be performed. Lateral and axial calcaneal **x-rays** are appropriate initially.

Obtaining baseline **lab work** is more controversial. A CBC and differential, ESR, and anti-streptolysin O (ASO) titer are the tests most likely to yield information. Obtaining an ESR before the child is started on nonsteroidal medications is recommended for baseline.

13. How should the child be treated initially?

Initial treatment may not only be therapeutic but diagnostic as well. **Immobilization** with crutches and non–weight-bearing are initial measures. If the child is noncompliant, a below-knee or above-knee **cast** for 2–3 weeks is in order.

Oral **nonsteroidal drugs** are indicated, including naproxen (10 mg/kg/day divided into two doses 12 hr apart), tolmetin (15 mg/kg/day divided into three doses), and ibuprofen (20 mg/kg/day divided into three doses. In the absence of preexisting gastrointestinal disease, these medications are usually well-tolerated.

14. If these simple measures fail to resolve the pain by the end of 3 weeks, what should be considered next?

A **total-body bone scan** should be obtained to identify any latent pathology at the site of pain. The total-body component will also provide a skeletal survey of other areas for unsuspected bone and joint lesions. These tests may suggest a more appropriate diagnosis or lead to further testing and imaging.

15. What are some of the considerations when planning to reconstruct syndactyly?

There must be a genuine reason for the reconstruction; cosmetics alone is not sufficient. Asymmetrical growth of one of the paired toes is the most common reason. Often, the middle phalanx in one or both sets of bones is truncated or lacks a growth plate.

Side-to-side fusion of the bones needs to be identified. Although not a contraindication to syndactyly reconstruction, this complex syndactyly has a higher incidence of long-term growth abnormality with time.

If tissues are carefully handled, vascular complications are rare. Adequate skin coverage is a bigger concern. For a few selected cases, creative flapping may allow complete coverage with the skin available from the adjacent toes. Often, the surgeon must harvest skin from another site to cover defects that result from the separation.

16. A 5-year-old boy is in the emergency room 3 hours after sustaining an inversion injury of the right ankle. The emergency room physician has diagnosed a lateral ankle sprain and prescribes Ace bandaging and acetaminophen with codeine. What do you think?

The tensile strength of the collateral ligaments is almost always greater than the shear or traction strength of the fibular growth plate. Although ligament damage may occur in this age group, the likelihood of a Salter I or II growth plate injury is much higher.

Careful palpation of the collaterals will reveal ligament injury. If there is pain on palpating the distal fibular growth plate, and there is no pain on palpating the lateral collateral ligaments, a diagnosis of growth plate injury is more appropriate.

If so, the child should be treated with rigid immobilization for 4 weeks. The parents should be warned that growth plate arrest can occur.

17. What is the most common cause for in-toeing gait in children over 2 years of age?

Abnormal femoral anteversion (antetorsion). The proximal neck–transcondylar axis angle is increased so that the femoral head is significantly advanced anterior to the coronal plane. In order for the femoral head to seat anatomically in the acetabulum, the distal femur must internally rotate on the transverse plane. This gives the child an obligate intoed gait.

18. Name the three clinical signs of femoral anteversion (antetorsion) in a 3-year-old child.

- With the hip in the extended position, internal rotation is $> 50°$ and external rotation is $< 25°$.
- The child can sit on the floor in the W-sitting (reverse tailor) position.
- Femoral antetorsion on direct or indirect measurement exceeds $25°$.

19. What are the two most common tarsal coalitions? How are they best imaged?

Calcaneonavicular and middle facet subtalar coalitions. Lateral and external oblique foot x-rays will demonstrate calcaneonavicular coalitions well. Subtalar coalitions are best imaged with coronal CT studies. If a CT study is not immediately available, plain lateral x-rays may show poorly visualized posterior facets, dorsal talar beaking, and the "halo" sign. Although they are not pathognomonic, these findings strongly support the diagnosis. Harris-Beath x-rays are also useful when CT studies cannot be immediately obtained.

20. What extrapedal problems may be associated with calcaneovalgus deformity of the feet?

Many cases of calcaneovalgus deformity occur in isolation, without comorbidity, but this is not always the case. Some are associated with buttocks breech presentation. For this reason, every infant with calcaneovalgus should be examined for knee subluxation and hip dislocation.

On occasion, calcaneovalgus is caused by paralysis of the posterior leg compartment muscles. It is important to examine the low back for cutaneous signs of spinal cord abnormality. Evidence of motor loss at and below the level of S1 should be sought. There is likely to be sensory loss at and below S1 as well.

21. How are Barlow's and Ortolani's tests done?

These tests are used to identify developmental hip dysplasia and dislocation.

Ortolani's test is performed with the infant supine, the thighs flexed at right angles to the trunk, and one side of the pelvis stabilized. The opposite hip is abducted, and the examiner makes an attempt to relocate a dislocated hip. If this can be accomplished, the examiner can feel the femoral head relocate.

Barlow's test is a provocative test to dislocate an unstable hip. The position is the same as for Ortolani's test, but the thigh is adducted while the examiner pushes the proximal femur laterally. If the test is positive, the examiner can feel the femoral head slip out of the acetabulum.

22. What is the Apgar score?

It is a numerical assessment of neurologic depression and intrapartum stress measured at 1 and 5 minutes after birth according to the following ratings. A score of 10 is ideal.

	Score		
PARAMETER	0	1	2
Heart rate	Absent	< 100 bpm	> 100 bpm
Respiratory effort	Absent	Slow, irregular	Good, crying
Muscle tone	Limp	Some extremity flexion	Active motion
Reflex irritability	Absent	Grimace	Grimace and cough/sneeze
Color	Blue and pale	Pink body, blue extremities	Totally pink

23. Describe the three classes of juvenile rheumatoid arthritis.

I. **Systemic onset**
   Associated with daily fever, macular rash, pleuritis, carditis, arthritis, hepatomegaly, splenomegaly, and generalized lymphadenopathy.

II. **Pauciarticular disease**
   Type 1: Occurs most frequently in girls around age 2 years, with knee and ankle involvement, iridocyclitis, rheumatoid factor (RF)-negative and ANA-positive.
   Type 2: Occurs around age 8 years, with lower extremity joint involvement, usually RF- and ANA-negative. Boys may develop into ankylosing spondylitis.

III. **Polyarticular disease**
   Type 1: Girls who are RF-negative and who some minor constitutional findings.
   Type 2: Adolescent girls who are RF-positive and who develop significant arthritis.

24. How many different techniques are available for tendo-Achilles lengthening?

1. Lengthening in continuity by fiber-sliding (e.g., Hoke, White procedures)
2. Z-lengthening (either in sagittal or coronal plane)
3. Selective lengthening of gastrocnemius at its aponeurosis (Baker, Vulpius, Strayer procedures)
4. Tendo-Achilles advancement (Murphy procedure)

25. What are the most common pedal "toddler" fractures?

"Toddler" fractures are fractures of cancellous bone seen in walking infants and very young children. There is always an injury, but it may be impossible to confirm if the injury was not witnessed by an adult. Initially, x-rays are negative, but after about 14–18 days, the healing fracture can be seen as an area of increased density.

The most common is fracture of the **posterior calcaneus**. This must be distinguished from a stress fracture, although the age and activity of the child point away from this latter diagnosis. Osteopenia from neuromuscular disease and unyielding equinus deformity increase the likelihood of this injury.

Cancellous fracture of the **proximal subarticular** cancellous bone of the **cuboid** is another frequent fracture site. Like the fractured calcaneus, the initial x-rays are negative.

Fracture of the cancellous **first metatarsal metaphysis** is another common toddler fracture. Differential diagnosis includes Salter I fracture of the first metatarsal growth plate, complex Salter II injuries, and the metaphyseal buckle (torus) fracture, which is sometimes called the "bunkbed" fracture.

26. What is the juvenile Tillaux fracture?

It is a variation of a Salter III fracture of the anterolateral part of the distal tibial epiphysis. It is caused by external rotation of the foot on the leg and occurs in children whose distal tibial epiphyseal plates are almost closed. The fracture occurs when the anterior inferior tibiofibular ligament pulls away the only portion of the epiphysis which can still fracture through the growth plate.

27. What is a "triplane" fracture?

This fracture occurs in the distal tibia of a child whose growth plate is closing. It has an intra-articular component which extends proximally in the *sagittal* plane from the articular surface to the physis. It then changes direction *transversely* in the physis and then changes direction again to extend *coronally* in the tibial metaphysis.

28. When should such injuries suggest child abuse?

The examiner should be appropriately suspicious of **all** injuries in infants and children. A careful history is followed by an equally careful and complete physical exam. Suggestive findings include:

History:
Injuries from unknown or undocumented causes
Conflicting stories from family members
Inappropriate concern by family members
Delay in seeking treatment
Absence of immunizations
Injuries inconsistent with the child's physical development

Physical exam:
An injury that does not fit the story
Bruises in various stages of healing
Wounds or lesions that have an identifiable shape
Burns on both feet and legs
General neglect and malnutrition
Elective mutism
Fracture patterns

Transverse metaphyseal	Multiple fractures
Spiral or oblique	Fractures of different healing stages
Metaphyseal chips	Rib fractures

29. How should early acute hematogenous osteomyelitis be worked up?

As the name implies, acute hematogenous osteomyelitis is the stage before the child becomes systemically ill. Diagnosis is made through a high index of suspicion with the following signs:

1. Pain over a metaphysis that is out of proportion to the history and clinical findings.
2. Lack of constitutional findings (except for mild hyperpyrexia)
3. Negative plain x-ray findings

Work-up should include the following:
1. CBC and differential
2. ESR
3. Bone scan to localize the lesion
4. MRI if doubt exists

Antibiotic therapy should be started as soon as the diagnosis is suspected.

BIBLIOGRAPHY

1. DeValentine SJ: Foot and Ankle Disorders in Children. New York, Churchill Livingstone, 1992.
2. Pizzutillo PD: Pediatric Orthopaedics in Primary Practice. New York, McGraw-Hill, 1997.
3. Rockwood CA, Wilkins KE, Beaty JH (eds): Fractures in Children, 4th ed. Philadelphia, Lippincott-Raven, 1996.
4. Schindler A, Mason DE, Allington NJ: Occult fractures of the calcaneus in toddlers. J Pediatr Orthop 2:201–205, 1996.
5. Tachdjian MO: The Child's Foot. Philadelphia, W.B. Saunders, 1984.

15. GERIATRICS

Jimmy Gregory, D.P.M.

1. What percentage of the U.S. population is over age 65?
According to the American Association of Retired Persons, 12.5% of the population, or over 30 million people, are over age 65. By the year 2000, approximately 35 million Americans will be age 65 and over.

2. List some of the physical and physiologic changes that occur with normal aging.
Changes associated with normal aging include:
Decreased cardiac function
Decreased nerve conduction
Diminished hearing and visual acuity
Decreased muscle mass
Impaired ability to eliminate waste products

3. On the cellular level, why does aging occur?
The exact mechanism is unknown, but some theories include:
1. An age-related decrease in the ability of DNA to repair itself may lead to multiple genetic injuries.
2. Cellular lipids are oxidized to lipofuscin, an age-related pigment, which accumulates in the heart and brain leading to functional deterioration.

4. What is the difference between senility and dementia?
Senility refers to the normal aging process. **Dementia** is a syndrome involving loss of intellectual function of sufficient severity to interfere with social and occupational functioning.

5. What is the most common cause of dementia?
Alzheimer's disease, which is the degeneration of brain tissue. It may occur at any age but is most commonly seen in older persons.

6. How does delirium differ from dementia?
Delirium is the loss of cognitive function. It is characterized by nonsensical or rambling speech, inability to maintain attention, and usually of acute onset.

7. What age-associated skin changes decrease the rate of wound repair?
1. There is a decrease in the inflammatory response, proliferative phase, and remodeling phase of wound healing which has been demonstrated by measuring wound closure times, epidermal turnover rates, and collagen deposition.
2. Microscopically, there is flattening of the epidermodermal junction which results in diminished nutrient transfer, decreased melanocytes necessary for ultraviolet protection, and decreased vitamin production.
3. Thinning of the dermis results in decreased vascularity which decrease hair bulk, eccrine glands, as well as pacinian and Meissner's corpulses responsible for pressure perception and light touch.

8. Classify foot problems in geriatric patients into general categories.
1. Skin and nail disorders
2. Circulatory changes
3. Neurologic disorders
4. Acquired deformities
5. Degenerative changes

9. What are two common causes of radiographic osteopenia in older persons? What are the radiographic features?

Osteoporosis, which is a decrease in bone mass, and **osteomalacia**, which is due to vitamin D deficiency, are two common causes. The radiographic features of osteoporosis and osteomalacia are trabecular bone resorption and intracortical tunneling.

10. What is the significance of peripheral vascular disease in the geriatric population?

Peripheral vascular disease is present in 20% of the geriatric population. Vascular disease may be arterial or venous in nature and predisposes individuals to ulceration, infection, delayed wound healing, and gangrene.

11. What are the most common nail disorders in the geriatric population?

Onychauxis, onychogryphosis, onychomycosis.

12. Define onychauxis.

Onychauxis is thickening of the toenail (see figure), which may be caused by trauma, previous infection, or systemic disease.

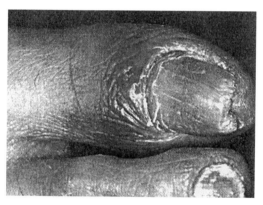

Onychauxis, thickening of the toenail. (From Birrer RB, DellaCorte MP, Grisafi PJ: Common Foot Problems in Primary Care. Philadelphia, Hanley & Belfus, 1992.)

13. What is the difference between onychorrhexis and Beau's lines?

Onychorrhexis is common in older persons and is evident by longitudinal striations in the nail plate. **Beau's lines** are transverse furrows in the nail plate and represent some pathologic disturbance of the nail matrix.

14. Can abnormalities in common laboratory tests be attributed to normal aging?

No. An abnormal CBC or abnormal serum electrolyte levels should not be discounted simply because of age. Abnormal values should be investigated regardless of patient age.

15. What changes of aging are seen in skin?

The major skin changes seen are dryness, uneven pigmentation, wrinkling, and laxity.

16. What is the recommended conservative treatment of hyperkeratosis in geriatrics?

The vast majority of hyperkeratotic lesions in geriatrics can be treated with debridement, emollients or mild keratolytics, padding, and accommodative shoes.

17. Which diseases place patients at risk for decubitus ulcers?

Spinal cord injury, neurologic defects, diabetes mellitus, impaired venous or arterial circulation.

18. List the factors contributing to the development of decubitus ulcers.
Pressure, friction, shear forces, and moisture.

19. Where do the majority of foot decubitus ulcers occur?
The heel and lateral malleolus.

20. What is the recommended treatment of decubitus ulcers?
1. Relief of pressure
2. Cleansing and debridement
3. Topical wound dressing

21. The majority of neurologic foot disorders are due to which two underlying disorders?
Diabetic neuropathy and stroke.

22. What are the most common foot deformities following a stroke?
Equinus, cavovarus hindfoot, clawtoes.

23. What is the most common form of arthritis in the geriatric population? What are its clinical findings?
Osteoarthrosis, or degenerative joint disease, is the most common form of arthritis in geriatrics. Clinical findings may include pain with joint motion and an appropulsive gait if it is affecting the first metatarsophalangeal, midtarsal, subtalar, or ankle joint.

24. Why does the elderly population have such a high rate of arthritis?
• Decreased bone mineral content
• Decreased muscle strength
• Decreased connective tissue elasticity
• Decreased cellular metabolism
• Decreased cellular reproduction

25. What is metatarsalgia? Why is it more common in geriatrics?
Metatarsalgia is used to describe a diffusely painful area in the foot plantar to the metatarsal heads. Many factors may cause metatarsalgia, but in geriatrics it is most frequently due to fat pad atrophy.

26. What disorders are responsible for heel pain in older persons?
1. Plantar fasciitis/heelspur
2. Fat pad atrophy
3. Stress fracture

27. Discuss the differential diagnosis for infracalcaneal heel pain and retrocalcaneal heel pain in the geriatric patient.
The differential diagnosis for infracalcaneal heel pain includes plantar fasciitis/heel spur syndrome, bursa secondary to fat pad atrophy, and plantar nerve entrapment. The differential diagnosis for retrocalcaneal pain includes Achilles tendinitis, retrocalcaneal exostosis or bursa, and Haglund's deformity.

28. Where does the posterior tibial tendon usually rupture?
In an area just posterior and distal to the medial malleolus. Rupture occurs because of chronic irritation in a vascularly compromised area.

29. What are the two primary goals when considering surgery in the geriatric patient?
Relief of pain and restoration of function.

30. Why is the elderly patient at increased risk of infection?

With advancing age, there is a decline in the production of antibodies in response to infections. An infection may remain hidden due to the inability of the immune system to manifest normal signs of infection.

31. A bunion deformity that fails a course of conservative treatment in a geriatric patient can be treated surgically by what procedures?

1. Silver bunionectomy
2. McBride or modified McBride bunionectomy
3. Keller arthroplasty

BIBLIOGRAPHY

1. American Association of Retired Persons: A Profile of Older Americans, 1990. Washington, DC, American Association of Retired Persons, 1991.
2. Espinoza DV, Doty S (eds): Age-related changes in elderly individuals. Clin Podiatr Med Surg 10(2):7, 1993.
3. Helfand AE: Disorders Associated with Aging: Principles and Practices of Podiatric Medicine. New York, Churchill Livingstone, 1990, p 549.
4. Tepelidis NT: Wound healing in the elderly. Clin Podiatr Med Surg 8(4):817, 1991.
5. Karpman RR: Foot problems in the geriatric patient. Clin Orthop 316:59, 1995.
6. Kosinski M, Ramcharitar S: In-office management of common geriatric foot problems. Geriatrics 49(5):43, 1995.

16. FOOT BIOMECHANICS

James M. Losito, D.P.M, F.A.C.F.A.O.M., F.A.C.F.A.S.

1. Name three forms of lower extremity compensation for ankle equinus.

Genu recurvatum, subtalar joint pronation, and midtarsal joint pronation all may occur in an attempt to keep the heel purchasing the ground prior to propulsion. Through excessive pronation, subtalar joint dorsiflexion occurs in lieu of limited ankle joint dorsiflexion. If the heel remains on the ground throughout stance, the equinus is considered to be totally compensated. An early heel-off occurs when the equinus deformity is only partially compensated.

2. How can you differentiate gastrocnemius equinus from soleal equinus?

By measuring the amount of ankle joint dorsiflexion first with the knee extended and then with the knee flexed (Silfverskiold test). If ankle joint dorsiflexion is limited with the knee extended, but more motion is present upon flexion of the knee, a gastrocnemius equinus is present. If there is no difference with the knee flexed or extended, then a combined gastrocnemius-soleus equinus is present.

3. How is a diagnosis of an anterior ankle impingement exostosis made clinically?

Limitation of ankle joint dorsiflexion (equinus) with the knee flexed and extended, accompanied by an abrupt end to range of motion. A stress lateral radiograph may confirm the diagnosis. Anterior ankle pain is the most common presenting symptom.

4. Explain the concept of planal dominance as it relates to pes planus.

The sagittal plane axis ("pitch") of the subtalar joint has an average angulation of 42°. If this axis is lower, the subtalar joint has an increased capacity for frontal plane motion (inversion-eversion). If the subtalar axis is high, more transverse plane motion of the subtalar joint is available. This concept explains why, in many flatfoot deformities, the frontal-plane (everted calcaneus) or transverse-plane (abducted forefoot) component tends to dominate.

5. What forefoot or rearfoot abnormalities may contribute to lateral ankle instability?

Forefoot valgus, plantarflexed first ray, and rearfoot varus. Forefoot valgus and plantarflexed first ray result in compensatory subtalar joint supination upon forefoot loading. With this laterally directed force (supination), lateral ankle instability may occur. A rearfoot varus results in an excessively inverted position of the heel upon loading, with the potential for lateral ankle instability.

6. What effect does femoral anteversion have on the subtalar joint during gait?

Excessive pronation. Any internal transverse-plane abnormality results in increased weight-bearing on the lateral column with resulting subtalar and midtarsal joint pronation. The patella will internally rotate upon heel contact, and the gait is in-toed.

7. What is considered the normal range of ankle joint dorsiflexion and plantarflexion?

The normal adult value, reached by age 15, is 10° of dorsiflexion and 20° of plantarflexion, with the knee extended. The Silfverskiold test is then performed (flex the knee), which takes the gastrocnemius off of stretch, usually producing more dorsiflexion.

8. How can a forefoot varus deformity be clinically differentiated from a forefoot supinatus deformity?

A forefoot varus is a primary structural deformity in which the forefoot is in a rigid, inverted position relative to the rearfoot. A forefoot supinatus deformity is a flexible, acquired positional adaptation in which the forefoot is inverted relative to the rearfoot. In the forefoot varus, the forefoot is in a fixed, nonreducible inverted position. The supinatus deformity is flexible and clinically reducible with gentle dorsal pressure.

9. How does the subtalar joint compensate for a forefoot varus deformity as compared to a forefoot supinatus deformity?

In a forefoot varus deformity, subtalar joint pronation occurs so that the forefoot may purchase the ground. A forefoot supinatus is an acquired deformity which is secondary to some pronatory force (e.g., equinus, rearfoot varus, etc.).

10. Describe a UCBL orthosis and its indications.

A UCBL (University of California Biomechanics Laboratory) orthosis typically consists of a semirigid plate of polypropylene that has a deep heel seat and a high medial flange and lateral clip. The device is flat-posted (0° motion), and any forefoot deformity is balanced. The indications include flexible pes planus, tarsal coalition, posterior tibialis tendon dysfunction, and neuromuscular diseases (e.g., cerebral palsy).

11. Which materials are considered appropriate for use directly against an insensitive foot?

Plastizote # 1 is the best material due to its heat-moldability. This increases the surface area of contact. PPT (Peron) is suitable but is not heat-moldable. Spenco and Viscolas are also acceptable, but like PPT, are not moldable.

12. What is the significance of hemorrhagic callus formation?

When a hematoma forms beneath or between layers of hyperkeratotic skin, it is referred to as a hemorrhagic callus. It indicates severe microtrauma is occurring, consistent with the loss of the patient's proprioceptive protective threshold. Consequently, a hemorrhagic callus is a preulcerative condition requiring accommodation.

13. Describe some of the potential etiologies of a functional hallux limitus.

An abnormally long first metatarsal, metatarsus primus elevatus, hypermobility of the first ray, or excessive subtalar joint pronation are potential causes. Any force that dorsiflexes the first metatarsal will cause jamming at the metatarsophalangeal (MTP) joint upon dorsiflexion of the hallux. Consequently, a functional hallux limitus may lead to the development of a structural hallux limitus. A rectus foot type may predispose to the development of hallux limitus.

14. What type of shoe modification is indicated in the management of hallux limitus or following a first MTP joint fusion?

A metatarsal rocker bar. The bar should be placed just proximal to the fused or painful joint, thus reducing extension and weight-bearing forces across the joint. A rigid-soled shoe will also limit the flexion/extension requirements of the affected joint and may be useful.

15. Describe foot and ankle function when the malleolar torsion is low or negative.

Low or negative malleolar torsion is a transverse-plane abnormality that results in compensatory subtalar and midtarsal joint pronation during gait. Decreased dorsiflexion of the ankle joint during the stance phase of gait occurs secondary to the increased subtalar joint pronation.

16. What is the correct range for malleolar torsion in an adult?

The adult range for malleolar torsion is 18–23° external and is best observed radiographically. Malleolar position is the clinical measurement, with a normal adult value of 13–18° external, reached by approximately 7–8 years of age.

17. Which muscle is the most efficient pronator of the subtalar joint?

The peroneus brevis. The brevis takes its origin at the styloid process of the fifth metatarsal and is a pure stance-phase muscle.

18. What are the most significant clinical findings in a patient with talocalcaneal coalition?

Limited and painful subtalar joint range of motion. The total range of subtalar motion in such a patient is usually < 15°. The foot may appear flat with an everted heel and peroneal spasm. The patient age (14–17 years old) and radiographs confirm the diagnosis.

19. What is the correct order of midtarsal and subtalar joint compensation for a flexible forefoot valgus deformity upon loading?

First, the longitudinal axis of the midtarsal joint supinates, followed by supination of the oblique axis of the midtarsal joint. If the forefoot has not yet fully purchased the ground, the subtalar joint inverts. This explains why forefoot valgus is commonly seen along with an inverted rearfoot (varus).

20. What is the most common lesion pattern observed in patients with forefoot valgus?

Plantar keratomas under the first and fifth metatarsal heads. The lesion plantar to the first metatarsal head is secondary to predominantly vertical forces, as the everted forefoot contacts the ground. The lesion plantar to the fifth metatarsal head is a consequence of shearing forces as the midtarsal and subtalar joints supinate, allowing the lateral border of the foot to contact the ground.

21. Which orthotic, with modifications, would be indicated in the patient with metatarsalgia and painful plantar tylomas with a cavus foot?

The orthotic plate should be flexible to attenuate the increased forces that plague the cavus foot type. A metatarsal raise, or "cookie," should be placed on the distal edge of the orthotic plate just proximal to the metatarsal heads. This reduces weight-bearing forces on the metatarsal heads. A forefoot extension with lesion accommodation may also be useful.

22. Tibial and femoral stress fractures are most often associated with which foot type?

A cavus foot type is very stable but does not absorb shock well due to its rigid structure and limited capacity for subtalar joint pronation. Consequently, forces are transmitted proximally with very little attenuation occurring at the foot.

23. Which biomechanical or structural factor(s) may influence the development of a hallux abductovalgus deformity?

Excessive subtalar joint pronation results in hypermobility of the first ray, which in turn can lead to deformity at the first MTP joint. The peroneus longus looses its plantarflexory vector of pull on the first ray when the subtalar joint is pronated, resulting in hypermobility of the first ray during gait. An adductus foot type predisposes to the development of hallux valgus.

24. What compensation occurs when there is a foot-drop or slap present?

Vaulting of the contralateral limb to gain ground clearance and circumduction of the affected limb. Knee and hip flexion occurs on the affected limb, hence the term "steppage" gait.

25. Describe a Trendelenburg type gait.

A Trendelenburg gait is secondary to weakness of the gluteus medius and is characterized by a hip-drop during the stance phase of gait on the opposite side of the affected muscle.

26. Which lower leg muscle functions as the primary decelerator at heel contact during normal gait?

The tibialis anterior undergoes eccentric contraction at heel contact, resulting in deceleration and preventing a foot slap. Concentric contracture occurs during the swing phase to allow for toe clearance.

27. Describe the relationship between the development of pes planus and shoe gear.

Wearing shoes during childhood plays little if any role in the development of the medial longitudinal arch and may actually interfere with normal arch development. Many studies have shown that the mean arch height is higher in feet which developed unshod compared to those who wore shoes. However, children should be encouraged to wear shoes when outdoors, primarily for protection.

28. Describe the position and motion of the ankle, subtalar joint, talus, and tibia at heel contact during normal walking.

At heel contact, the subtalar joint is in a supinated position, with the tibia externally rotated. The ankle joint is neutral or slightly plantarflexed. As heel contact progresses, the subtalar joint pronates, the tibia internally rotates to the femur, and the talus plantarflexes and adducts.

29. What is considered the normal range for subtalar joint pronation during the contact phase of normal gait? What percentage of the gait cycle does this represent?

At heel contact, the subtalar joint should pronate approximately 10° during the first 8–10% of stance phase during normal gait. Pronation of the subtalar joint "unlocks" the midtarsal joint, allowing for hypermobility and an increased capacity for adaptation to changes in terrain. Pronation of the subtalar joint beyond 8–10% of stance during walking gait is considered excessive.

30. Compare the function of the subtalar joint during running as compared to walking. What defines the "double-float phase"?

During running, there is an increased rate, amount, and duration of subtalar pronation as compared to walking. During running, the subtalar joint pronates from heel strike up to 20% of stance. Maximum pronation occurs at approximately 40% of the cycle and may occur up to 85% of the stance phase. Additionally, the base of gait is significantly decreased during running as compared to walking.

The "double-float phase," which occurs only in running, is the period during which both feet are off of the ground. One leg is in the "foot-descent" stage of the swing phase and the other leg is in the "follow through" stage of the stance phase.

BIBLIOGRAPHY

1. Cavanagh PR: The biomechanics of lower extremity action in distance running. Foot Ankle 7:197–217, 1987.
2. Colsgiuri S, Marsden LL, Naidu V, Taylor L: The use of orthotic devices to correct plantar callus in people with diabetes. Diab Res Clin 28(1):29–34, 1995.
3. Cornwall MW, McPoil TG: The influence of the tibialis anterior muscle activity on rearfoot motion during walking. Foot Ankle Int 15(2):75–79, 1994.
4. Coughlin MJ: Hallux valgus: Causes, evaluation and treatment. Postgrad Med 75:174–187, 1984.
5. Green DR, Carol A: Planal dominance. J Am Podiatr Med Assoc 74(2):98–103, 1984.
6. Hillstrom HJ, Perlberg G, Siegler S, et al: Objective identification of ankle equinus deformity and resulting contracture. J Am Podiatr Med Assoc 81:519–520, 1991.
7. Liu XC, Fabry G, et al: The ground reaction force in the gait of intoeing children. J Pediatr Orthop 4(1):80–85, 1995.
8. Nigg BM: Biomechanical analysis of ankle and foot movement. Med Sci Sports Exerc 23:22–29, 1987.
9. Nyska M, McCabe C, Linge K, et al: Effect of the shoe on plantar foot pressures. Acta Orthop Scand 66(1):53–56, 1995.
10. Rodgers MM: Biomechanics of the foot during locomotion. In Grabiner MD (ed): Current Issues in Biomechanics. Champaign. IL, Human Kinetics Publishers, 1993, pp 34–36.
11. Root ML, Orien WD, Weed JH: Normal and Abnormal Function of the Foot. Los Angeles, Clinical Biomechanics Corp., 1977, pp 154.
12. Roy K, Scherer P: Forefoot supinatus. J Am Pediatr Med Assoc 76:390–394, 1986.
13. Rzonca E, Levitz S, Lue B: Hallux equinus and the stages of hallux limitus and rigidus. J Am Podiatr Med Assoc 74:390–393, 1984.
14. Sachithanandam V, Joseph B: The influence of footwear on the prevalence of flat foot: A survey of 1846 skeletally mature persons. J Bone Joint Surg [Br] 77(2):254–257, 1995.
15. Sanfililppo MS, Stess RM, Moss K: Dynamic plantar pressure analysis: Comparing common insole materials. J Am Podiatr Med Assoc 82:507–512, 1992.
16. Sobel EC, Levitz SJ: Torsional development of the lower extremity—Implications for in-toe and out-toe treatment. J Am Podiatr Med Assoc 81:344–356, 1993.
17. Sommer HM, Vallentyne SW: Effect of foot posture on the incidence of medial tibial stress syndrome. Med Sci Sports Exerc 27(6):800–804, 1995.
18. Valmassy RL (ed): Clinical Biomechanics of the Lower Extremities. St. Louis, Mosby, 1996.
19. Wu K: Foot Orthoses: Principles and Clinical Applications. Baltimore, Williams & Wilkins, 1990.

17. FOOT AND ANKLE TRAUMA

Kim Felder-Johnson, D.P.M., and Alex Reyzelman, D.P.M.

1. What is a Jones fracture?

It is a fracture of the proximal fifth metatarsal diaphysis approximately 1.5 cm from the tip of the tuberosity. It has a potential for nonunion and must be distinguished from the oblique avulsion fracture of the tuberosity of the fifth metatarsal, which tends to heal without complication.

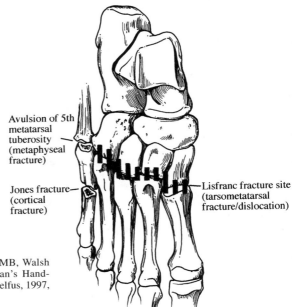

Avulsion of 5th metatarsal tuberosity (metaphyseal fracture)

Jones fracture (cortical fracture)

Lisfranc fracture site (tarsometatarsal fracture/dislocation)

Fractures of the foot. (From Mellion MB, Walsh WM, Shelton GL: The Team Physician's Handbook, 2nd ed. Philadelphia, Hanley & Belfus, 1997, with permission.)

2. What is a march fracture?

A march fracture is a stress fracture of a metatarsal. It carries this name because of its frequent occurrence in military personnel.

3. What are the main principles in dealing with fractures and dislocations of the ankle?

1. Reduction of the injury should be performed as soon as possible.

2. The reduction must be maintained during the healing period with either external immobilization such as a cast or internal fixation devices.

3. All joint surfaces must be reduced anatomically to help diminish the risk of posttraumatic arthritis.

4. What is the ankle syndesmosis?

It is the relationship or articulation between the distal tibia and fibula, and is maintained by the interosseous membrane, the anterior/inferior tibiofibular ligament, the posterior inferior tibiofibular ligament, the posterior talofibular ligament, and the inferior transverse ligament.

5. What complications may occur following ankle fractures or dislocations?

Posttraumatic arthritis, reflex sympathetic dystrophy (RSD), neurovascular injury, nonunion, malunion, and infection (particularly if the fracture was open or if operative intervention was used).

6. What is a worrisome complication of fractures of the talar neck?

Avascular necrosis (AVN) of the talar body.

Several questions in this chapter have been modified from McMullen ST: Foot and ankle trauma. In Brown DE, Neumann RD: Orthopedic Secrets. Philadelphia, Hanley & Belfus, 1995.

7. What is the radiographic appearance of AVN of the talus?

There is increased density of the avascular body compared with the surrounding bone, which is vascular and undergoing disuse resorption. Hawkin's sign is the presence of subchondral osteopenia and excludes the diagnosis of AVN. Bone scanning or magnetic resonance imaging may also be helpful in the diagnosis of AVN.

8. Which x-ray views are necessary when evaluating an injured ankle?

Anteroposterior, lateral, and mortise views. The mortise view is taken with the leg internally rotated approximately 15–20 degrees, which aligns the beam perpendicular to the intermalleolar line.

9. What is a pylon fracture?

It is a distal tibial metaphyseal fracture with extension into the joint surface, usually with extensive comminution.

10. When evaluating a person with a calcaneus fracture, you must consider injuries to what other areas?

It is important not to overlook potential spinal injuries. A typical mechanism in both fractures is axial loading. Other associated fractures include femoral neck fractures and tibial plateau fractures.

11. What is the orientation of the primary fracture line in intra-articular calcaneal fractures?

The calcaneus initially fractures into two main fragments; anteromedial and posterolateral, which are produced by a fracture line running obliquely from plantar-medial to dorsolateral.

12. What are two commonly identified fracture patterns in intra-articular calcaneal fractures?

The joint depression, which is more common, and tongue type.

13. For what should all patients who sustain a calcaneal fracture be examined?

Seventy percent of patients with calcaneal fractures have associated lower extremity injuries. Compression fractures of the spine occur in 10% of these patients. Compartment syndrome of the foot can occur in approximately 10% of all calcaneal fractures.

14. What are the common mechanisms of ankle fractures?

Adduction, abduction, external rotation, and vertical loading.

15. How are ankle fractures classified?

The two most common are the Lauge-Hansen and the Danis-Weber AO classification systems.

16. What is the Lauge-Hansen classification?

The Lauge-Hansen classification is based on the suspected mechanism of injury. In each category, the injury begins in a specific anatomic location and progresses sequentially about the ankle, creating the injury patterns described.

Supination adduction (SA)
    I. Transverse avulsion type fracture of the fibula below the level of the tibial plafond
    II. Vertical fracture of the medial malleolus
Supination external rotation (SER)
    I. Disruption of anterior tibiofibular ligament
    II. Spiral oblique fracture of the distal fibula originating near the level of the tibial plafond
    III. Disruption of posterior tibiofibular ligament or fracture of posterior malleolus
    IV. Oblique fracture of medial malleolus or rupture of deltoid ligament
Pronation adduction (PA)
    I. Transverse fracture of medial malleolus or rupture of deltoid ligament
    II. Rupture of syndesmotic ligaments
    III. Short horizontal or oblique fracture of the fibula above the level of the ankle joint

Pronation external rotation (PER)

    I. Transverse fracture of the medial malleolus or disruption of the deltoid ligament

    II. Disruption of anterior tibiofibular ligament

    III. Oblique fracture of the fibula approximately 4–5 cm above the level of the tibial plafond

    IV. Rupture of posterior tibiofibular ligament or avulsion fracture of posterior lateral tibia

Pronation dorsiflexion (PD)

    I. Fracture of medial malleolus

    II. Fracture of anterior margin of tibia

    III. Supramalleolar fracture of fibula

    IV. Transverse fracture of posterior tibial surface

17. Using the Lauge-Hansen classification, what is the most common mechanism of ankle fracture?

Supination-external rotation. Sixty to eighty percent of ankle fractures are of this type.

18. What is the Danis-Weber AO classification system?

It is based on the level of the fibula fracture.

Type A, fibula fracture below syndesmosis

    1. Isolated fracture

    2. With associated fracture of medial malleolus

    3. With associated posterior medial tibia fracture

Type B, fibular fracture of level of syndesmosis

    1. Isolated

    2. With associated medial malleolus or deltoid ligament injury

    3. With associated medial lesion and fracture of posterior lateral tibia

Type C, fibular fracture above syndesmosis

    1. Isolated fibular fracture

    2. Comminuted fibular fracture

    3. Proximal fracture of the fibula

19. What is an injury to the tarsal metatarsal joint area called?

This joint is known as Lisfranc's joint (see figure in Question 1). Injuries may include disruption of the ligaments supporting the joints and associated fractures. For subtle injuries, displacement may be seen only on a weight-bearing oblique view of this region. Anatomic reduction is mandatory.

20. What are the most common mechanisms responsible for tarsometatarsal injuries?

Twisting abduction force can abduct the forefoot on the tarsus. This is seen in motor vehicle and horseback accidents. Axial loading of a fixed foot can occur when a heavy object falls on the heel or from a missed step off a curb. Direct crushing blow to the dorsum of the foot is the third common mechanism of injury to Lisfranc's joint.

21. How are talus fractures classified?

The Hawkins classification system is used:

Type I: Nondisplaced vertical fracture of the talar neck

Type II: Displaced fracture of the talar neck with subluxation or dislocation of the subtalar joint with the ankle joint remaining intact

Type III: Displaced fracture of the talar neck with dislocation of the body of the talus from both the subtalar and ankle joints

The risk of AVN increases as the amount of the displacement increases.

22. LARD and LATAS are acronyms for evaluating and describing fracture and dislocation injuries. What components of the evaluation do these describe?

L-length, A-angulation, R-rotation, D-displacement and L-location, A-alignment, T-type, A-articular, S-stability are the components of the evaluation for the assessment of fractures and dislocations. Assessment of these components not only aids in the description but in the decision process for the treatment course.

23. How are talar body fractures classified?

Sneppen described the following classification system: type 1, osteochondral/transchondral fracture; type 2, coronal, sagittal, or horizontal shear fracture; type 3, fracture of the posterior talar process; type 4, fracture of the lateral process; type 5, crush injury of the talar body.

24. What is the treatment for talar body fractures?

While each case must be assessed and managed on an individual basis, the general treatment protocol is based on the type of fracture identified. Type 1 fractures are managed like Berndt-Hardy lesions. If the fracture is nondisplaced, a below-the-knee cast is used for 4–6 weeks, non-weightbearing. If there is a displaced fragment, this is removed and treatment is the same. Type 2 fractures are treated with open reduction and internal fixation and below-the-knee casting for 6–8 weeks, non-weightbearing. Type 3 fractures are casted for 6–8 weeks non-weightbearing in a below-the-knee cast. Type 4 fractures are closed, reduced if nondisplaced, then placed in a below-the-knee cast with well-padded pressure against the lateral process. If the fracture is displaced, open reduction and internal fixation are performed, followed by a below-the-knee cast for 6–8 weeks. Type 5 fractures undergo a pantalar arthrodesis followed by casting in a position of function for 12–16 weeks. All of the fractures are initially assessed for neurovascular status, length, angulation, rotation, displacement, location, alignment, articular involvement, type, and stability before treatment is performed.

25. What is a Watson-Jones Type 2 navicular fracture and what is an associated injury seen with this type of fracture?

An avulsion of the tuberosity. The mechanism of injury resulting in this type of avulsion fracture can result in a compression fracture of the calcaneocuboid joint.

26. Why can ice be contraindicated in a digital crush injury?

Often in a digital crush injury there is vascular compromise. Ice placed on a digit with vascular compromise can result in vasoconstriction, which may result in further tissue loss or necrosis, increasing the potential risk of gangrene or amputation.

27. What is the treatment protocol for an open fracture?

The initial treatment involves debridement and lavage. Anesthesia is obtained, and the wound is debrided of foreign bodies, contaminants, and devitalized tissue. The wound should be copiously irrigated. Removal of any loose osseous fragments with further irrigation should be performed. Fractures should be stabilized and vascular repair performed if required. Cultures should be taken before administering antibiotics. Depending on the injury and contaminants, double or triple antibiotic coverage should be instituted. Closure of the wounds should be delayed if the injury is greater than 6 hours old, or if the injury falls into the type II (in some cases) and type III (all cases), until after the 5th–7th day following local wound care and antibiotics.

BIBLIOGRAPHY

1. Hawkins LG: Fractures of the neck of the talus. J Bone Joint Surg 52A:991–1002, 1970.
2. Jones R: Fracture at the base of the fifth metatarsal by indirect violence. Ann Surg 35:697–700, 1902.
3. Lauge-Hansen N: Fractures of the ankle combined experimental-surgical and experimental-roentgenologic investigations. Arch Surg 60:967–985, 1950.
4. Manoly A II: Compartment syndromes of the foot: Current concepts. Foot Ankle 10:340–344, 1990.
5. Myerson MS: Experimental decompression of fascial compartments of the foot with a basis for fasciotomy in acute compartment syndrome. Foot Ankle 8:308–314, 1988.
6. Rockwood CA Jr, Greene DP, Buckholz RW, et al (eds): Rockwood and Green's Fractures in Adults, 4th ed. Philadelphia, Lippincott-Raven, 1996.

18. PODIATRIC SPORTS INJURIES

Kenrick J. Dennis, D.P.M., and Paul S. Bishop, D.P.M.

1. What are the most common causes of heel pain in athletes?

Plantar fasciitis, or heel spur syndrome, comprises approximately 30% of the overuse injuries seen in a podiatric sports medicine practice. The most important other consideration in the differential diagnosis is a stress fracture of the calcaneus.

The athlete will describe an insidious onset of pain which is increased on first weight-bearing and point to the origin of the plantar fascia. They commonly describe the injury as a "stone bruise." The objective exam shows pain on direct palpation of the medial calcaneal tubercle. An equinus deformity at the ankle joint is a common sequelae. If pain is present on medial to lateral compression of the calcaneus, the practitioner must be suspicious of stress fracture and order appropriate x-rays, and possibly a bone scan, to confirm the diagnosis.

2. Describe conservative care for plantar fasciitis.

Initial treatment should include ice, nonsteroidal anti-inflammatory medications, wearing a good supportive shoe, exercise to tolerance, and aggressive Achilles tendon stretching. If the pain is not at least 50% improved within 2 weeks, an x-ray should be taken and an injection of 4–6 mg of a short-acting steroid (e.g., dexamethasone) given. A functional orthotic may be considered if a significant biomechanical contribution is identified. A total of three local steroid injections may be utilized, spaced every 2–3 weeks, if pain persists.

Surgical intervention should not be considered until the patient has failed at least 6 months of conservative care.

3. What are the important considerations in the evaluation and treatment of an inversion ankle sprain?

The primary goal in the early evaluation of an inversion ankle sprain is to rule out fracture, particularly a high fibular fracture as well as distal fractures of the metatarsals (Jones' fracture). Once fracture is ruled out, initial treatment must focus on edema control. This may be as simple as ice, compression, and elevation at home, but may include the use of an Unna's boot or some other removable compression device. Crutches should be used until weight-bearing is painfree.

Early active mobilization is now supported in the literature as the treatment of choice. An athlete may return to sport when he or she can accomplish 20 toe-raises on the affected ankle without pain.

4. What is turf toe? How do you treat it?

"Turf toe" is one of those diagnoses used to describe myriad clinical presentations. In its purest definition, turf toe refers to a sprain of the ligaments of the first metatarsophalangeal (MTP) joint. However, in its generic use, it may be used to describe pain associated with hallux limitus or sesamoid pathology.

Evaluation must focus on ruling out fracture. There is normally pain on all range of motion of the joint, with point tenderness and edema surrounding the MTP joint. Treatment includes rest, ice, and compression of the painful joint until gross swelling resolves. The great toe may be splinted with athletic tape as the athlete returns to sports (see figure, top of next page). A functional orthotic, with a Morton's extension, may be necessary for long-term treatment.

5. Define sesamoiditis.

The great toe sesamoid bones are prone to injury in any sport involving impact on a dorsiflexed MTP joint. It is a common injury in a rigid forefoot valgus foot type.

Turf Toe Taping

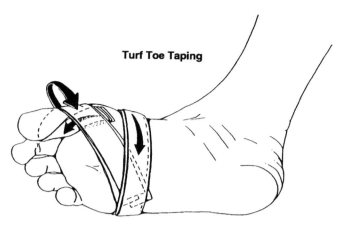

Taping to limit motion of MTP joint in treating turf toe. (From Mellion MB, Walsh WM, Shelton GL: The Team Physician's Handbook. Philadelphia, Hanley & Belfus, 1997, with permission.)

Pain is present on direct palpation as well as forced dorsiflexion of the first MTP joint. Bilateral x-rays should be taken to help differentiate a fracture from a bipartite sesamoid. Bone scan should be made available to any athlete desiring early definitive diagnosis.

Treatment may range from a simple felt "dancer's pad," to short-leg walking cast, to surgical excision. A patient who has not responded to conservative care may benefit from a single inter-articular injection of 1 ml of dexamethasone. Any time surgical correction is planned, the patient must be thoroughly informed as to potential postoperative transverse-plane complications.

6. What is the treatment of subungual hematoma?

Subungual hematoma ("runner's toe") in the athlete is most commonly the result of chronic repetitive pressure to the nail plate—i.e., a "bruised" toe nail. The primary etiology is a shoe that is slightly short (there should be at least a thumb's width distance between the longest toe and the end of the shoe).

If there is not a significant history of trauma (e.g., having the toe stepped on, or just complet-ing a marathon), radiographs should be taken (lateral view with the great toe dorsiflexed) to rule out a subungual exostosis.

If the toe is not painful, no treatment is one alternative. If the nail is loose, total avulsion is indicated. Drainage would be indicated for a painful and "tense" nail that is intact. After a sterile prep, the nail is easily drained by using an 18-gauge needle between the thumb and index finger and lightly "drilling" two to three holes in the nail plate. Compression dressing and soaks are re-quired, and the patient should understand that he or she may need to drain the nail two to three times. The patient should be made aware that the nail will spontaneously avulse in 6–8 weeks as a new nail grows in.

7. What specifically are shin splints?

The term *shin splints* is one of those all-inclusive terms and may include any pathology distal to the knee and proximal to the midfoot. It most commonly includes posterior tibial muscle injury, anterior tibial muscle injury, and stress fracture. The primary etiology for this injury is some type of training error. Throughout evaluation, one must consider training surface, shoes, foot type, and leg-length differences. Point tenderness over the anterior tibial crest warrants radi-ographs and possibly a bone scan to rule out stress fracture.

Treatment includes nonsteroidal anti-inflammatory drugs (NSAIDs), ice, physical ther-apy, strengthening of the affected muscle, modification of training, and possibly a functional orthotic device. Left untreated, a mild case of anterior or posterior tenosynovitis will escalate into a stress fracture.

8. Describe the presentation of tibialis posterior dysfunction.

The posterior tibial tendon is a major arch-supporting structure of the foot. The muscle originates on the posterior aspect of the tibia, becomes a tendon in its distal third, courses under the medial malleolus in the flexor compartment, and inserts into the navicular tuberosity. The tendon may give off many insertion slips into the plantar aspect of the cuneiforms and medial metatarsals. Its function is to act as a stirrup to reinforce the medial longitudinal arch.

Injury to the posterior tibial tendon is usually the result of overuse in athletes. Typically, the patient presents with pain medially in the arch, which may extend proximally along the course of the tendon posterior to the medial malleolus. The patient may also complain of plantar arch pain mimicking plantar fascia pain. The medial arch may be slightly lower on the affected side, especially if there is a traumatic tear or rupture of the tendon. Edema can best be observed from behind the patient. While you look at the feet from behind, the affected side will have more toe visible over the lateral border of the foot.

The foot may be pronated or even apropulsive throughout gait, as the tendon cannot supinate the foot in midstance. The tendon integrity may also be tested by asking the patient to stand on the toes. With posterior tibial tendon dysfunction, the heel cannot invert on heel raise, and in the case of rupture, a heel lift may not be possible.

Diagnostic studies include MRI, tenogram, and ultrasound. MRI is the most sensitive and specific and has the benefit of being noninvasive.

9. How is tibialis posterior dysfunction treated?

Early treatment should include NSAIDs, ice, and medial arch support (e.g., rigid functional orthotic). All patients are strongly discouraged from using nonsupportive shoegear or going barefoot. More advanced tendon injury may require cast immobilization for 4–6 weeks and possible surgical repair. This injury must be diagnosed and treated early so as not to progress into more complicated sequelae.

10. How do you diagnose a stress fracture?

A stress fracture is the result of chronic repetitive force being applied to a bone. The elastic properties of bone allow it to flex to some extent; however, repetitive stress without time to heal between episodes leads to weakening of the bone. The periosteum becomes inflamed, and new bone formation begins. With this in mind, radiographic evidence of stress fracture is not apparent for at least 14–21 days after the pain begins.

The most common areas for stress fracture in the foot and ankle are the metatarsal bones, as well as the distal tibia and fibula. This injury often occurs about 6 weeks after beginning a new training program and presents as an insidious onset of pain and swelling with no specific traumatic event. Any athlete who comes to the office with pain in the forefoot, with dorsal edema and point tenderness on metatarsal shift palpation dorsally, must be presumed to have a stress fracture until proven otherwise. Definitive diagnosis is by technetium bone scan.

11. What is Achilles tendinitis?

Inflammation of the paratenon about the Achilles tendon is a common and often debilitating injury to the athlete. If left untreated, it may lead to partial or complete rupture of the Achilles tendon. The injury is most commonly seen in the cavus foot with equinus, but it may also be caused by excessive subtalar pronation in the planus foot type.

There is normally tenderness to compression of the tendon abut 2 cm proximal to its insertion in the calcaneus. Sometimes, crepitus can be felt while moving the ankle through its range of motion. Gross swelling around the insertion indicates the absolute necessity of early aggressive treatment. Definitive diagnosis of tendon pathology is obtained via MRI.

Treatment includes ice, heel lifts, soft-tissue massage, physical therapy, NSAIDs, cast immobilization, and surgical release of any scar tissue. Local injections of steroid are contraindicated.

12. How can an athlete prevent blisters on the feet?

Blisters are a common result of any chronic repetitive movement in which friction is involved. Therefore, a decrease in friction will lead to a decrease in blisters—that may be easier said than done! Friction points are often caused by an ill-fitting shoe. The proper length of any athletic shoe is at least a thumb's width distance from the end of the longest toe to the end of the shoe while standing (with a pair of sports socks on). The shoe should also have a flex point in the forefoot that is consistent with the MTP joint of the athlete.

Keeping the feet dry is another important preventive measure. A sock that thoroughly "wicks" moisture away from the foot is important. For long events, the athlete may even consider changing socks and/or shoes during the event.

If a blister is caused by friction, decreasing the friction should help to prevent blister formation. If a blister is predictable for a certain duration or intensity of activity, the athlete should consider placing a generous portion of Vaseline over the hot spot prior to putting on socks before the event.

13. Are blister dressings effective in preventing blisters?

Over-the-counter blister dressings (e.g., Spenco Second Skin) certainly have a place in the treatment of the recurrent blister. The key to success with such products is meticulous application. All too often, they are applied in haste, only to move during the event and lead to even more problems. Directions on the label must be followed to the letter.

14. Do athletes need to wear cotton socks?

Not really. The goals of a sock are to pad the foot and remove perspiration and moisture away from the skin. The latter is more important for most athletes. Densely padded acrylic socks appear to wick fluid and resist compaction better than cotton socks in recent reviews. Two pairs of socks do not appear to prevent blisters. If two pairs of socks are to be worn, the shoe needs to be fitted originally with both socks on.

When fitted, seams in socks need to be smooth and not located over bony prominences. If socks become wet, either by perspiration or a damp environment, they need to be changed.

15. What are the risks associated with a fifth metatarsal fracture?

Fracture of the base of the fifth metatarsal is a common complication of an inversion ankle sprain. As the peroneus longus and brevis fire in an attempt to overcome the inversion force, the peroneus brevis may avulse a portion of its attachment on the fifth metatarsal base. Accurate evaluation is critical to an athlete's return to sports.

An avulsion fracture of the fifth metatarsal base which has minimally displaced is treated simply with compression, surgical shoe, and activities as tolerated. A **Jones' fracture**, which is a fracture approximately 1.5 cm distal to the tip of the fifth metatarsal base, has an extremely high chance of nonunion if not treated appropriately. A displaced Jones' fracture requires open reduction and internal fixation, while a nondisplaced Jones' fracture may possibly be treated with a short-leg non–weight-bearing cast.

16. What are the differences in indications for hard and soft orthotics?

A functional orthotic device serves to control abnormal motion of the foot. The key to successful orthotic treatment is in obtaining an accurate impression of the foot and in constructing the appropriate orthotic device.

In general, a **rigid functional orthotic** is used for a foot type and injury pattern that involve pathologic motion about the subtalar/midtarsal joint complex. So, a ligamentous strain, tenosynovitis, or capsulitis, which is caused by the foot going through an excessive amount of motion, may benefit from a rigid functional orthotic. A rigid device normally remains effective for

7–10 years, during which time the foot structure normally changes slightly, rather than the device wearing out.

If the injury pattern is one due to excessive force, a **soft orthotic device** would be indicated. In a more rigid cavovarus foot type with a symptom complex due to increased forces (e.g., stress fractures, knee/hip pain), a soft orthotic may be indicated. The goal in this case is to help absorb shock but also to introduce motion (in contrast to the planus foot type) into this rigid foot. Patients must be cautioned that a soft orthotic will wear out in 12–18 months and require replacement.

17. How often should athletes replace their shoes?

Any wear in a shoe will only magnify and accelerate an already-unstable foot structure. So, always think "shoes" if a new injury does not seem to have a simple answer. A shoe is worn out if:
- Any shoe that is over 6 months old that is used for exercise 3 or more times per week.
- Obvious holes or tears in the upper.
- A worn outer sole. If the black outsole has worn through to the white midsole, the shoe will not support the foot when it contacts the ground.
- A broken-down midsole. This can be determined by placing the shoes on a flat surface and looking at the shoe from the back. If any tilt can be perceived in the back of the shoe, it is time to replace it. Once the shoe tilts into this abnormal position, the shoe will throw the foot into this pathologic alignment every time the foot hits the ground.

18. What should an athlete look for in shoe fit?

An ill-fitting shoe is one of the most common causes of chronic aches and pains in the athlete. Some tips to achieve a proper fit include:
- Purchase shoes late in the day in case the foot has swollen somewhat during the day.
- Try on shoes with the same sock that is intended to be worn while exercising.
- Make sure there is at least a thumb's width distance between the end of the longest toe and the end of the shoe.
- When the shoe is laced, no part of the foot should bulge over the side of any part of the shoe.
- The shoe needs to bend or flex where the ball of the foot bends. (Such a shoe is much harder to find than one might think.)
- There should be no slippage of the heel when walking. The heel counter should fit snugly and securely.
- Make sure the two shoes are symmetric.
- Run fingers along the inside of the shoe to make sure there are no prominent seams or other irregularities.
- Place the shoes on a counter top and look at them from behind. The heel counters should sit perpendicular to the counter top. Any tilt indicates that the shoe was glued incorrectly and will throw the foot into an abnormal position during exercise.

BIBLIOGRAPHY

1. Black JR, Bernard JM, Williams LA: Heel pain in the older adult. Clin Podiatr Med Surg 10:113–119, 1993.
2. Burks RT, Morgan J: Anatomy of the lateral ankle ligaments. Am J Sports Med 22:72–77, 1994.
3. Campbell P, Lawton JO: Heel pain: Diagnosis and management. Br J Hosp Med 52:380–385, 1994.
4. Chandler TJ, Kibler WB: A biomechanical approach to the prevention, treatment, and rehabilitation of plantar fasciitis. SportsMed 15:344–352, 1993.
5. Clanton TO, Ford JJ: Turf toe injury. Clin Sports Med 13:731–740, 1994.
6. Conti S, et al: Clinical significance of magnetic resonance imaging in preoperative planning for reconstruction of posterior tibial tendon ruptures. Foot Ankle 13:208–214, 1992.
7. Detmer DE: Chronic shin splints: Classification and management of medial tibial stress syndrome. Sports Med 3:436–446, 1986.
8. Eiff MP, Smith AT, Smith GE: Early mobilization versus immobilization in the treatment of lateral ankle sprains. Am J Sports Med 22:83–88, 1994.

9. Herring KM, Richie DH: Comparison of cotton and acrylic socks using a generic cushion sole design for runners. J Am Podiatr Med Assoc 83:515–521, 1993.
10. Johnson K, Strom D: Tibialis posterior tendon dysfunction. Clin Orthop 239:196–206, 1989.
11. Moore MP: Shin splint: Diagnosis, management, prevention. Postgrad Med 83:199–209, 1988.
12. Mueller T: Acquired flatfoot secondary to tibialis posterior dysfunction: Biomechanical aspects. J Foot Surg 30:2–11, 1991.
13. Palamarchuk HJ, Kerzner M: An improved approach to evacuation of subungual hematoma. J Am Podiatr Med Assoc 79:566–568, 1989.
14. Quill GE: Fractures of the proximal fifth metatarsal. Orthop Clin North Am 26:353–361, 1995.
15. Rodeo SA, O'Brien S, Warren RF, et al: Turf toe: An analysis of metatarsophalangeal joint sprains in professional football players. Am J Sports Med 18:280–285, 1990.

19. SPORTS INJURIES AND COMPARTMENT SYNDROME

Jeffrey A. Ross, D.P.M., F.A.C.F.A.S.

1. What is a compartment syndrome?

A compartment syndrome is defined as a condition in which an elevated tissue pressure exists within a closed fascial space, resulting in reduced capillary blood perfusion and compromised neuromuscular function. Compartment syndromes may be acute or chronic.

2. What are some of the differential diagnoses when evaluating chronic leg pain in athletes?

Chronic compartment syndrome
Medial tibial stress syndrome
Stress fractures
Gastrocnemius strain
Nerve entrapment syndromes
Venous disease arterial occlusion
Fascial herniations
Tendinitis
Radiculopathies

3. What are some of the atypical causes of leg pain?

Occult trauma
Infections
Systemic conditions
Upper/lower motor neuron lesions
Neoplasms
Rheumatic conditions
Superficial/deep vein thrombophlebitis

4. When does a chronic exertional compartment syndrome occur?

It results from abnormally high intramuscular pressure during exercise or shortly thereafter.

5. Describe the physiologic events in a chronic compartment syndrome.

Circulation to the microvasculature is impeded, creating a compromised condition of the intracompartmental musculature. Intra- and extracellular fluid accumulation within the fascial space occurs. Venous and lymphatic compromise contributes to increased tissue pressure, creating further vascular compromise.

6. Which type of athlete is most affected by this condition?

In a study by Detmer et al., of the 100 consecutive operative cases of chronic compartment syndrome, approximately 70% involved runners.

7. In sports, what are the two most common conditions likely to produce an acute compartment syndrome of the leg?

Tibial fracture and muscle rupture.

8. Define tibial stress syndrome.

Tibial stress syndrome is an inflammatory condition characterized by pain commonly localized to the posterior medial tibial crest and uncommonly to the anterior crest.

9. Name the anatomical structure that attaches along the crest of the tibia.

The crests of the tibia are attachment sites for the deep fascia of the leg, which extend from the knee to the ankle.

10. Describe the anterior and posterior compartment fascia.

The anterior compartment fascia extends from the anterior peroneal septa and encompasses the anterior crest of the tibia. The deep posterior compartment fascia inserts into the posterior-medial crest of the tibia and generally intersects the deep transverse fascia, soleus fascia, and superficial posterior compartment fascia to form the intermuscular septum (see figure).

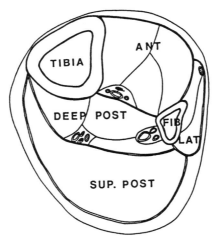

The four compartments of the leg. (From Mellion MB, Walsh WM, Shelton GL: The Team Physician's Handbook, 2nd ed. Philadelphia, Hanley & Belfus, 1997, with permission.)

11. How is tibial stress syndrome classified?
Tibial stress syndrome is classified by duration, location, and severity of symptoms.

Duration	Location	Severity of Symptoms
Acute, < 6 hrs	Posterior-medial	Grade I (mild)
Subacute, 2–6 hrs	Anterior	Grade II
Chronic, > 6 hrs	Combined	Grade III
		Grade IV (severe)

12. Name the four requisites for making a diagnosis of compartment syndrome.
1. A limiting anatomical envelope
2. Increase in tissue pressure
3. Compromised circulation
4. Neuromuscular dysfunction

13. What techniques can be used to measure intracompartmental tissue pressures?
Needle-manometer
Wick catheter
Rorabeck's slit catheter
McDermott's solid-state transducer intracompartmental (STIC) catheter (for the dynamic measurement of intracompartmental pressure)

14. What is the advantage of the wick-catheter technique developed by Scolander?
Its principal advantage is the avoidance of the need for continuous infusion of saline in an already compromised compartment. The wick catheter also can be used for continuous monitoring of intracompartmental pressures during exercise.

15. What are the criteria used to diagnose a chronic compartment syndrome?
The chronic compartment syndrome has also been described as an exertional compartment syndrome. Pedowitz developed criteria that include any one of the following:
1. Preexercise pressure greater than 15 mmHg
2. 1-min postexercise pressure of > 30 mmHg
3. 5-min postexercise pressure of > 20 mmHg

16. What type of pathology is frequently seen anatomically in compartment syndrome?

Muscle herniations through fascial defects have been found at a higher rate in compartment syndrome patients (approx. 30–60%) and can be a source of chronic pain with or without related nerve entrapment or compartment syndrome.

17. Name two major nerves involved with a lower-leg compartment syndrome.

Two commonly involved nerves that show signs of compressive neuropathy are the superficial and deep peroneal nerves.

18. What noninvasive method is effective in determining abnormal compartment pressures?

Magnetic resonance imaging is advantageous because it can provide a noninvasive means of assessing intracompartmental pressures simultaneously in all compartments.

19. Compression of the tibial nerve in the retromalleolar region is referred to as what type of syndrome?

Proximal tarsal tunnel syndrome.

20. What is another entity that mimics a compartment syndrome?

Intermittent claudication (or limping) refers to a symptom complex characterized by pain in the muscles of the lower extremity with exercise.

21. What must be considered when determining treatment alternatives for the athlete?

The goals of the athlete must be considered. If the athlete can reduce activities to a tolerable symptom level, then surgery is not indicated.

22. What are the aims of the four-phase treatment program for tibial stress syndrome?

Phase 1—decrease pain and inflammation
Phase 2—decrease and prevent scar tissue and decrease tension forces acting on the bone
Phase 3—strengthen the fascia-bone inferface and surrounding soft-tissue structures
Phase 4—return the athlete to his or her desired activity

23. How can a practitioner help to prevent an athlete from developing tibial stress syndrome?

1. Determine proper shoe selection with patient's own particular biomechanical considerations
2. Maintain flexibility and range of motion through specific stretching exercise
3. Strengthen weak muscle groups
4. Use temporary or prescription orthotics when indicated
5. Establish a reasonable training program that is consistent with the goals and abilities of the athlete

24. When addressing compartment syndrome with a patient, what should you discuss?

Patients should be thoroughly informed that they are at risk for developing an acute exertional compartment syndrome.

25. What type of conservative treatment can be recommended?

Prolonged rest	Orthotic therapy
Modifying the offending activity	NSAIDs
Stretching exercise	Diuretics
Altering the training program	Physical therapy
Shoe modifications	

26. Which type of surgical treatment is indicated for chronic compartment syndrome?

Surgical decompressive fasciotomy of the affected compartment has a 90% probability of producing significant improvement, if not complete recovery (see figure).

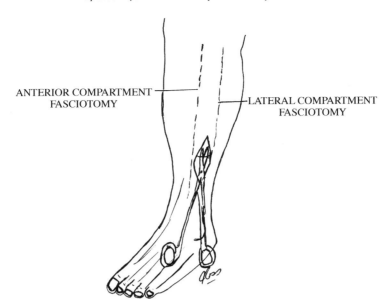

ANTERIOR COMPARTMENT
FASCIOTOMY

LATERAL COMPARTMENT
FASCIOTOMY

27. Why can a failure occur in a fasciotomy for chronic compartment syndrome?

Inadequate fasciotomy or missed diagnosis (i.e., failure to recognize the isolated tibialis posterior compartment syndrome and to institute adequate decompression of this compartment). Neuromuscular damage might also produce a poor result.

28. Name a significant postoperative complication of fasciotomy.

Decreasing muscle strength, with reported deficits of up to 20% for the released compartment's muscles.

29. What is the double-incision technique performed in chronic compartment syndrome?

The double-incision technique, as proposed by Mubarak and Owen, incorporates an anterolateral incision made midway between the tibia and fibula.

30. For acute compartment syndromes, which type of fasciotomy is recommended?

Fasciotomies are performed as open procedures under direct vision. All of the wounds remain open throughout the length of the compartment and are managed with sterile dressings.

31. How is chronic compartment syndrome treated?

The treatment for chronic compartment syndrome is subcutaneous fasciotomy, and the skin is closed primarily.

32. Should a fascial defect be closed?

No. It has been shown that increased intracompartmental pressures exist after fascial closure. It has even been shown that acute compartment syndromes may be produced when these fascial defects are closed during surgical treatment for chronic compartment syndrome.

33. When can an athlete be allowed to return to full athletic activities?

The following criteria should be met:
1. Absence of pain and tenderness in the leg
2. Full return of flexibility and strength
3. Ability to demonstrate running capability to allow for resumption of individual's sport activities.

34. When is surgical decompression indicated in an acute compartment syndrome?

The following are surgical indications for acute compartment syndrome:

1. Clinical signs of acute compartment syndrome with demonstrable motor or sensory loss
2. Elevated tissue pressure > 35 mmHg
3. Interrupted arterial circulation to an extremity for > 4 hours

BIBLIOGRAPHY

1. Almadahl S, Due J, Sandal F: Compartment syndrome with muscle necrosis following repair of hernia of tibialis anterior. Acta Clin Scand 153:695, 1987.
2. Amendola A, Rorabeck CH, Bellett D, et al: The use of magnetic imaging in exertional compartment syndromes. Am J Sports Med 18:29–34, 1990.
3. Andrish JT: The leg. In DeLee J, Drez D (eds): Orthopaedic Sports Medicine: Principles and Practice, vol 2. 1994, pp 1612–1618.
4. Bouche RT: Chronic compartment syndrome of the leg. J Am Podiatr Med Assoc 80:633–648, 1990.
5. Clanton TO, Solcher BW: Chronic leg pain in the athlete. Clin Sports Med 743–749, 1994.
6. Detmer DE: Chronic shin splints: Classification and management of medial tibial stress syndrome. Sports Med 3:436–446, 1986.
7. Fronek J, Mubarak S, Hargens A, et al: Management of chronic exertional anterior compartment syndrome of the lower extremity. Clin Orthop 220:217–227, 1987.
8. Garfin SR, Tipton CM, Mubarak SJ, et al: The role of fascia in the maintenance of muscle tension and pressure. J Appl Physiol 51:317–320, 1981.
9. Marens M, Backaert M, Vermaut G, Mulear J: Chronic leg pain in athletes due to a recurrent compartment syndrome. Am J Sports Med 12(2):148–151, 1984.
10. Matsen FA: Etiologies of compartment syndrome. In Compartmental Syndromes. New York, Grune & Stratton, 1980.
11. Mubarak S, Owen C: Double-incision fasciotomy of the leg for decompression in compartment syndromes. J Bone Joint Surg 59A:184, 1977.
12. Pedowitz R, Hargens A, Mubarak S, Gershuni D: Modified criteria for the operative diagnosis of chronic syndrome of the leg. Am J Sports Med 18(1):35–40, 1990.
13. Rorabeck C, Bourne R, Fowler P, et al: The role of tissue pressure measurement in diagnosing chronic anterior compartment syndrome. Am J Sports Med 16:224–227, 1988.

20. GOUT

Stephen C. Wan, D.P.M., F.A.C.F.A.S.

1. Gout is the most common form of inflammatory joint disease in men of what age group?

Over 40.

2. Who makes up the largest group of gout patients—underexcretors or overproducers?

Underexcretors more effectively retain uric acid and so are more often affected.

3. Why are postmenopausal women also commonly affected by gout?

Estrogen increases uric acid excretion, and so postmenopausal women become underexcretors.

4. Why is the first metatarsophalangeal (MTP) joint often the first joint to be affected in acute gouty attacks?

At body temperature, the concentration of monosodium urate in plasma is approx. 6.8 mg/dl. The temperature at the first MTP joint is approx. 30°C, and at this temperature, the concentration of monosodium urate is roughly 4.0 mg/dl. Therefore, urate crystals precipitate much easier into this joint. This predisposing condition is further exacerbated by the increasing tendency of this joint's exposure to repeated microtrauma (including increased abnormal weight-bearing stress).

5. Any rapid change in the uric acid levels in the body can precipitate acute gouty attack—true or false?

True.

6. Discuss the exacerbating factors of acute gout.

Typically the exacerbating factors can be classified into two categories: those that increase and those that rapidly decrease uric acid levels:

Increase uric acid	Rapidly decrease uric acid
Sustained alcohol consumption	High-dose aspirin use
High purine intake	Use of uricosurics or allopurinol
Diuretic use	Sudden stoppage of alcohol consumption
Low-dose aspirin intake	
Excessive cell turnover (e.g., myelo-proliferative diseases, some cancers)	
Hypertension	
Intrinsic renal disease	
Cyclosporine use	

The presence of aspirin, uricosurics, or allopurinol on this list in no way suggests that these agents should *not* be used to combat acute gouty attacks, but merely points out that the engagement of these factors may occasionally produce the opposite clinical effect, however temporary.

7. Name the classic triad that constitutes podagra.

Rapid onset of significant pain, erythema, and edema at the first MTP joint.

8. Do patients who are more susceptible to acute gouty attacks triggered by surgery, minor trauma, and acute illnesses usually have an underlying history of hyperuricemia?

Yes.

9. What are the common methods of diagnosing gout?

1. Clinical history and physical examination—prior history of gout and hyperurecemia; clinical presentation of podagra, and rapid relief of pain with nonsteroidal anti-inflammatory drugs (NSAIDs).
2. Serum uric acid level
3. X-rays
4. Synovial fluid analysis—needle-shaped monosodium urate crystals with negative birefringence under polarized microscopy.

10. Why do serum uric acid determinations and x-rays, in and of themselves, have limited value in establishing a diagnosis of gout?

As many as 25–30% of patients suffering from gout can have a normal serum uric acid level during an acute attack. In the early stages of the disease, x-rays reveal only soft-tissue swelling. It is in the advanced stages of the disease that the typical presentation of juxta-articular erosion and sclerotic margins become evident.

11. What are the most common treatments for acute gouty attacks?

1. Colchicine, oral or intravenous
2. NSAIDs
3. Intra-articular corticosteroids

12. Discuss the appropriate use and cautionary aspects of NSAIDs in gout.

Generous dosing of NSAIDs, particularly indomethacin (50 mg tid to qid), is highly effective in the rapid reduction of clinical signs and symptoms. Appropriate dosing should be carried out during the first week, with gradual tapering during the second week. Gastrointestinal and other side effects should be monitored prudently in elderly patients, particularly those with renal dysfunction.

13. What is the mode of action of colchicine in gout?

Colchicine inhibits the phagocytosis of urate crystals by neutrophils and interferes with the transport of phagocytosed materials to the lysosomes. Its interference with the chemotactic response also reduces joint inflammation.

14. How should colchicine be used in the treatment of acute gout?

Colchicine is generally administered as 1 mg orally as an initial dose, followed by 0.5 mg every 2 hours, until gastrointestinal discomfort or diarrhea develops, or until a total dose of 8 mg has been given. Relief of clinical gouty signs and symptoms is reached within 2 days, provided that the patient is willing to endure the GI discomfort.

This drug may be given intravenously if there is the desire to avoid GI side effects, but the risk of toxicity is much greater than with the oral route. An IV initial dose of 2 mg may be administered, followed by two separate doses of 1 mg at 6-hour intervals, with the total dose not exceeding 4 mg within the first 24 hours.

15. What precautions in patient selection, dosing, and drug interaction need to be exercised when administering colchicine?

The doses should be reduced by at least 50% in the elderly and in patients with renal and hepatic dysfunction. The risk of renal, hepatic, and CNS injury is especially elevated with intravenous therapy. The concomitant use of colchicine with cimetidine or erythromycin increases the plasma and tissue levels of colchicine and the danger of toxic side effects.

16. What precaution is needed before administering an intra-articular injection of corticosteroids into an acute gouty joint?

The presence of joint sepsis must first be ruled out.

17. What are the goals of management of gout?
- Relieve the signs and symptoms of acute attack
- Reduce uric acid levels
- Reduce and, if possible, eliminate the factors that produce gout

18. Discuss the difference in clinical effectiveness between allopurinol and uricosurics.

Allopurinol is a xanthine oxidase inhibitor and is the drug of choice for urate overproducers. It blocks the final step in urate synthesis, thereby reducing the production of urate. It is most effective for patients with markedly elevated levels of uric acid, a history of frequent gouty attacks, history of renal insufficiency, and the tophaceous phase of gout.

Uricosurics (e.g., probenecid) act by increasing renal excretion of uric acid and are effective in the treatment of uncomplicated cases of gout. Patients with history of renal dysfunction are therefore unsuitable candidates for these medications. Urolithiasis is a potential risk of therapy.

19. List some of the side effects of allopurinol.

Although side effects and allergic reactions are rarely encountered with the use of allopurinol, when they occur, they may be serious and life-threatening. The rate of occurrence is < 1/1000 cases. They include:

Bone marrow suppression	Hepatitis
Stevens-Johnson syndrome	Urticaria
Acute renal failure	Vasculitis
Fever	

20. Which drug interactions must be considered in the use of probenecid?

Probenecid prolongs the half-life of penicillin, heparin, salicylates, and indomethacin. In addition, salicylates reduce the effectiveness of probenecid.

21. Discuss the appropriate dosing of allopurinol in the treatment of gout.

A dose of 300 mg/day is effective in restoring the urate concentration to normal in acute attacks. To avoid exacerbation of acute gout due to sudden and rapid changes in uric acid levels, start with a lower dose initially (100 mg/day), with incremental additions until the desired dosage level is reached. For example, a dosage of 100 mg/day for the first week, 200 mg/day for the second week, and reaching 300 mg/day by the third week will gradually restore the urate concentration to normal without the nuisance of additional exacerbation during the acute phase of attack. The long-term maintenance dosage in patients with normal renal function is 300 mg/day, with appropriate adjustment of dosage in those with decreased glomerular filtration rate.

22. Discuss the appropriate dosing of the most commonly used uricosuric drugs (probenecid and sulfinpyrazone).

Probenecid is effective at the dose of 1–2 g/day. Sulfinpyrazone is best started at an initial dose of 50–100 mg twice daily with a gradual increase to 200 mg twice daily.

In prescribing uricosurics, maintenance of high urine volume is recommended. Patients should be advised to maintain adequate intake of fluids. In addition, an alkaline urine level can be achieved with 1 g of sodium bicarbonate three times a day.

23. What is the goal of urate-lowering therapy?

The goal of treatment is to reduce the serum urate concentration to about 6 mg/dl and perhaps even lower in cases of tophaceous gout. Periodic monitoring is preferred. Intermittent treatment or the cessation of drug therapy may lead to recurrence of acute attacks within 6 months and the formation of tophi within 3 years. Urate-lowering drug therapy is therefore life-long.

BIBLIOGRAPHY

1. Cohen MG, Emmerson BT: Crystal arthropathies: Gout. In Klippel JH, Dieppe PA (eds): Rheumatology. London, Mosby, 1994, pp 7.12.1–7.12.16.
2. Janson RW: Gout. In West SG (ed): Rheumatology Secrets. Philadelphia, Hanley & Belfus, 1997.
3. Kelley WN, Schumacher HR Jr: Gout. In Kelley WN, Harris ED Jr., Ruddy S, Sledge CB (eds): Textbook of Rheumatology, 4th ed. Philadelphia, W.B. Saunders, 1993, pp 1291–1336.
4. Pratt PW, Ball GV: Gout: Treatment. In Schumacher HR Jr (ed): Primer on the Rheumatic Diseases, 10th ed. Atlanta, Arthritis Foundation, 1993, pp 216–219.
5. Sells LL, German DC: An update on gout. Bull Rheum Dis 43:4–6, 1994.

21. ARTHRITIDES

Thomas F. McCloskey, D.P.M.

1. Articular disease can be grouped into six broad classifications. What are they?

1. Infectious
2. Connective tissue disease (SLE, mixed, scleroderma, dermatomyositis)
3. Crystal deposition (gout, pseudogout)
4. Osteoarthritis
5. Neuropathic
6. Inflammation of the synovium (rheumatoid arthritis, psoriatic arthritis, ankylosing spondylitis, Reiter's syndrome)

2. Name the bacteria that is most commonly associated with infectious arthritis in infants and children.

Hemophilus influenzae. Others commonly involved include *Staphylococcus aureus, Streptococcus pyogenes,* and Gram-negative bacilli.

3. Infectious arthritis may be caused by several mechanisms. Name them.

Direct invasion

Immunologic process triggered by a distant infection (for example, Reiter's syndrome, acute rheumatic fever)

Hematogenous spread

4. Discuss the common characteristics of a patient with systemic lupus erythematosus (SLE).

The typical patient is a female between the ages of 15 and 45 years. Although SLE can occur at nearly any age, the incidence of disease clearly increases in women of child-bearing age. The female-to-male ratio during these ages may be > 8:1, but during childhood or after menopause, the ratio is closer to 2:1. This pattern strongly suggests that sex hormones influence the probability of developing or expressing SLE, a conclusion that is supported by studies in animals models of lupus. It should be emphasized that although males develop disease less frequently, their illness is not milder than in females. Also, the incidence of SLE is about 2–4 times greater in blacks and hispanics than in whites in the United States.

5. Describe the criteria used in the classification of SLE.

Any person having 4 or more of the following 11 criteria, serially or simultaneously, during any interval of observation is considered to have SLE for the purposes of clinical studies.

Criterion	Definition
1. Malar rash	Fixed erythema, flat or raised over the malar eminences, tending to spare the nasolabial folds
2. Discoid rash	Erythematous raised patches with adherent keratotic scaling and follicular plugging; atrophic scarring may occur in older lesions
3. Photosensitivity	Skin rash as a result of unusual reaction to sunlight, by patient history or physician observation
4. Oral ulcers	Oral or nasopharyngeal ulceration, usually painless, observed by physician
5. Arthritis	Nonerosive arthritis involving two or more peripheral joints, characterized by tenderness, swelling, or effusion

Table continued on following page.

Criterion	Definition
6. Serositis	Pleuritis: convincing history of pleuritic pain or rub heard by physician or evidence of pleural effusion, *or* Pericarditis documented by EKG or rub or evidence of pericardial effusion
7. Renal disorder	Persistent proteinuria > 0.5 gm/day or > 3+ if quantitation not performed, *or* Cellular casts (red cell, hemoglobin, granular, tubular, or mixed)
8. Neurologic disorder	Seizures in the absence of offending drugs or known metabolic derangements, e.g., uremia, ketoacidosis, or electrolyte imbalance, *or* Psychosis in the absence of offending drugs or known metabolic derangement, e.g., uremia, ketoacidosis, or electrolyte imbalance
9. Hematologic disorder	Hemolytyic anemia with reticulocytosis, *or* Leukopenia < 4000/μl on two or more occasions, *or* Lymphopenia < 1,500/μl on two or more occasions, *or* Thrombocytopenia < 100,000/μl in the absence of offending drugs
10. Immunologic disorder	Positive LE cell preparation, *or* Anti-DNA: antibody to native DNA in abnormal titer, *or* Anti-Sm: presence of antibody to Sm nuclear antigen, *or* False-positive serologic test for syphilis known to be positive for at least 6 months and confirmed by TPI or FTA-ABS
11. Antinuclear antibody (ANA)	An abnormal titer of ANA by immunofluorescence or an equivalent assay at any point in time and in the absence of drugs known to be associated with "drug-induced lupus"

Adapted from Tan EM, et al: The 1982 revised criteria for the classification of systemic lupus erythematosus. Arthritis Rheum 25:1271–1277, 1992.
TPE = *Treponema pallidum* immobilization test; FTA-ABS = fluorescent treponemal antibody absorption test.

6. The crystals of gout are made up of what substance?

Monosodium urate (MSU). The deposition of MSU crystals occurs due to hyperuricemia.

7. Discuss the etiology of hyperuricemia.

Primary gout. There is either an inherited overproduction of uric acid due to a problem in purine synthesis or a problem with renal uric acid excretion, or a combination of these processes.

Secondary gout. This form of gout is acquired from underlying conditions such as polycythemia, multiple myeloma, or sickle cell or other hemoglobinopathies.

8. The first metatarsophalangeal joint is more commonly affected in gout. Discuss some of the theories for this.

In 75% of patients with gout, the first MPJ is affected with attacks occurring most commonly at night. Some feel that this area of the body cools more quickly, allowing the crystals to come out of solution. Acute gout of the first MPJ joint is called podagra.

9. Discuss the common characteristics of the patient with gout.

• 25% have a positive family history
• Males predominate, 80–85% of patients are middle-aged
• Postmenopausal women
• 5–28/1000 males, 1–6/1000 females

10. Define pseudogout.

Synovitis caused by calcium-containing salts (calcium pyrophosphate, calcium hydroxyapatite and calcium orthophosphate) found in cartilage affecting one or more joints. It mimics gout but the crystal is calcium pyrophosphate dihydrate. Symptoms are the same as for any acute arthritis.

11. What joint is most commonly affected by pseudogout and how does it appear on radiographs?

The knee joint is most commonly affected. Radiographs demonstrate multiple areas of calcification linearly arranged in the cartilage.

12. Discuss the radiologic findings of gout.

Soft-tissue swelling around the affected joint in early acute cases.

C-shaped, punched-out subchondral lesions may be seen with severe cystic destruction noted late in the disease.

In chronic gout, there are tophi and bony erosions. Tophi produce irregular soft-tissue densities—occasionally calcified.

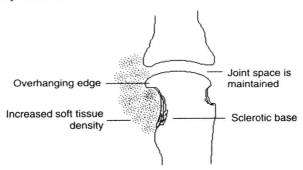

Radiologic changes in a patient with gout. (From Mehta A: Common Musculoskeletal Problems. Philadelphia, Hanley & Belfus, 1997, with permission.)

13. What are Heberden's nodes?

Bony protuberances at the margins and dorsal surfaces of the DIP joints of the fingers associated with osteoarthritis.

14. Define osteoarthritis.

The name itself implies an inflammatory process; however, this is not accurate. This is a non-inflammatory disease process primarily of weightbearing joints. It is characterized by deterioration of the articular cartilage and the formation of new bone at joint margins and subchondral areas.

15. Where are Bouchard's nodes located?

The proximal interphalangeal joints of the fingers.

16. Which joints are most affected by osteoarthritis?

The facet joints of cervical and lumbar spine areas, hips, knees, interphalangeal joints of fingers, first metatarsophalangeal joint of the great toe.

17. What is neuropathic arthropathy (Charcot joints)?

This is a chronic, progressive degenerative process that affects one or more peripheral and/or vertebral articulations. It represents a complication of neurologic disorders that cause a disturbance in sensory innervation.

18. There are three stages in the formation of a Charcot joint. What are they?

1. Joint subluxation, osteoporosis, cortical defects
2. Osteolysis, fracture, periosteal elevation or new subperiosteal formation
3. Healing stage—reconstructive, decreased swelling, and bony ankylosis

19. What are the most common neurologic diseases that cause Charcot joints?

Diabetes, alcoholism, congenital indifference to pain, myelomeningocele, syringomyelia, syphilitic tabes dorsalis, Charcot-Marie-Tooth disease, peripheral nerve injury, amyloid neuropathy.

20. There are two primary types of findings in Charcot joints. What are they? Discuss them.

1. Atrophic—"pencil-in-cup" deformation, resorption of bone end. Usually affects upper extremities.

2. Hypertrophic—Joint space narrowing with bony sclerosis. Fracture and articular surface fragmentation occurs with new periosteal bone formation. Joint subluxation occurs.

21. Rheumatoid arthritis affects which joints most commonly?

Any joint is possible but the metacarpophalangeal joints and the proximal interphalangeal joints (PIPJ) of the hand are the most common.

22. Describe swan-neck and boutonniere deformities.

The swan-neck deformity involves hyperextension at the PIPJ and flexion of the distal interphalangeal joints (DIPJ). The boutonniere deformity is a flexion of the PIPJ and extension of the DIPJ.

23. What are the diagnostic criteria of rheumatoid arthritis?

Four of the following must be present to make the diagnosis.
1. Morning stiffness of greater than 1 hour
2. 3 or more joints involved
3. Arthritis of the hands
4. Nodules
5. Radiographic findings
6. Serum rheumatoid factor (Rf) is positive
7. Symptomatic arthritis of the same joints right and left

24. Discuss the roentgenographic changes in rheumatoid arthritis.

Early in the course of the disease there may be no articular change. Later changes include juxta-articular osteopenia, marginal joint erosion, and uniform joint narrowing.

25. Although lab testing may be inconclusive, discuss the role that the lab plays in the diagnosis of rheumatoid arthritis.

At least 85% of patients will have elevated levels of Rf. This serves as a good confirmatory test but is poor in early screening. Rheumatoid arthritis is primarily diagnosed by history and physical examination, but ESR, c-reactive protein, and Rf may help confirm the diagnosis.

BIBLIOGRAPHY

1. Hawkins ES, Beilstein DP: Pedal manifestations of systemic lupus erythematosus. Clin Podiatr Med Surg Jan. 1988, pp 1–16.
2. Levy LA: Arthritis. In Levy LA, Hetherington VJ (eds): Principles and Practice of Podiatric Medicine. New York, Churchill Livingstone, 1990, pp 363–367.
3. Mann RA, Coughlin MJ (eds): Surgery of the Foot and Ankle, 6th ed. St. Louis, Mosby, 1993.
4. Rodnan GP, Schumacher HR (eds): Primer on the Rheumatic Diseases, 8th ed. Atlanta, Arthritis Foundation.
5. Stiles RG, Resnick D, Sartoris DJ: Radiologic manifestations of arthritides involving the foot. Clin Podiatr Med Surg Jan 1988, pp 1–16.
6. Waxman J: Clues to differentiating between osteoarthritis and rheumatoid arthritis. J Musculoskel Med 10:3, 1993.
7. West SR: Rheumatology Secrets. Philadelphia, Hanley & Belfus, 1997.

22. DIABETES

Larry A. Suecof, D.P.M.

GENERAL CARE

1. Define diabetes mellitus.

Diabetes mellitus is a syndrome characterized by hyperglycemia and a disturbance of carbohydrate, fat, and protein metabolism. It is associated with an absolute or relative deficiency of insulin secretion or action. Diabetics are prone to many complications, which can be characterized as microvascular, macrovascular, or neuropathic. The long-term results of these pathologies are ocular, neurologic, and cardiovascular.

2. Outline the clinical classification of diabetes mellitus.

There are three clinical classes of diabetes mellitus:
   Diabetes mellitus (DM)
   Impaired glucose tolerance (IGT)
   Gestational diabetes mellitus (GDM)
There are four clinical subclasses of diabetes mellitus:
   Insulin-dependent diabetes mellitus (IDDM, Type I)
   Non-insulin-dependent diabetes mellitus (NIDDM, Type II)
   Secondary and other types of diabetes (associated with certain conditions and syndromes)
   Malnutrition-related diabetes mellitus

3. What commonly used drugs adversely affect glucose tolerance?

Thiazide diuretics	Glucocorticoids
Estrogen/progesterone	Nicotinic acid (niacin)
Diphenylhydantoin	Catecholamines
Pentamidine	Certain antihypertensives

4. Describe the features of insulin-dependent diabetes mellitus (IDDM, Type I).

Prone to ketosis, these patients manifest insulin deficiency due to islet cell loss. The etiology of IDDM is heterogeneous, with genetic, autoimmune, and viral factors all theorized to contribute to the origin of the disease. IDDM usually occurs (although not always) before age 30. It starts with an abrupt onset, requiring prompt medical treatment. Most of these patients are lean and have experienced the classic triad associated with the onset of diabetes. Microvascular complications tend to predominate, with the leading cause of death being microangiopathy (renal failure), although these patients also may develop significant macrovascular complications. Type I DM accounts for 10% of all patients with DM.

5. Describe the features of non-insulin-dependent diabetes mellitus (NIDDM, Type II).

Type II patients are ketosis-resistant, with the disease occurring at any age but usually > 45 years. Patients tend to be overweight, and the onset and progression of the disease tend to be slow. NIDDM accounts for 90% of all cases of DM. Due to the insidious nature of this disease, these patients are the main focus of screenings for diabetes.

In general, Type II diabetes is characterized by diminished tissue sensitivity to insulin and impaired beta cell function. At this time, it is impossible to determine the primary defect in the cause of this disease. Although these patients do develop microangiographic and neuropathic complications, macrovascular disease develops in a large percentage, with up to 55–75% succumbing to cardiovascular disease.

6. What are the acute diabetic complications that require immediate action?

1. Diabetic ketoacidosis (DKA)
2. Hyperglycemic, hyperosmolar nonketotic states (HHNS)
3. Hypoglycemia

Diabetic ketoacidosis consists of the triad of hyperglycemia, ketosis, and acidosis. HHNS is defined by severe hyperglycemia and increased serum osmolarity. Patients with HHNS are generally encountered with depressed sensorium relative to DKA; it is usually found more frequently in elderly patients or in newly diagnosed diabetics. HHNS tends to be quite insidious in onset.

7. What are the signs of hypoglycemia and how are they treated?

Hypoglycemia Symptoms and Treatment

STATUS	SYMPTOM	TREATMENT
Mild	Glucose 50–60, tremor, palpitations, sweating, hunger	10–20 gm glucose (40–80 cal) orally (4 oz unsweetened fruit juice)
Moderate	Headache, mood change, irritability drowsiness	20–40 gm glucose, repeat if necessary 1 mg glucagon, if appropriate
Severe	Unresponsiveness, convulsions	Glucagon IV glucose D50 (10–25 gm) over 1–3 min IV at 5–10 gm/hr until recovery

8. Explain the relevance of hemoglobin A1c (glycated hemoglobin).

In normal hypoglycemic subjects, a small proportion of hemoglobin A is attached nonenzymatically to a carbohydrate moiety. This glycated hemoglobin can be divided into A1a, Alb, Alc. This occurs continuously through the life of the red blood cell. The amount of the glycosylated hemoglobin reflects glycemic control over a 6–12 week period in both Type I and Type II diabetes mellitus. The drawback to A1c measurements is the lack of standardization between assays from different laboratories.

9. What are the major findings of the DCCT (Diabetes Control and Complications Trial)?

The DCCT tested whether the complications of DM are related to the degree of hyperglycemia. The study lasted approx. 7 years and showed a 60% reduction in risk between the intensively treated groups and the conventionally treated group as relates to diabetic nephropathy, neuropathy, and retinopathy. The intensely treated group showed a delayed onset and slowed progression of these complications. They had an average blood glucose of 155 mg/dl and hemoglobin HbA_{1-c} of approx. 7.2%.

10. How do the sulfonylurea drugs work in treating NIDDM?

One of three classes of drugs used to treat NIDDM, the sulfonylureas include tolbutamide, tolazamide, chlorpropamide, glypizide, and the new agent glimepride. Most current studies suggest that these drugs increase endogenous insulin secretion as their major antidiabetic effect. These drugs probably also act peripherally, at the insulin receptor site, and in the liver, where they may reduce the accelerated rate of hepatic glucose production seen in Type II diabetics.

11. Name the different types of insulin available for treatment of Type I and Type II DM. Compare their time course of action.

Insulin preparations are generally classified by species of derivation (beef, pork, human) and duration of action (short, intermediate, interacting). Human insulin is least antigenic, followed by pork and then beef. Human insulin may act quicker and last a shorter time than the animal insulins. Although insulins are classified into short, intermediate, and long preparations, their actual effects do not always coincide with such simple descriptions.

Insulin Type	Onset	Duration
Short-acting (regular)	0.5–2 hrs	3–6 hrs
Intermediate (lente, NPH)	3–6 hrs	12–20 hrs
Long-acting (ultra-lente, protamine zinc)	6–12 hrs	18–36 hrs

12. How should a Type II patient be managed perioperatively?

Optimal blood glucose levels perioperatively range between 140–240 mg/dl, although there is no increase in postoperative risk up to 270 mg/dl. Levels < 140 mg/dl require special vigilance by the anesthetist and surgeon preoperatively. If the patient has generally good insulin control, one may opt to give the patient a hypoglycemic agent in the morning with a small amount of water on the day of surgery. If the patient is very tightly controlled, with glucoses between 110–140, the oral agent may be withheld prior to surgery and given only when the patient is eating postoperatively. Chlorpropamide should be withheld 24 hours before surgery.

13. What are the options for treating the IDDM patient perioperatively?

For Type I patients, use one-half to two-thirds of the normal morning dose given as NPH or lente (holding regular insulin) prior to surgery. Glucose is then infused as a 5% solution, and the glucose levels are monitored every 2–4 hours until surgery. If the surgery is performed earlier in the day, the patient may receive the balance of insulin postoperatively. If the surgery is performed later in the day, put the patient on insulin coverage until the next morning. If a patient uses an evening dose of insulin and is taking oral nutrition by dinner, use the normal evening insulin dose.

Variable rate insulin infusion is another technique preferred by many today. Regular insulin in NSS at a concentration of 1 U/ml is infused IV via a pump at a rate of 0.5–1 U/hr. Rates are adjusted in steps of 0.3 U/hr according to the sliding scale of glucose measurements. Glucose is supplemented at 5–10 gm/hr and the physician's choice of IV fluid.

LOWER-EXTREMITY VASCULOPATHY

14. What is the pattern of macrovascular disease affecting the lower extremity in the diabetic patient?

Macrovascular disease in the diabetic has a great predilection for the tibioperoneal trunk (infrapopliteal). Forty percent of these patients have palpable popliteal pulses, and 80% of the patients presenting with this distribution have diabetes mellitus. The foot arteries, from the dorsalis pedis through the digital arteries, are frequently spared. Despite the increased frequency of infrapopliteal disease, inflow disease (aortoiliac) is not unusual, and indeed the femoral artery still remains the most common site of occlusion in the diabetic, just as in the nondiabetic. Sparing of the vessels of the foot are the rule rather than the exception, leading to an overall long-term limb salvage of up to 90%.

15. How frequent is vascular disease in the diabetic patient? What is its impact?

Peripheral vascular disease is four times more common in diabetics than in nondiabetics, with an overall prevalence of 10% in the U.S. population. Forty-five percent of diabetics will have peripheral vascular disease after 20 years. After 13 years with the disease, 61% of men and 32% of women will manifest medial calcific sclerosis.

Diabetes is responsible for approx. 50,000 amputations per year in the United States, and 50% of all nontraumatic amputations in this country are in diabetics. After their first below-knee amputation, 42% of patients will lose the contralateral limb within 1 year, and up to 56% will lose the contralateral limb by the third to fifth year. Between 11–40% of patients will die within the first year of their below-knee amputation, and by the fifth year, 39–68% of patients will have died due to comorbid conditions.

16. **List the signs and symptoms of macrovascular disease.**
    1. Intermittent claudication of the thigh, calf, or arch of the foot
    2. Dry, scaly skin (frequently seen with autonomic neuropathy as well)
    3. Diminished pulses at any level of the lower extremities
    4. Atrophic subcutaneous tissue and skin
    5. Absence of hair
    6. Prolonged venous filling time (not reliable in chronic venous insufficiency)
    7. Dependent rubor
    8. Pallor on elevation
    9. History of acute or recurrent distal cholesterol embolization

17. **Is occlusion of the small vessels the mechanism leading to foot ulceration or gangrene in diabetics?**

It is a misconception that diabetic patients have an occlusive microvascular lesion, and this misconception could doom the diabetic patient who has a vascular or neuropathic foot lesion to unnecessary early amputation. Neither histologic nor in vivo studies provide evidence that capillary closure (small vessel/capillary occlusion) is a major factor contributing to foot ulceration.

Rather, it is far more likely that functional changes develop in the diabetic foot microcirculation in parallel with neuropathy and occlusive arterial disease (macrovascular), and it is these functional abnormalities that are ultimately responsible for failure of microvascular function. Sympathetic nerve damage resulting in unregulated arteriovenous shunting, impaired autoregulation of microvascular blood flow/pressure, hyperglycemia-mediated endothelial dysfunction, abnormal rheology, and abnormal white cell function all combine to suggest a functional microvascular lesion as opposed to a structural microvascular lesion. When one superimposes a proximal arterial occlusion on an already abnormal circulation, this will additionally compound and worsen the situation.

18. **Which patients are most likely to present with the classic "small-vessel" patchy gangrene associated with palpable pedal pulses?**
    1. Transplant patients
    2. Diabetics on long-term corticosteroids
    3. Diabetics with end-stage renal disease
    4. Occasionally, patients with very-long-term IDDM who present with an occluded posterior tibial vessel, palpable dorsalis pedis, poor collateralization, and enlarging heel necrotic ulceration

19. **How does medial calcific sclerosis affect the diabetic lower extremity?**

Medial calcific sclerosis, or medial calcinosis, frequently involves diabetic arteries at all levels but may spare the foot. In it, the intima and media are affected, but this lesion is not occlusive in nature. When one sees calcification in the arteries in a young patient, the patient is likely to be diabetic.

This lesion is problematic when interpreting noninvasive pressure studies by giving false elevation of systolic pressures. The lesion can also complicate the vascular surgeon's attempts at distal vessel anastomosis.

20. **What techniques are available to evaluate vascular disease and amputation level?**
    The most common techniques in use are:
    1. Noninvasive Doppler measurements
    2. Ankle brachial index
    3. Pulse volume recording
    4. Segmental pressure measurements in the lower extremity
    5. Systolic toe pressures
    6. Transcutaneous oxygen (PT_{CO_2})
    7. Arteriography (gold standard)

Additional methods include:
1. Fluorescein/fluorometry
2. Laser Doppler flowmetry
3. Skin temperature assessment
4. Xe-133 radial isotope clearance

21. Ankle brachial index and systolic toe pressures are common ways to evaluate the diabetic patient noninvasively. How useful are these parameters for predicting healing of ulcers or amputation?

The **ankle brachial index** (ABI) in predicting success of wound, ulcer, or amputation site healing in the foot is frequently unreliable. This is usually due to falsely elevated systolic pressures resulting from increased medial calcinosis of the arteries. This problem is seen in up to 50% of diabetic patients. Generally, an ABI of 0.45 or less leads to a poor prognosis in terms of wound healing in the foot. In diabetics, medical calcinosis may falsely elevate the ABI and make it useless in determining wound healing prognosis.

Toe systolic pressures, on the other hand, have been reported to be more reliable in the prediction of wound healing/amputation site healing. Systolic toe pressures of ≥ 30 usually heal, while pressures ≥ 45 are consistent with primary healing in 85% of patients. It should be noted that decreased vascular resistance secondary to autonomic neuropathy may make these numbers less reliable.

NEUROPATHY

22. What percentage of patients with diabetes develop peripheral neuropathy?

60–70%. One long-term study of over 4400 patients, followed for 36 years using absent ankle reflexes and decreased vibratory perception in the distal foot, found that 60% of patients had neuropathy at 25 years into their disease. Seven percent of diabetics had neuropathy on the presentation of their disease.

23. Define diabetic neuropathy.

Diabetic neuropathy is peripheral, somatic, or autonomic nerve damage attributable to diabetes, being multifactorial in origin.

24. How does one classify the different neuropathic processes?

There are multiple classifications of diabetic neuropathy. One convenient way to classify the diseases is as follows:
1. Polyneuropathy (including distal sensory motor, proximal motor, symmetrical and asymmetrical, truncal, and distal motor)
2. Focal and multifocal neuropathies (mononeuropathy and mononeuropathy multiplex)
   a. Cranial (ophthalmoplegia)
   b. Truncal asymmetrical
   c. Limb plexus mononeuropathy (peroneal neuropathy, etc.)
   d. Multiple mononeuropathies
   e. Entrapment neuropathies (carpal tunnel, tarsal tunnel syndrome)
3. Autonomic neuropathy (cardiovascular, GI, GU, miscellaneous)

25. Explain hyperglycemic neuropathy.

This polyneuritis is present at the time of diagnosis of the patient presenting with hyperglycemia. The patient presents with tingling, paresthesias, pain, and dysesthesia distally in the extremity. It frequently subsides in the first 3–6 months of treatment.

26. What are the features of treatment-induced neuropathy?

Exacerbation of a distal sensory polyneuritis may follow insulin treatment. This condition may be painful, and slow recovery is the rule. A careful history and physical are required to help make an appropriate diagnosis.

27. What is the most common type of neuropathy accompanying diabetes? Describe its symptoms.

Distal sensory polyneuropathy is the most common neuropathy encountered in the long-term diabetic patient. Symptoms range from mild, distal numbness and tingling at the level of the toes (frequently worse at night and bedtime) through complaints of severe, sharp stabbing pains, crushing or squeezing pain, or severe remitting dysesthesias. Frequently patients complain that it feels as if a tourniquet has been tied around their feet and ankles or that their feet feel like tree trunks or stumps when they are walking.

28. How does one diagnose diabetic sensory motor neuropathy in an office setting?

The diagnosis and staging of sensorimotor diabetic neuropathy are based on:
1. Clinical symptoms
2. Clinical signs
3. Quantitative sensory testing
4. Electrophysiology

29. Are there any standardized ways to quantify clinical symptoms and signs at the bedside?

Dyck has developed the neuropathy symptom score (NSS) that is a useful tool to quantify clinical symptoms of neuropathy. The neuropathy disability score (NDS) is another such technique described by Dyck, which allows the physician to quantify clinical signs at the bedside using simple clinical tools. These tools are a pin for pain perception, cotton wool for touch perception, cold perception with a tuning fork that has been immersed in cold water, and vibration with a tuning fork with a vibration of 128 Hz.

30. What is esthesiometry?

Esthesiometry, or the cutaneous perception threshold (CPT), uses Semmes-Weinstein monofilaments to help diagnose loss of protective sensation (evidence of peripheral neuropathy). Lack of perception of the 5.07 filament (10 gm of pressure) is consistent with loss of protective sensation, and these patients should be considered at high risk for ulceration.

31. Some patients presenting with diabetic neuropathy are characterized as having "small fiber disease" or "large fiber disease." What is meant by this?

Patients with diabetic peripheral neuropathy present with varying degrees of pain and sensory loss. **Small fiber disease** refers to pain that is a burning, twisting, or crushing of the involved lower extremities. It is usually worse at resting, especially at bedtime, and is usually improved during ambulation. The nerve fibers involved are generally the small white myelinated A-delta fibers or unmyelinated C-fibers. The pain may be all-consuming and difficult to control. The neurologic exam is relatively normal, frequently with intact reflexes and normal vibration, light touch, and proprioception.

Large fiber disease presents as an insidious loss of sensation in the feet and lower extremities. The onset may be so prolonged that patients frequently do not realize the loss of lower-extremity protective sensation, despite the fact that they might be severely insensate. These patients have large fiber signs (A-β) with significant loss of vibration sensation, proprioception, and deep tendon reflexes.

Note that large and small fiber disease usually coexist together, mixing the clinical picture.

32. Autonomic neuropathy is found in a significant number of patients with peripheral sensory motor neuropathy. What are the consequences of peripheral autonomic neuropathy in the lower extremities?

1. Impaired neurogenic control mechanisms
2. Increased arteriovenous shunting
3. Reduced capillary blood flow
4. Impaired postural vasoconstriction
5. Impaired cutaneous responses to reactive hyperemia

33. What are the clinical signs of peripheral autonomic neuropathy seen on a physical exam?
1. Anhydrosis or hyperhydrosis
2. Neuropathic edema
3. Bounding lower-extremity pulses
4. Hot, hyperemic feet
5. Poorly healing wounds in a hyperperfused foot

34. Which medications are useful in controlling painful diabetic neuropathy?
Nonnarcotic analgesics (acetaminophen, aspirin)
Mild narcotic analgesics (propoxyphene) or synthetic narcotic analgesics (tramadol)
Tricyclic antidepressants (e.g., amitriptyline, desipramine)
Phenothiazines (alone or combined with tricyclics)
Antiepileptic drugs (gabapentin, diphenylhydantoin, and carbamazepine)
Selective serotonin reuptake inhibitors (paroxetine, fluoxetine, sertraline)
Atypical antidepressants (trazodone, bupropion)
Topical agents (capsaicin 0.25%/0.75%)
Narcotic analgesics (codeine, oxycodone, hydromorphone)

35. What vitamins and nutritional supplements may have an impact on diabetic neuropathy?
γ-Linoleic acid, α-lipoic acid, B-complex vitamins (B_6, B_{12}), pycnogenol, other antioxidant supplements.

IMMUNOLOGIC AND INFECTIOUS COMPLICATIONS

36. What are the main contributors to poor wound healing in the diabetic?
• Infection
• Pressure
• Ischemia
• Immunologic/cytophysiologic defects
• Nutrition

37. What immuno/cytophysiologic defects may impair healing?
Deficiency in chemotaxis of neutrophils and decreased phagocytosis
Glycation of collagen and intracellular accumulation of sorbitol
Abnormalities in intracellular metabolism
Inadequate production of local growth factors
Impaired bacterial killing

38. Name the most common organisms infecting superficial diabetic wounds.

Staphylococcus aureus	*Enterococcus*
Staphylococcus epidermidis	*Klebsiella/Enterobacter* spp.
Group A and B streptococci	*Pseudomonas* spp.
Proteus spp.	*Bacteroides* and other anaerobes
Escherichia coli	

39. When infections are monomicrobial, which organisms are likely involved?
Staphylococcus aureus and streptococci.

40. When infections are polymicrobial, what organisms are usually involved?
Frequently gram-positive organisms such as staphylococci and streptococci mixed with gram-negative bacilli such as *Proteus* species, *Escherichia coli*, *Enterobacter*, and *Pseudomonas*. Anaerobes may also be found in these types of wound infections. Overall, mixed polymicrobial infections account for only a minority of wounds seen in daily practice.

41. In which clinical presentations is a mixed infection most likely?
1. Presence of necrotic tissue
2. Sequestered pus in an anatomic deep space
3. Crepitus in deep tissues
4. Foul smell in wound
5. Long-term complicated infections treated with multiple courses of antibiotics

42. Why are superficial swab specimens of ulcerations to be avoided?
Multiple studies have pointed out the unreliability of superficial swabs as opposed to aspiration, curettement, or deep biopsy. Culture of swabbings appears to be reliable in only 17–50% of cases.

43. Which antibiotics would be the best choice in the treatment of a superficial, mild diabetic foot ulcer without bone involvement (Wagner grade 1 or 2)?
An oral antibiotic, generally a first-generation cephalosporin or penicillinase-resistant penicillin. An alternative to these would be erythromycin or clindamycin.

44. With a moderate or severe ulceration (Wagner grade 3–5), what would be the most appropriate way to manage wound infection and sepsis?
One must be sure to provide adequate drainage, adequate soft-tissue debridement, and adequate antibiotics. Antibiotic therapy should be aimed at gram-positive coverage for staphylococci and streptococci and gram-negative coverage for Enterobactericiae as well as *Pseudomonas* and anaerobes. Monotherapy for these patients could include piperacillin/tazobactam (Zosyn) or ticarillin/clavulanate (Timentin), or one may choose double antibiotic therapy such as ampicillin/sulbactam (Unasyn) and ceftazidime (Fortaz). One rarely needs to use aminoglycosides for *Pseudomonas* or *Proteus* infections, unless the patient has signs of gram-negative sepsis. One should always remember to modify or reduce antibiotics after appropriate sensitivities have been obtained.

45. What is the drug of choice in treating a methicillin-resistant staph infection?
Intravenously, the drug of choice is **vancomycin**. In less-aggressive infections or local cellulitis, minocycline is the drug of choice. Alternate drugs are sulfamethoxazole/trimethoprim, ciprofloxacin, and occasionally, clindamycin.

JOINT AND BONE COMPLICATIONS

46. What are the common bone and joint manifestations in diabetes mellitus?
1. Limited joint mobility
2. Plantar fibromatosis
3. Charcot arthropathy
4. Intrinsic minus foot
5. Osteoarthritis
6. Gout and hyperuricemia

47. Limited joint mobility is well-substantiated in the diabetic population, with an incidence of 8–40% in insulin-dependent patients. What is the distribution of affected joints?
Limited joint mobility is found in multiple joints throughout the body. Both the hands and feet are affected, as well as other large joints.
Delbridge notes limited range of motion at the level of the subtalar joint and the first metatarsophalangeal joint. This limitation of motion in the rear foot has obvious implications in terms of shock absorption and accommodation throughout the rest of the foot. The overall result is abnormally high pressures and a permissive role in the formation of ulcerations of the feet.

48. Define the intrinsic minus foot. Discuss the clinical importance of this syndrome.
The intrinsic minus foot refers to the atrophy of the intrinsic muscles secondary to neuropathy, with the resulting hammering or clawing of the toes and its sequelae. This includes increased plantar pressures under the metatarsal heads secondary to dorsiflexion at the MTP joint and

destabilization of the toes along with distal migration of the fat pad. The implications of the syndrome are an increased frequency of ulceration along the dorsal aspect of the toes and the ball of the foot. The cause of this condition is chronic sensory motor polyneuropathy.

49. Define the Charcot foot (diabetic neuropathic osteoarthropathy).

Neuropathic arthropathy has a multifactorial etiology that results in fractures, effusions, and ligamentous laxity, followed by erosion of articular cartilage, fragmentation, luxation, disintegration, and collapse of the foot. Minor acute trauma and moderate repetitive stresses have been implicated in the origins of this condition.

50. What factors contribute to neuropathic arthropathy?

Symmetrical polyneuropathy with loss of protective sensation and/or vibratory sensation along with autonomic neuropathy and trauma are probably the most common contributing factors. Additional factors include mechanical stress (e.g., after great toe amputation), fractures of the foot secondary to trauma, equinus deformity, immunosuppressive/corticosteroid administration (in transplant patients), and corticosteroid-induced osteoporosis.

51. When should one consider a diagnosis of Charcot foot?

Whenever a clinician encounters a warm edematous foot in a patient with neuropathy without a portal of entry, the diagnosis of Charcot foot should be entertained. The clinical appearance may be one of acute erythema and edema, or minimal erythema might be seen and warmth and swelling may be the primary initial signs. X-rays are frequently negative in the early stages (sometimes up to 6–8 weeks), and technetium imaging is quite sensitive for this condition, yielding a fairly characteristic picture of diffuse global uptake and increased activity in all three phases. The ESR is usually only minimally elevated, although comorbid conditions may cloud the picture with this marker. The white cell count is also usually normal, although a mild leukocytosis might be seen.

DERMATOPATHOLOGIC COMPLICATIONS

52. Which skin diseases occur with increased incidence in diabetes mellitus?

Dermatophytosis	Syndrome of limited joint mobility and waxy skin
Erythrasma	Yellow skin syndrome
Onychomycosis	Necrobiosis lipoidica diabeticorum
Anhydrosis/hyperhydrosis	Bullosa diabeticorum

53. What are the important features of bullosa diabeticorum?

This condition usually occurs on the dorsum of the foot, including the toes, but may include the plantar aspects of the toes and ball of the foot as well. The size of the bullae ranges from 5 mm up to 15–20 cm, and as the bullae enlarge, they become more flaccid. There generally is not surrounding erythema, although this at times may be seen. The bullae may be intraepidermal or subepidermal, and they are particularly problematic in the patient with vascular disease, due to the large areas of skin that may be involved with resulting necrosis.

54. How frequently do ulcerations of the foot occur in diabetics?

Up to 15% of diabetics will develop ulcerations in their lifetime. Ulcerations superficial to the glenoid ligament (Wagner grade 1 and 2) can be healed 90% of the time without surgical intervention. Lesions from the glenoid down to the level of bone (Wagner grade 3 or 4) have a healing rate of 50% or less. Most of these patients will likely need surgery for correction of their problem.

55. What percentage of ulcers will recur following nonsurgical cure?

Edmonds reported a 26–83% recurrence in 2 years, depending on the patient's post-ulcer follow-up and care. Other authors report recurrence in 19.6–40% of patients, most within 8–22 months following healing.

56. When should one soak diabetic ulcerations?

Soaking can lead to maceration and further infection. Bacteria may be driven further into the tissues on soaking as well. Patients with neurovascular conditions are at particular risk during soaking, due to increased tissue demands when soaking in higher temperatures.

57. Which topical solutions are the preferred antiseptic to prevent foot wounds from becoming infected?

Virtually none of the over-the-counter antiseptics/antibacterials are without cytotoxicity to fibroblasts. This list includes betadine, acetic acid, hydrogen peroxide, and Dakin's solution. In general, there is no substitute for appropriate debridement and addition of a normal saline moist dressing in maintaining wounds for healing. It is common to use betadine and Dakin's solution in one-quarter strength in helping to maintain an antiseptic environment for the wound without dessication or cytotoxicity. When hydrogen peroxide is used as a cleansing agent, one-fourth to one-half strength should be used.

58. What are the main reasons that ulcers fail to heal?

1. An inability to control abnormally high pressures
2. Local or diffuse infection
3. Inadequate perfusion

59. What are the permissive factors in ulcer formation?

Neuropathy (somatic and autonomic)   High pressures (intrinsic and extrinsic)

Vascular disease (macrovascular   Limited joint mobility
    and microvascular)

60. What intrinsic factors may modify the body's resistance to ulceration?

1. Sensory and autonomic neuropathy
2. Soft-tissue resistance and viscoelastic properties
3. Intrinsic alterations of the foot which heighten or focus environmental stress (bony prominence)

61. Name the extrinsic factors that are important in ulcer formation.

1. Direct mechanical disruption (e.g., stepping on a foreign object)
2. Alterations in tissue perfusion from continuous low pressure (tight shoes)
3. Inflammatory autolysis secondary to repetitive moderate stress
4. Thermal stress, both hot and cold
5. Chemical stresses (keratolytics)
6. Shearing forces

62. What techniques can the clinician use in helping to diagnose osteomyelitis at the base of an ulcer?

The diagnosis of osteomyelitis at the base of an ulcer can be a difficult one to make. The following techniques may help in diagnosis:

1. A thin stainless steel smooth probe. The smooth metal easily passes through soft tissues to the deepest part of the wound and will probe bone if it is exposed.
2. X-ray evaluation (standard foot views)
3. Radionuclide imaging or MRI
4. Ancillary laboratory tests (CBC, ESR)
5. Bone biopsy, which is the gold standard for definitive diagnosis in the face of conflicting clinical and laboratory information.

63. When is radionuclide imaging necessary in the diagnosis of osteomyelitis?

Three- or four-phase bone scans are highly sensitive but relatively nonspecific in diagnosing osteomyelitis. Scans are positive quite early in the disease, well before x-rays become positive.

Additionally, bone scans may be positive when a simple periostitis or cortical osteomyelitis is evident without penetration into the medullary canal. This condition is frequently missed on x-ray.

Technetium white cell (HMPAO) and indium-labeled white cell scans have helped to increase the specificity of these scans in diagnosis, although there are still false-positives. Problems with spatial resolution as well as problems with cellulitis affecting adjacent, contiguous ulcerations may confound the diagnosis using these scans. The diagnosis of osteomyelitis with a contiguous ulceration may require bone biopsy.

64. What techniques can be used to heal superficial ulcerations (Wagner class 1 or 2) in an ambulatory setting?
Bed rest/crutch walking/wheelchair
Felted foam therapy, pressure relief
Total contact casting
Total contact splinting
Patellar tendon weight-bearing prosthesis
Healing sandal with appropriate total contact orthotic (Plastozote)

65. For an ulceration deep to the tendon with involved bone or joint (Wagner grade 2 or 3), what questions are important in determining an appropriate treatment regimen?
1. Is this a local process, without pus and minimal tendon/bone involvement?
2. Is there associated cellulitis in the soft tissues of the foot?
3. Is the patient febrile?
4. Is the patient exhibiting signs of systemic toxicity (nausea, vomiting, fevers, malaise, uncontrollable blood sugars)?

66. If neither pus nor cellulitis is involved and the patient manifests a localized ulceration that tracks to joint or bone, what would be an appropriate approach to management?
First and foremost, one must evaluate the patient's vascular status. If the patient has signs of significant vascular inflow or outflow disease, consultation with a vascular surgeon should be first and foremost. Even when perfusion is adequate, definitive surgical intervention is usually still considered since these conditions rarely clear up with oral or intravenous antibiotics. Osteomyelitis and chronic septic joints are surgical diseases.
When dealing surgically with these types of ulcers, the following techniques are usually utilized:
Excision of ulceration and infected joint/bone and soft tissue with primary closure
Local tissue rearrangement using local flap procedures
Various free flaps
Skin grafting (rarely used in plantar ulcerations)

67. When dealing with a deep tracking infection associated with pus, cellulitis, and systemic toxicity, what is the most appropriate treatment regimen?
Immediate hospitalization, which will allow for metabolic control, appropriate culture and sensitivities with Gram stain, institution of broad-spectrum IV antibiotics (as these infections are frequently polymicrobial), and early surgical debridement and appropriate drainage. Depending on the the patient's vascular status, the vascular surgeon should become involved early with an eye toward revascularization if there is any question as to the perfusion of the foot.

68. Once the physician has controlled all the important parameters to allow for appropriate ulcer healing, what techniques may be useful to augment the secondary healing of ulceration?
1. Wound dressings (NSS, one-quarter strength betadine or Dakin's, hydrocolloids, hydrogels, alginates)
2. Drug therapy (pentoxifylline, vitamin C, zinc)
3. Platelet-derived growth factors
4. Adjunctive hyperbaric oxygen therapy

BIBLIOGRAPHY

1. American Diabetes Association: Clinical Practice Recommendations, 1996. Diabetes Care 19(suppl 1): 1996.
2. Ferando D, Masson E, Deves A, et al: Relationship of limited joint mobility to abnormal foot pressures in diabetic foot ulceration. Diabetes Care 14:8, 1991.
3. Flynn MD, Tooke JE: Aetiology of diabetic foot ulceration: A role for microcirculation? Diabetic Med 8:320, 1992.
4. Gentzkow GD, Iwasaki SD, Hurshon KS, et al: Use of Dermagraft: A cultured human dermis to treat diabetic foot ulcers. Diabetes Care 19:350, 1996.
5. Helm PA, Walker SC, Pulliam GF: Recurrence of neuropathic ulcers following treatment and total contact casting. Arch Phys Med Rehabil 72:967, 1991.
6. Kozak, Hoar, Rowbotham, et al: Management of Diabetic Foot Problems. Philadelphia, W.B. Saunders Co., 1984.
7. Lavery L, Dennis KJ: The Diabetic Foot. Clin Podiatr Med Surg Jan 1995.
8. Levin M, O'Neil L, Bowker J: The Diabetic Foot, 5th ed. St. Louis, Mosby Year Book, 1993.
9. Lipsky B, Pecoraro R, Larson S, et al: Outpatient management of uncomplicated lower extremity infections in diabetic patients. Arch Intern Med 150:790, 1990.
10. Lipsky B, Pecoraro R, Wheat LJ: The diabetic foot: Soft tissue and bone infection. Infect Dis Clin North Am 4(3):409–432, 1990.
11. Lolgerfo FW, Coffman JD: Vascular and microvascular disease in the diabetic foot: Implications for foot care. N Engl J Med 311:1615–1619, 1984.
12. Palumbo PJ, Melton LJ: Peripheral vascular disease and diabetes. In Harris MI, Hamman RF (eds): Diabetes in America. Bethesda, MD: National Institute Arthritis, Diabetes, and Digestive and Kidney Diseases [NIH publ. no. 85-1468.] 1985, vol XVI, pp 1–21.
13. Peters A, Kerner W: Perioperative management of the diabetic patient. Exp Clin Endocrinol Diabetol 103:213–218, 1995.
14. Steed DL, Diabetic Ulcer Group Study: Clinical evaluation of recombinant human platelet derived growth factors for treatment of lower extremity diabetic ulcers. J Vasc Surg 21:71, 1995.
15. Thomson FJ, Veves A, Ashe H, et al: A team approach to diabetic foot care—The Manchester experience. Foot 2:75–82, 1991.
16. Uccioli L, Monticone G, Durola L, et al: Autonomic neuropathy influences great toe blood pressure. Diabetes Care 17:284, 1994.

23. CHARCOT OSTEOARTHROPATHY

Lee J. Sanders, D.P.M

1. Who was J.-M. Charcot?

Jean-Martin Charcot (1825–1893) was a great French neurologist who brought attention to the arthropathies associated with tabes dorsalis (neurosyphilis). His meticulous studies of patients at the Salpêtrière, the "grand asylum of human misery" in Paris, enabled him to depict for the first time a distinct pathologic entity, the arthropathy of ataxia. He believed that lesions of the spinal cord were responsible for the enormous bone and joint destruction associated with tabetic arthropathies. He described a sudden and unexpected arthropathy that often began without apparent cause. Sharp, shooting pains in the extremities often preceded the joint affection. There was a sudden onset of generalized swelling of the limb with rapid changes in the articular surfaces of the joint, extensive looseness of the ligaments, and frequent occurrence of dislocations.

2. Why is Charcot's name associated with neuropathic joints?

Charcot's brilliant contribution to the understanding of neuropathic joints was publicly recognized in 1882, when it was written that "these bone and joint changes constitute a distinct pathological entity. They deserve the name of 'Charcot's joint.'" Accordingly, this term has been perpetuated to describe bone and joint changes associated with all neuropathic arthropathies.

3. Is this condition of importance today?

Yes, specifically in relation to the **diabetic foot**.

4. What are some commonly cited disorders with the potential for producing Charcot's joint?

Diabetes mellitus (the leading cause)	Syringomyelia
Chronic alcoholism	Spina bifida
Hansen's disease	Meningomyelocele
Peripheral nerve injuries	Congenital insensitivity to pain

5. In addition to Charcot's work in tabetic arthropathies, what are some of his other neurologic discoveries?

Charcot may be better known for his descriptions of amyotrophic lateral sclerosis, multiple sclerosis, progressive muscular dystrophy (Charcot-Marie-Tooth disease), Parkinson's disease, and hysteria, and his studies in cerebral localization. Among Charcot's eminent students were Joseph Babinski, Pierre Marie, Georges Gilles de la Tourette, and Sigmund Freud.

6. How do you identify the acute Charcot foot?

Early recognition is facilitated by careful history and physical examination. Look for areas of erythema, swelling, increased skin temperature, deformity, or instability of the foot and ankle. Early changes (mild erythema and swelling) affecting the tarsometatarsal joints may appear to be early osteoarthritis. Local skin temperature elevation is noted and may precede collapse of the foot. Areas of increased warmth correspond to areas of inflammation or hyperemia, which are at risk for bony resorption and ulceration. A localized increase in skin temperature greater than 2–3° C should be considered a significant finding portending imminent osteoarthropathy.

7. What are the diagnostic criteria for Charcot's arthropathy?

The diagnosis of the acute neuropathic joint depends primarily on the clinical suspicion of this disorder. Patients demonstrate loss of protective sensation, absent deep tendon reflexes, and diminished vibratory sense. They are generally afebrile, with normal white blood cell counts and no shift in differential. A mild elevation in ESR may be noted. The most specific diagnostic tools for distinguishing between the acute Charcot joint and osteomyelitis in the diabetic foot are careful clinical and radiologic examinations. Indium-111 scans (high negative-predictive value for osteomyelitis) and MRI may be of value. Bone biopsy should be reserved for those cases that are equivocal, when there has been a chronic nonhealing wound or soft-tissue infection contiguous to bone.

8. Are there early radiographic findings that may alert the clinician to the diagnosis of the Charcot foot?

Early radiographic changes in the midfoot may include a small fracture at the base of the second metatarsal, disruption of the second metatarsal-cuneiform joint, or lateral deviation of the metatarsal bases on the cuneiforms. Resorption of the distal metatarsal bones and osteolytic destruction of the tarsal bones with subsequent collapse of the arch are characteristic findings. Fragmentation of bone frequently accompanies dislocations.

9. What factors contribute to the development of noninfective bone and joint destruction in individuals with diabetes?

Peripheral neuropathy with loss of protective sensation, autonomic neuropathy with increased peripheral blood flow, mechanical stress and trauma appear to be the key component factors leading to neuropathic osteoarthropathy. Other factors may include nonenzymatic glycosylation of collagen, decreased cartilage growth activity, corticosteroid-induced osteoporosis, or other metabolic abnormality that may weaken bone.

10. List some high-risk clinical characteristics of a diabetic individual who is at risk for the development of Charcot's arthropathy.

The average age reported for the onset of diabetic neuropathic osteoarthropathy is 57 years. Most patients are in their fifth or sixth decade of life, with an average duration of diabetes of 15 years. Type I diabetics may be younger, with an average age of 33 years and duration of diabetes of 20 years. High-risk patients demonstrate loss of protective sensation, absent deep tendon reflexes at the ankle, and diminished or absent vibratory sensation.

11. Is bilateral involvement common?

Bilateral involvement has been described in 5.9%–39.3% of reported cases. Subtle radiographic changes may be noted in the contralateral foot.

12. Are there specific patterns of bone and joint involvement? Is ulceration associated with any of these patterns?

There are five characteristic anatomic patterns of bone and joint destruction observed in neuropathic diabetics (see figure on next page).

I—**Forefoot** (metatarsal heads, MTP joints, phalanges, and interphalangeal joints). Radiographic findings are often atrophic and destructive, mimicking osteomyelitis. Plantar ulceration is an associated finding.

II—**Tarsometatarsal joints.** Characterized by disruption of the TMT joints, often with collapse of the midfoot. Plantar ulceration frequently develops at the apex of the collapsed cuneiforms or cuboid.

III—**Naviculocuneiform, talonavicular,** and **calcaneocuboid joints**. Characterized by dislocation of the navicular or disintegration of the naviculocuneiform joints. Very early findings may be subtle, evidenced by osteolytic changes at the naviculocuneiform joints. This pattern can be seen by itself or associated with other patterns of involvement.

IV—**Ankle joint.** Occurs infrequently and accounts for only 3–10% of reported cases, but neuropathic arthropathy of the ankle joint almost always results in severe deformity and instability. This pattern may also be associated with involvement of the subtalar joint.

V—**Calcaneus** (calcaneal insufficiency avulsion fracture). Neuropathic osteopathy of the calcaneus is characterized by an avulsion fracture of the posterior process of the calcaneus. This is the least commonly reported pattern of involvement.

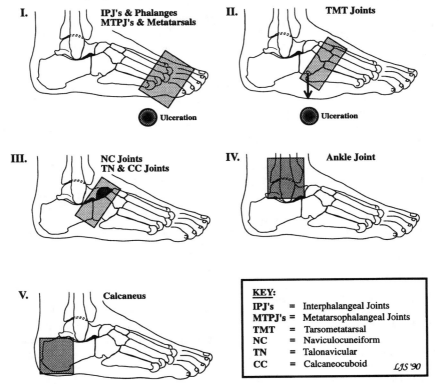

Anatomic patterns of bone and joint destruction in diabetics with neuropathic osteoarthropathy of the foot and ankle. Patterns I and II are frequently associated with bony deformity and ulceration. The most frequent joint involvement is seen in patterns I, II, and III, with the most severe structural deformity and functional instability associated with patterns II and IV. (From Sanders LJ, Frykberg RG: Diabetic neuropathic osteoarthropathy: The Charcot foot. In Frykberg RG (ed): The High Risk Foot in Diabetes Mellitus. New York, Churchill Livingstone, 1991, p 308; with permission.)

13. How should the acute Charcot foot be managed?

Management is based on the joints affected, the degree of involvement (e.g., deformity, fractures, bone fragmentation, and instability), and presence of concurrent ulceration and infection.

The acute destructive phase of this condition, **the stage of development**, is characterized radiographically by joint effusions, edema, subluxation, detritus, intra-articular fractures, and fragmentation of bone. At this time, the foot should be treated conservatively with elevation and a well-padded compression dressing, followed by cast immobilization. The period of immobilization varies among cases, but the rule of thumb is at least 3–4 months.

14. What clinical and radiographic changes are noted during the reparative phase of healing?

With rest and cast immobilization, there is a reduction of swelling, absorption of fine debris, and healing of fractures. This reparative phase of healing marks the **stage of coalescence**.

Clinically, there is a lessening of swelling and erythema and normalization of skin temperature. Stability of the foot may or may not be achieved.

15. What constitutes the final phase of bone healing?

In the final phase of bone healing, the **stage of reconstruction**, further repair and remodeling take place, with proliferation of new bone. There is decreased joint mobility and increased stabilization of the foot. Fusion and rounding of large fragments are late findings.

16. Are current therapies effective?

Therapies for the treatment of the Charcot foot are discouraging and fail to address the underlying disease process. Recent studies have demonstrated that drugs that inhibit osteoclastic bone resorption may have a role in the treatment and prevention of Charcot's arthropathy. Selby and associates, using the bisphosphonate pamidronate in six diabetic patients with active disease, noted a significant reduction in bone turnover as judged by alkaline phosphatase activity.

17. Does electrical bone stimulation enhance healing of neuropathic fractures?

At present, there are no published prospective, randomized, controlled clinical trials to support the use of electrical bone stimulators for the treatment of Charcot joints.

18. When should surgical management be considered?

Surgical management should be delayed until the acute inflammatory condition has subsided. This is evidenced by reduction of edema, erythema, skin temperature, and radiographic evidence of healing. At this time, unstable joints and deformities that predispose to shearing stress and ulceration may be corrected. The goal is to obtain a durable, plantigrade foot for ambulation.

19. What are the criteria for surgical intervention?

Criteria for surgical intervention include instability of the foot or ankle, deformity, chronic ulceration, progressive joint destruction (despite conservative care), adequate circulation, and no active infection. The patient should be medically stable and compliant and have the potential for returning to an active lifestyle.

Open reduction with internal fixation should be reserved for unstable joints, typically the TMT, pantalar, tibiotalar, tibiotalocalcaneal, and talocalcaneal joints. Operative management is technically demanding with a high rate of complications.

BIBLIOGRAPHY

1. Charcot J-M: On some arthropathies apparently related to a lesion of the brain or spinal cord. January 1868. [Transl. by Hoché G and Sanders LJ.] J Am Podiatr Med Assoc 82:403–411, 1992 [Reprint].
2. Charcot JM: Sur quelques arthropathies qui paraissant dépendre d'une lésion du cerveau or de la moelle épinière. Arch Physiol Norm Pathol 1:161, 1868.
3. Eichenholtz SN: Charcot Joints. Springfield, IL, Charles C Thomas, 1966.
4. Sanders LJ, Frykberg RG: Diabetic neuropathic osteoarthropathy: The Charcot foot. In Frykberg RG (ed): The High Risk Foot in Diabetes Mellitus. New York, Churchill Livingstone, 1991, pp 297–338.
5. Sanders LJ, Frykberg RG: The Charcot foot. In Levin ME, O'Neal LW, Bowker JH (eds): The Diabetic Foot, 5th ed. St. Louis, Mosby Year Book, 1993, pp 149–180.
6. Selby PL, Young MJ, Boulton AJM: Bisphonates: A new treatment for diabetic Charcot neuroarthropathy? Diabetic Med 11:28–31, 1994.

24. AUTOIMMUNE DISEASES

Major Mary Cook, D.P.M., and Kim Felder-Johnson, D.P.M.

1. Mrs. Jones is a 45-year-old patient with a 20-year history of rheumatoid arthritis. Her disease has been maintained with 7.5 mg prednisone per day for the past year. She is scheduled for a panmetatarsal head resection to alleviate chronic metatarsalgia. How should she be managed perioperatively?

Perioperative management would include administering 100 mg IV hydrocortisone preoperatively, followed by 100 mg 8 hours postoperatively. The prolonged use of exogenous steroids will cause a suppression of the HPA (hypothalamus-pituitary-adrenal axis). This suppression can last as long as one year after stopping the drug and interferes with the patient's normal response to stressful situations. Therefore, whenever these patients are in stressful situations, they will require increase of steroid for coverage. This coverage is needed only until the stressful situation is over; tapering is not necessary unless coverage is required for three or more days. Suddenly stopping the steroid could lead to withdrawal reactions as serious as cardiovascular collapse.

2. Management of patients with rheumatoid arthritis is aimed at relief of pain, reduction of inflammation, and preservation of muscle and joint function. Simple analgesics are usually considered first, followed by the nonsteroidal anti-inflammatory drugs. However, it is often necessary to use combination therapy. The drug classes typically used include penicillamines, gold salts, corticosteroids, and antimalarials. Which of these drug classes is not considered a "specific" drug for rheumatoid arthritis?

The corticosteroids are not specific in the treatment of rheumatoid arthritis. Although most patients will respond to corticosteroids, this class of drug will not alter the natural progression of the disease. Penicillamines, gold salts, and antimalarials will produce a gradual suppression of the disease process. The mechanism of action is unknown, the side effects are many, but used cautiously with careful monitoring these drugs prove beneficial to the rheumatoid arthritis patient.

3. Which autoimmune disease is characterized by diminished lacrimal and salivary gland secretion?

Sicca complex (dry eyes and mouth) is characteristic of Sjögren's syndrome. Sjögren syndrome, which may be seen as a primary disorder or in association with another connective tissue disorder, commonly involves major and minor salivary glands as well as lacrimal glands. These include parotid and submandibular glands.

4. Keratoderma blennorrhagicum is the characteristic cutaneous manifestation of which autoimmune disease?

The once-thought triad of urethritis, arthritis, and conjunctivitis in Reiter's syndrome has been expanded to a tetrad that include keratoderma blennorrhagicum. This cutaneous disorder often begins on the soles of the feet as small red to yellowish brown vesicles or papules.

5. Myasthenia gravis is an autoimmune disorder causing a progressive weakness with exertion, ptosis, diplopia, difficulty chewing or swallowing, respiratory difficulties, or some combination of these problems. Which gland is usually malfunctioning in this condition?

The thymus gland. Myasthenia gravis is associated with either thymic hyperplasia or a thymoma. Anticholinesterase drugs provide symptomatic relief, but do not alter the course of the disease. Thymectomy usually leads to remission or some degree of symptomatic relief. Corticosteroids are indicated for patients who have not responded to the other mentioned treatments.

147

6. The differentiation of systemic lupus erythematosus (SLE) from other diseases primarily involving connective tissue may be difficult. What is the best screening test for SLE?

The best screening test is ANA. Among the autoantibodies expressed in patient sera, those directed against components of the cell nucleus (ANA) are the most characteristic of SLE and are found in over 95% of patients.

7. Which two autoantibodies are unique to SLE and are included in the serologic criteria for the classification of this disease?

Multiple ANA specificities occur in SLE but two are virtually specific for this disease. Antibodies to double-stranded DNA and an RNA-protein complex termed Sm are found essentially only in SLE patients.

8. Patients who are seronegative (no rheumatoid factor in the serum) tend to have a different illness from patients who are seropositive. What are some of the differences?

There is an increased prevalence of the B-cell alloantigen HLA-DR4 in patients who have seropositive rheumatoid arthritis but not in those who are seronegative. Seropositive patients tend to have more severe disease, more erosions, and more extra-articular features.

9. What is pannus?

Pannus is a chronic proliferative lesion consisting of a mass of fibroblastic, vascular, and inflammatory cells. The mass accumulates at the margin of the synovial membrane-cartilage border, driven by cellular interactions based in the synovial membrane and the soluble mediators generated in the synovial fluid. The mass can cause local erosions of cartilage and bone or produce enzymes that degrade collagen and proteoglycans in the cartilage.

10. What is boutonniere deformity and what disease is it commonly associated with?

Boutonniere deformity is a digital deformity that results from chronic swelling or rupture of the extensor hood at the proximal interphalangeal joint. The deformity exhibits dorsiflexion at the metatarsophalangeal joint, plantarflexion at the proximal interphalangeal joint, and hyperextension of the distal interphalangeal joint. This deformity is commonly associated with rheumatoid arthritis.

11. What cutaneous lesions might be observed in a patient with systemic lupus erythematosus (SLE)?

The characteristic cutaneous lesion of SLE is a malar "butterfly" rash on the face. Other cutaneous lesions seen with lupus include discoid lesions; erythematous, firm, maculopapular lesions of the face, exposed neck areas, upper chest, and elbows; ulcerations of the oral and buccal areas, mucous membranes, and anterior nasal septum; mottled erythema of the palms; and generalized alopecia.

12. What does the acronym CREST stand for and which of the collagen vascular diseases is it most commonly associated with?

CREST syndrome is most commonly seen with scleroderma. Each letter of the acronym represents a disorder seen with the syndrome:

C = Calcinosis
R = Raynaud's phenomenon
E = Esophageal dysfunction
S = Sclerodactly
T = Telangiectasia

13. A 35-year-old man is being evaluated for plantar fasciitis. He has been complaining of lower back pain and heel pain for a few months. He related that he had been evaluated in back clinic several months ago and was told that he had degenerative joint disease consistent

with his age and prior athletic lifestyle. He relates that his heel pain has somewhat improved with conservative therapy but that his lower back and joints are more painful and stiff for longer periods of time on a daily basis, usually in the morning. He was referred back to orthopaedics for further evaluation with pre-clinic spine films. You pulled up the radiology report just to follow up the outcome and noted that prior spine films demonstrated squaring of the superior and inferior margins of the vertebral bodies. The latest films demonstrated some degenerative arthritis and inflammation of the sacroiliac joints bilaterally. In addition, the radiologist had written in quotes "bamboo spine." What would you clinically suspect and what test might help your diagnosis at this point?

Sacroiliitis is classic and always seen with ankylosing spondylitis. The squaring of the superior and inferior aspects of the vertebral bodies is the result of inflammatory disease at the site of the insertion of the outer fibers of the annulus fibrosus or enthesopathy. This is a phenomenon frequently seen on early radiographic evaluation of ankylosing spondylitis. The late changes of this process produce the classic "bamboo spine." This finding is rare. The lab test to consider would be HLA-B27. This is expensive and should not be done routinely, since the diagnosis is typically based on clinical and radiographic findings.

14. What is the triad typically associated with Reiter's syndrome?

Reiter's syndrome was originally described by Dr. Hans Reiter in 1916. His description included a triad of conditions which included arthritis, urethritis, and conjunctivitis. Today Reiter's syndrome is defined as a seronegative arthropathy that follows urethritis, cervicitis, or dysentery.

15. What are three clinical features, which may be the reason for initial presentation, seen in a patient with Reiter's syndrome?

• Sausage digit (also seen with psoriatic arthritis)
• Achilles tendinitis or insertional swelling
• Plantar fasciitis
• Low back pain

16. What pedal manifestations might be seen in a patient with psoriatic arthritis?

The distal interphalangeal joints may present with periarticular swelling and flexion deformities. The digit may have a sausage-like appearance. Nail changes include onycholysis, discoloration, fragmentation, and pitting. Skin lesions may include macular, papular plaques with scaling.

17. What is morphea and what condition is it associated with?

Morphea is a cutaneous condition that presents as erythematous, violaceous plaques with inflammatory borders. Plaques may become sclerotic and waxy or ivory. Histologically, these lesions result from new collagen deposition in the dermis and septae of the subcutaneous tissue. Microscopically, there are infiltrates of lymphocytes, plasma cells, and histiocytes. Morphea is seen with localized scleroderma.

18. A 34-year-old male presents with a complaint of his toes turning black. History was significant for a 24-pack-year history of smoking and symptoms consistent with Raynaud's phenomenon. The patient relates that his toes have been turning black for the last few weeks becoming more progressive. He denies trauma or injury to his feet. On clinical exam the patient has cyanotic-appearing fingers and toes. There is dry gangrene to the hallux and the second and third toe of the left foot, and to the fourth and fifth toes of the right foot. His feet are cool to the touch and shiny. There is no palpable pedal pulse. What would a working diagnosis include and what study might you consider ordering?

A working diagnosis should include thromboangiitis obliterans, or Buerger's disease. This is an inflammatory obliterative disease that affects small and medium-sized arteries and veins of the distal extremities. Buerger's disease usually affects young males under the age of 40 who are heavy smokers. There is a genetic predisposition for the disease and prevalence of HLA-AP and B5. These patients also demonstrate cell-mediated hypersensitivity to type I and II collagen and antibodies to these antigens. The symptoms as described above result from impaired arterial supply and segmental thrombophlebitis. Angiography can be performed to assess the severity of the disease. Treatment consists of stressing to the patient the need to cease smoking, sympathectomy, and vasodilating agents.

19. What might the urinalysis of a patient with systemic lupus erythematosus (SLE) demonstrate if there is renal involvement.

Glomerulonephritis is often seen in advanced cases of SLE. Urinalysis would show excessive cellular cysts and sediment and profuse proteinuria.

20. What are Grotton's papules and what autoimmune disease are they associated with?

Grotton's papules are violet, flat-topped hyperemic lesions that appear on the interphalangeal joint surfaces in patients with dermatomyositis.

21. A patient presents with a complaint of a wart on the bottom of his foot. He relates that he had a similar lesion in the dorsolateral aspect of his foot. This went away on its own over several months. On examination, a violaceous, macular lesion is noted on the central-lateral sole of the patient's foot. It is nontender and slightly raised. Examination of the lower legs demonstrates four similar lesions in a linear pattern on the contralateral leg. Further questioning of the patient reveals previous hospitalization for pneumonia and a positive history of IVDA and homosexuality. The remaining clinical exam is unremarkable. What is your diagnosis and what test might you order? What might your test reveal?

The lesion is clinically consistent with Kaposi's sarcoma. The lesion presents as a macular vascular tumor, slowly progressive in nature. History of regression can be seen with this lesion, but is rare. Tests should include HIV and skin lesion biopsy. The blood test might reveal positive HIV. The skin biopsy, if positive for Kaposi's sarcoma, may demonstrate a discrete intradermal nodule with vascular channels lined by atypical endothelial cells, copious extravasated erythrocytes, and hemosiderosis deposition.

Note: The opinions and assertions contained herein are the private views of the authors, and are not to be construed as the official policy or position of the U.S. Government, the Department of Defense, or the Department of the Air Force.

BIBLIOGRAPHY

1. Farthing CF, Brown SE, Staughton RC: A Color Atlas of AIDS, 2nd ed. St. Louis, Mosby, 1988.
2. Geha RS, Rosen FS: Case Studies in Immunology: A Clinical Comparison. New York, Gordon Publishing/Current Biology, 1996.
3. O'Shea JJ, et al: Immune Disorders. Springhouse, PA, Springhouse Corporation, 1995.
4. Roitt I: Immunology, 4th ed. St. Louis, Mosby, 1996.
5. West SG: Rheumatology Secrets. Philadelphia, Hanley & Belfus, 1997.

25. VASCULAR PROBLEMS

Anthony S. Kidawa, B.S., D.P.M.

1. Where in the lower extremities do atheromatous plaques tend to develop?

These lesions typically develop at arterial bifurcation sites, including the distal abdominal aorta, common iliac, common femoral, popliteal, and the trifurcation into the tibial and peroneal trunks. In addition, the superficial femoral may develop a thrombus at the adductor hiatus due to a life-long compression by this muscle.

2. How can the level of an occlusive arterial lesion be predicted by symptoms or signs?

The symptom of claudication involves the musculature one joint distal to the proximal primary lesion. A secondary lesion further down the extremity will further reduce the perfusion and may present when walking a shorter distance or as nocturnal pain. If the flow dynamics are markedly disturbed, a tertiary lesion may develop, causing rest pain even on dependency, with attendant dependent rubor, trophic skin and nail changes, and ischemic skin ulceration.

3. How can one differentiate arteriogenic versus venogenic dependent rubor?

With elevation of the extremity (Samuel's test), arteriogenic rubor converts to pallored pedal skin, while venogenic dependent rubor converts to normal coloration.

4. Aside from atherosclerosis obliterans, what are other causes of claudication?

Deep thrombophlebitis of the tibial, popliteal, or femoral veins
Popliteal entrapment
Sciatica (neurogenic claudication)
Femoral or popliteal arterial calcification
Anemia (hypochromic, microcytic, sickle cell, thalassemia)

5. Does absence of pedal pulses always indicate an arterial deficit?

Pedal pulses may be absent with significant arterial occlusion of one thrombotic lesion or as the sum result of two lesser occlusive lesions. In addition, the pulses may be decreased due to systemic hypotension, systemic or venous ankle and pedal edema, lymphedema, significant lipoma formation, local inflammation, marked capsular effusion about the ankle or pedal joints, as well as general obesity.

6. Which noninvasive tests can be used to assess normal pulsations, pressures, and flow and to confirm a suspicion of an occlusive arterial lesion?

- Segmental pneumatic plethysmography reflects the large-vessel wall reactivity to pulsations.
- Segmental (including ankle) pressures indicate the presence of normal or decreased heads of pressure, depending on the degree of stenosis.
- Doppler insolation of arteries demonstrates normal flow dynamics versus aberrant eddy currents distal to thrombotic lesions.
- Digital photocell plethysmography demonstrates the pulsatility of the end arterioles comprising the glomus in the pulp of a toe.
- Digital pressures assess the head of pressure in the digital arteries.
- Thermography, skin thermometry, and percutaneous oximetry reflect the degree of cutaneous perfusion, whether by the primary arterioles or by collaterals, which may be present in cases of significant occlusion of the limb's named arteries.

7. What relationship is there between the pressures at various limb levels and the arm?

The systolic pressures should not decrease from one level to the next distal segment by > 20 mm Hg, or by 10 mm Hg as compared to the same level of the contralateral limb. The ankle/arm ischemic index in the normal person is 1.00–1.20.

8. Can the ankle ischemic index serve as an indicator for management of the arterially compromised patient?

An index of 1.00–0.90 may only warrant recommendations for walking exercise to assist in establishing collaterals and an aspirin daily to retard further plaque formation. An index of 0.90–0.50 should be treated with Trental (pentoxiphylline), while an index < 0.50 warrants revascularization. Wound healing following trauma or podiatric surgery may be retarded if the index is < 0.30.

9. What effects does Möckenberg's medial calcific sclerosis have on the results of noninvasive studies?

The below-knee and ankle pressures with resultant ankle ischemic indices are spuriously increased, while all other pulse and flow determinants are normal.

10. How and where is the arterial system compromised in the diabetic?

The macrocirculation to the level of the ankles is predisposed to form occlusive lesions, which adversely affect all the noninvasive arterial studies and cause symptoms of claudication, night cramps, or rest pain initially relieved by dependency or, with near-total occlusion, not even relieved by dependency. The microcirculation can concurrently develop arteriolosclerosis, leading to digital ischemia with still patent arteries more proximally in the limb. Either of these circumstances leads to autosympathectomization since there exists no further need for protective constriction.

11. If autosympathectomization has occurred, how can it be identified or confirmed?

The pedal skin no longer sweats, and there are no variations in temperature irrespective of the clothing or ambient temperature. By digital plethysmography, the vasovagal test evokes no additional pulse constriction, while the postocclusive reactive hyperemia test demonstrates no capacity for additional dilation of the microcirculation as reflected by no increase in digital pulsations.

12. What is the difference between Raynaud's phenomenon, Raynaud's syndrome, and Raynaud's disease?

The **phenomenon** is characterized by episodic digital skin palloring with paresthesias, possibly followed by cyanosis, and finally presenting with rubor and warmth as well as a throbbing sensation.

The **syndrome** is a repeated presentation of the phenomenon under circumstances of coldness or anxiety and is associated with a collagen disorder whether known or yet to be identified.

The **disease** state is diagnosed when the trilogy of colors with associated symptoms is noted for at least 2 years without the definition of an underlying collagen disease.

13. Which collagen diseases typically affect the microcirculation?

Rheumatoid arthritis	Giant cell arteritis
Systemic lupus erythematosus	Erythema nodosum
Systemic sclerosis	Erythema induratum
Polymyositis	Nodular vasculitis
Polyarteritis nodosa	Nonsuppurative panniculitis

14. What other disorders can mimic Raynaud's constrictive signs and symptoms?

Acrocyanosis in the vasoconstrictive stage and erythromelalgia or ergotism in the dilated stage. Reflex sympathetic dystrophy can present at various times with either the dilated or constricted stage.

15. What precautions are recommended to preclude vasospastic crises?

Avoidance of exposure to cold environment, such as wearing gloves or keeping the hands in pockets, wearing two or three pairs of socks on the feet, wearing rubber-soled shoes in wet and cold weather or rubbers in snow, as well as wearing multiple layers of clothes.

16. What medications are recommended to dilate the vasospastic patient?

Nitroglycerine 2% ointment applied as a ¾-inch strip to either the dorsum of the foot or anterior ankle under an extra large BandAid, to be changed every 5–6 hours upon exposure to the cold environment. Alternately, a calcium channel or β-blocker medication is recommended for short-term use outdoors or in the slow release form for all-day dilation.

17. In the diabetic, where do atheromatous lesions occur most frequently? What is their composition?

Atheromatous plaques typically develop in the coronary, cerebral, and large arteries of the extremities. Their composition includes cholesterol, lipids, calcium, platelets, erythrocytes, and smooth muscles.

18. Which factors in the diabetic should be controlled to minimize vascular complications?

Hyperglycemia	Smoking
Hyperinsulinemia	Hypertension
Hypercholesterolemia	Obesity
Hypertriglyceridemia	

19. What methods are employed to increase blood flow through collateral channels?

Avoidance of vasoconstriction through exposure to cold temperatures or usage of vasoconstrictor medications, cessation of tobacco smoking, increasing physical activity and walking to tolerance 2–4 times daily, and raising the head of bed by 12–16 inches.

20. Identify the clinical findings leading to the suspicion of an arteriovenous fistula.

Following a penetrating wound or a dislocated open or closed fracture, the following are noted: increase in limb length if injury occurs prior to epiphyseal closure, thrill and bruit, persistent increased skin temperature at site of injury, cardiomegaly and congestive failure, prominent distal varices, edema, indurative cellulitis, stasis pigmentation, and the possible concurrent presence of digital ischemia.

21. What factors should be recalled to determine the etiology of deep thrombophlebitis?

Severe trauma	Congestive cardiac or coronary failure with
Postop stagnation	dehydration
Infections	Cancer (e.g., pancreatic leading to hypercoagulability)
Blood dyscrasias (e.g.,	Postural pressure on deep veins
polycythemia vera)	Oral contraceptives
Pregnancy	Idiopathic

22. Which noninvasive modalities are used to document deep thrombophlebitis?

Doppler venous flow assessment demonstrates venous flow which may not be spontaneous, phasic with respiration, and augmentable upon compression of veins. **Plethysmography** (pneumatic, impedance, or mercury strain) demonstrates the limited venous capacitance of a thrombosed vein and retarded outflow on decompression. To view the thrombus directly, a duplex system is employed which reflects the Doppler signals from the vessel and images them in an anatomical form.

23. What are the normal maximal venous capacitance and outflow values?

The maximal venous capacitance is dependent on the size of an extremity, with the nonsymptomatic or nonthrombosed extremity serving as the standard. By comparison, a thrombosed limb demonstrates minimal additional capacitance since the venous tree is already congested. The normal venous outflow following release of a thigh tourniquet is < 3 seconds.

24. Identify the complications associated with iliofemoral venous thrombosis.

Phlegmasia alba dolens (edematous milk leg), associated with associated lymphatic obstruction

Phlegmasia cerulea dolens (edematous mottled blue discoloration), associated with high venous pressure resulting in arterial insufficiency.

25. List the symptoms of pulmonary embolism.

From most to least prevalent, the symptoms of pulmonary embolism are:

1. Dyspnea
2. Pleuritic chest pain
3. Apprehension
4. Cough
5. Hemoptysis
6. Diaphoresis
7. Syncope

26. What should be considered in the differential diagnosis of deep vein thrombosis?

1. Arthritis of knee or ankle
2. Nerve compression
3. Cellulitis
4. Ruptured Baker's cyst
5. Muscle spasm or tear
6. Muscle trauma
7. Muscle hematoma
8. Painful varices

27. Following injury, which leg compartment is typically involved? What are the clinical findings?

The anterior leg compartment is most frequently involved, presenting with initial changes in light touch sensation, followed by decreased motor function, increased compartment tension, pain on passive followed by active motion, and preservation of pulses until the end stage.

28. What are the typical sources of embolism presenting in the lower extremity?

Aside from detachment of a non-fibrin-bound plaque located proximal to the leg, the typical sources are cardiogenic, including those due to atrial fibrillation, left ventricular aneurysm, left ventricular thrombosis following myocardial infarction, valvular disease (either stenosis or incompetence), and prosthetic valves.

29. What complications can follow an embolic blockage of a limb artery?

The sequelae vary depending on time of consultation and diagnosis and include ischemic ulceration of leg, digital or pedal gangrene, a compartment syndrome, as well as metabolic changes including acidosis, hyperkalemia, and myoglobinuria.

30. Describe the clinical features leading to the diagnosis of erythromelalgia.

- Red painful extremities when the temperature rises above the critical point of 89–96° F, which are aggravated with dependency and relieved upon elevation.
- Pedal pain is aggravated with a tourniquet applied to the leg.
- The warmed skin area is swollen, painful, and puffy.
- Relief of signs and symptoms in a cool environment.

31. What are the treatment options for erythromelalgia?

Relief may be provided with avoidance of heat, use of light-weight socks, wearing of perforated shoes or sandals, and treatment with aspirin or serotonin-blocking agents (e.g., methylsergide).

32. Which techniques are available for revascularization of an arterially compromised lower extremity?

The surgical procedures employed depend on the skill of the surgeon as well as the degree and level of stenosis which alter the hemodynamics of flow and perfusion pressure. From the oldest to the latest techniques, the options include embolectomy, thrombectomy, excisional endarterectomy, bypass procedures using synthetic materials, reverse or in-situ long saphenous bypass, balloon angioplasty, as well as catheter-guided rotary thrombectomy or laser thrombus ablation.

33. What is the differential clinical finding leading to a diagnosis of lymphedema?

Although most forms of venogenic, cardiogenic, or systemic edema are pitting, lymphedema is nonpitting and presents with dermal hypertrophy that can lead to formation of mossy skin followed by tumor formations of varied proportions.

34. Can the pitting form of edema eventuate in nonpitting lymphedema?

When the excessive intracellular fluids found in pitting edema chronically compress against the lymphatic channels leading to their collapse, lymphedema starts to develop. This intermediate level is recognized when following the release of finger pressure over a bony surface, some pitting is still evident while the rest of the digital depression has immediate rebound. The latter is the nonpitting component, while the residual pitted depression is attributable to the initial form of pitting edema.

35. What are the treatment options for chronic lymphedema?

For prophylaxis against excessive lymphedema formation, custom-fitted support stockings of appropriate length are recommended with a compression of 40–50 mm Hg to be applied before arising from bed.

With recalcitrant advanced forms of edema formation, the use of sequential intermittent compression therapy applied at a pressure of 70–90 mm Hg for up to 1 hour at a time, as often as three times daily depending on the severity of edema.

BIBLIOGRAPHY

1. Coffman JD: Raynaud's Phenomenon. New York, Oxford, 1989.
2. LeClerc JR (ed): Venous Thromboembolic Disorders, Philadelphia, Lea & Febiger, 1991.
3. Ouriel K: Lower Extremity Vascular Disease. Philadelphia, W.B. Saunders, 1995.

26. NEUROLOGY: PART I

Jeanean Willis, D.P.M.

1. What causes muscle weakness?

It is caused by lesions of the motor neurons or primary muscle disease. True muscle weakness is uncommon. When examining the patient, the physician often misinterprets insufficient patient effort as muscle weakness, and insufficient effort is usually due to a patient's guarding against pain or fear of injuring the examiner.

2. Define muscle tone.

Muscle tone is the resistance that an examiner perceives when passively manipulating the limbs of a patient. It is regulated by reflex activity of the nervous system.

3. What is the difference between hypotonia and hypertonia?

Hypotonia is a decrease of resistance to passive manipulation. It is seen in lower motor neuron disease.

Hypertonia is an increase in resistance to passive manipulation of the limbs. It is seen in an upper motor neuron lesion.

4. Name the parts of a lower motor neuron or motor unit.

A lower motor neuron consists of the following parts:

Anterior horn cell   Axon
Ventral root   The muscle fibers or group innervated by that axon
In summary, the anterior horn cells and everything else outside of the spinal cord.

5. What is an upper motor neuron?

Also known as the corticospinal tract, the upper motor neuron consists of the spinal cord and brain.

6. Give examples of some upper and lower motor neuron diseases.

Upper motor neuron disorders
    Primary lateral sclerosis   Tropical spastic paraparesis
    Lathyrism   Epidemic spastic paraparesis
    Familial (hereditary) spastic paraparesis
Lower motor neuron disorders
    Spinal (bulbospinal muscular) atrophies   Cancer (?)
      (e.g., Werdnig-Hoffman disease)   Monoclonal gammopathy
    Poliomyelitis, post-polio syndrome
Combined upper and lower disorders
    Amyotrophic lateral sclerosis (ALS)

7. When does hypotonia occur?

It occurs once the ventral roots containing the motor nerve fibers to the limb are cut. It also results from transection of the dorsal roots that contain sensory fibers from the muscle.

8. When does hypertonia occur?

Hypertonia occurs in two forms—spasticity and rigidity:

In **spasticity**, there is an increase in the "clasp-knife" type of resistance to passive manipulation, and this is usually accompanied by an increase of the deep-tendon reflexes. The "clasp-knife" phenomenon indicates marked increase of resistance to passive manipulation occurring during the initial portion of the manipulation. As the manipulation proceeds, the resistance suddenly disappears.

In **rigidity**, there is a "cogwheel" type of resistance to passive manipulation, often without changes in the deep tendon reflexes.

9. What is a dermatome?

A dermatome is an area of skin supplied by a posterior root. For example, the lateral aspect of the leg and dorsum of the foot is mainly innervated by the L5 nerve root.

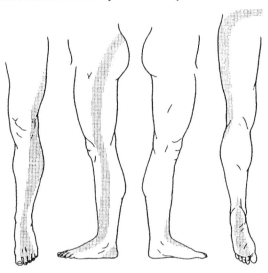

L5 dermatome. (From Wienir MA: Limb radicular pain and sensory disturbance. Spine State Art Rev 2:533–564, 1988, with permission.)

10. What does a positive Tinel's sign indicate?

Tinel's sign is a tingling sensation felt distally upon percussion of a nerve that is regenerating, most commonly due to nerve entrapment. The correct term is Hoffmann-Tinel sign.

11. What are paresthesias?

Spontaneous sensations of prickling, tingling, or numbness.

12. Does the use of sorbitol as a sugar substitute in diabetes promote the development of peripheral neuropathy?

No. The accumulation of sorbitol within the peripheral nerve is implicated in the genesis of peripheral neuropathy through activation of the polyol pathway. The sorbitol formed from glucose by the action of aldose reductase accumulates within the nerve because the neurolemma is impermeable to it. However, exogenously administered sorbitol is unable to enter the nerve.

13. How do you grade muscle strength?

Observation	Grade
No contraction	0/5
Trace contraction	1/5
Active movement with gravity eliminated	2/5
Active movement against gravity	3/5
Active movement against resistance	4/5
Full strength	5/5

14. How do you test vibratory sensation?

Using a 128-Hz tuning fork, lightly tap the fork with your hand and then place the fork on a bony prominence. Start distally and test bilaterally. Let the vibrations of the fork naturally decay. The patient should feel the vibration within 2–3 seconds of when the examiner no longer feels the vibration.

15. In what conditions is vibratory sensation impaired?

Diminished vibratory sensation is usually prominent in peripheral neuropathy and in spinal cord syndromes involving the dorsal columns. It can also be seen in lesions of the brainstem, thalamus, sensory cortex, and thalamocortical projections.

16. How do you assess proprioception?

Start with the hallux and hold the distal phalanx at the sides. With the patient's eyes closed, move the the toe up and down at small increments and ask the patient to describe each movement.

17. How do you assess temperature sensation?

As an adjunct to the pain evaluation, you can assess temperature sensation by simply placing a cold object, such as tuning fork, on the toes, and running the object up the medial and lateral aspect of the foot and legs bilaterally. The temperature should be present and symmetric.

18. What does it mean if a patient has a dissociated sensory loss?

A dissociated sensory loss, meaning that the patient has a loss of pain but not temperature or vibratory sensation and not proprioception, is an indication of a spinal cord or brainstem lesion.

19. What is a radiculopathy?

A pathologic abnormality of a nerve root, the most common being a herniated disc.

20. What is polyneuropathy?

It is a diffuse, symmetric involvement of peripheral nerves, but may affect motor, sensory, and autonomic fibers differentially.

21. What is sciatica?

Sciatica is a common term for radiculopathy, or "pinched nerve," as the nerve exits by the spinal column.

22. What does a positive Babinski reflex indicate?

A positive Babinski is elicited when the plantar aspect of the foot is stroked laterally, and the hallux extends or dorsiflexes and the lesser toes fan out. This indicates an upper motor neuron disorder.

23. Describe the scale for grading reflexes.

Observation	Grade
Absent response	0
Slight jerk or palpable contraction	1+
Average jerk	2+
Brisk jerk	3+
Hyperactive reflex or hyperreflexia (pathologic)	4+

A pathologic reflex is an indication of an upper motor neuron lesion.

24. Is itching a sign of neurologic impairment?

Yes, it can be. However, it is rare.

BIBLIOGRAPHY

1. Chusid JG: Correlative Neuroanatomy and Functional Neurology. Norwalk, CT, Lange Medical Publ., 1982.
2. Curtis B, Jacobsen S, Marcus E: An Introduction to the Neurosciences. Philadelphia, W.B. Saunders, 1972.
3. Gilman S, Newman S: Manter and Gatz's Essentials of Clinical Neuroanatomy and Neurophysiology. Philadelphia, F.A. Davis Co., 1987.
4. Glick T: Neurologic Skills. Boston, Blackwell Scientific Publ., 1993.
5. Guberman A: An Introduction to Clinical Neurology. Boston, Little, Brown & Co., 1994.
6. Mumenthaler M, Schliack H: Peripheral Nerve Lesions. New York, Thieme Medical Publ., 1991.

27. NEUROLOGY: PART II

Samuel J. Spadone, D.P.M.

1. What is the defining characteristic of a radiculopathy?

Symptoms and observable deficits (if any) are distributed in a **dermatomal pattern** and may be noted to involve one or more major nerve distributions. Typically vertebral signs and symptoms (back pain, changes in the intensity of symptoms with changes in posture, and pain on palpation of the adjacent vertebrae) are present. Signs and symptoms may be confined to a single dermatome (monoradiculopathy) or span several dermatomes (polyradiculopathy), although the dermatomes are not necessarily adjacent. Polyradiculopathy has a second accepted meaning: radiculopathy superimposed on a background of polyneuropathy.

2. What is the defining characteristic of a plexopathy?

Symptoms and observable deficits (if any) are distributed along the **course of nerves distal to the suspected site of involvement** in the plexus. No signs or symptoms are noted along the course of nerves originating proximal to the site of involvement. Nerves arising distal to the site of the suspected lesion may be uninvolved, especially if they do not serve the same dermatomes as those arising at the site of the lesion.

While the signs and symptoms of a plexopathy may be confined to a single dermatome, thus making distinction from radiculopathy difficult, the diagnosis is suggested by the absence of symptoms and signs in areas of the involved dermatome(s) served by nerves originating more proximally in the plexus than the site of the lesion. This said, plexopathies affecting the lower extremities are relatively uncommon, and other causes of the patient's presentation should be considered.

3. If a lumbosacral plexopathy is suspected, what are the most common etiologies that must be ruled out?

Tumors	Iatrogenic injury (e.g., surgical procedures)
Coagulopathies	Birth trauma (to the neonate)
Trauma	Ischemic disease
Pregnancy	

4. Because plexopathies involving the lower limbs are infrequent, what other etiologies must be considered?

Space-occupying lesion within the spinal cord

Inflammation of cauda equina (Elsberg syndrome)

Pseudopalsies induced by pain resulting from inflammatory disease of the hips and/or sacrioiliac joint

Limb girdle muscular dystrophy and other proximal myopathies (though the findings are purely motor in these cases)

Occlusion of the pelvic arteries (rarely seen in females)

5. A patient presents with distal bilaterally symmetric anesthesia in a stocking pattern. What is the most likely etiologic process?

This pattern is associated with length-dependent axonopathy which is usually associated with a metabolic etiology (e.g., diabetes, alcoholism, etc.).

6. Describe the characteristics of an upper motor lesion as noted on clinical examination.

Hyperreflexia, preservation of muscle mass (at least initially) and tone (possibly hypertonic or even spastic), without evidence of muscle fasciculation.

7. Describe the characteristics of a lower motor neuron lesion as noted on clinical examination.

Hypo- or areflexia, early and significant muscle atrophy, decreased muscle tone (flaccid paralysis), and muscle fasciculation.

8. How does a mononeuropathy differ from mononeuropathy multiplex?

Mononeuropathy is dysfunction of a single nerve and its terminal branches, whereas mononeuropathy multiplex is the dysfunction of multiple separate nerves and their terminal branches.

9. What is the clinical significance of mononeuropathy as opposed to mononeuropathy multiplex?

Mononeuropathy *may* be the earliest finding in a condition that eventuates in mononeuropathy multiplex or even polyneuropathy. However, mononeuropathy may be caused by entrapment, radiculopathy, trauma, or other *single* focal lesions.

Mononeuropathy multiplex is, by definition, caused by multiple lesions. In mononeuropathy multiplex, one must consider metabolic (bilateral symmetry may not be evident for 6 months or more), inflammatory, or ischemic etiologies. Multiple focal trauma accounting for the condition is unlikely and should be discernible from a careful history. Similarly, multiple nerve entrapments, while conceivable, are unlikely.

10. A patient presents with unilateral mononeuropathy multiplex (sensory and motor deficits) with distal sparing. What are the most likely etiologies of this condition?

Inflammatory neuropathy and ischemic neuropathy.

11. A patient presents with unilateral proximal weakness but an intact sensory examination. Distally, motor and sensory function is grossly normal. What is the most likely etiology of this condition?

An inflammatory myopathy. Myasthenia gravis cannot be excluded from the differential at this point.

12. How are traumatic nerve lesions classified?

There are two widely accepted classification systems, devised by Seddon and by Sunderland.

Seddon system:

1. **Neurapraxia**—A sudden, temporary block of nerve conduction without disruption of the mechanical integrity of the nerve. Full recovery is expected unless there is prolonged ischemic insult.

2. **Axonotmesis**—Transection of axons with preservation of the nerve sheaths, as may be seen in severe blunt trauma. Wallerian degeneration of the distal fibers is inevitable, but, given the presence of intact nerve sheaths, spontaneous recovery is possible and may be nearly complete.

3. **Neurotmesis**—Complete transection of the nerve including the Schwann cell sheaths. If there is minimal retraction of apposing ends of the severed nerve, spontaneous recovery without surgery may occur, but, given the elastic properties of nerves, dehiscence of the severed ends is the rule, and surgical reapproximation with or without grafting is often necessary. Full recovery of function is unlikely regardless of the treatment employed.

Sunderland's classification:

Type I—Blockage of conduction without axonal injury (analogous to Seddon's neuropraxia)

Type II—Injury to the axon with preservation of the nerve sheaths and fascicles (commonly seen in entrapment syndromes)

Type III— Injury to the axons and endoneurium with preservation of the perineurium

Type IV—Injury to the axon, endoneurium, and perineurium with preservation of the gross continuity of the nerve (e.g., the epineural tissue is intact)

Type V—Complete severance of the nerve (analogous to Seddon's neurotmesis).

Seddon's classification is simpler and, for this reason, perhaps better suited for use in the initial clinical assessment of patients. However, the additional information conveyed by Sunderland's criteria may be of considerable value when surgical repair of a nerve is contemplated, and for medicolegal reasons, the additional detail it provides may be desirable in documenting operative findings. Regardless of the classification system employed, lesions will often be mixed in nature, and treatment decisions are based on the predominance of the clinical manifestations.

13. Is the prognosis for regeneration better for distal or more proximal lesions?

All things being equal, the prognosis is better for recovery from **distal** traumatic lesions. Proximal versus distal must be qualified in this context: they are better thought of in terms of the distance between the lesion and the end organ(s) (e.g., muscles) innervated by the affected nerve rather than the distance between the lesion and the spinal roots. This is because the greater the distance between the site of injury and the end organ predisposes to at least two untoward events: mass innervation in which a single resprouting axon sends terminals to many motor fibers which it did not originally innervate, and an increased time to reinnervation. The latter is deleterious to full recovery because of the atrophy and structural changes which take place as a function of time without innervation.

14. What common condition can present with symptoms of pseudoclaudication, uni- or bilateral neuropathy, and/or radiculopathy?

Spinal stenosis. The prevalence of this condition is variously estimated to be from < 2% to as much as 6% of the population. The term *pseudoclaudication* is almost synonymous with *cauda equina syndrome*, which is a classic presentation of central canal stenosis in the lower lumbar region. As this condition can take different forms, different clinical manifestations occur.

15. In an otherwise healthy patient presenting with acute onset of bilateral paresthesia followed by ascending weakness in a symmetric fashion, what disorder must be considered in the differential diagnosis?

Guillain-Barré syndrome. This disorder is believed to be autoimmune-mediated, perhaps triggered by an infectious disorder. Most cases resolve spontaneously, but prompt referral to a neurologist is mandatory. Some patients will suffer aspiration, autonomic changes affecting cardiac output, and/or respiratory failure. Treatment with intravenous IgG or plasmapheresis may be beneficial in decreasing the duration and severity of the disease.

16. How do a neurofibroma and a neurinoma differ?

A **neurofibroma** is a **tumor** commonly (but not exclusively) seen in von Recklinghausen's disease. They are commonly multiple, usually but not always encapsulated, and composed of all the elements of the nerve tissue (neurons, Schwann cells, and fibroblasts) arranged loosely in myxoid stroma. Typically, the involved nerve runs through the lesion which makes resection of these tumors without transection of the nerve unlikely. Neurofibromas associated with the large nerves of the neck and extremities have a 3% chance of sarcomatous transformation, whereas malignancy rarely develops in more superficial peripheral tumors.

Neurinomas (schwannomas) are typically solitary encapsulated tumors eccentrically located on the course of the affected nerve such that the tumor may be resected without necessitating transection of the nerve. Histologically, these tumors are composed of proliferating Schwann cells and show alternating areas of high and low cellularity. These tumors rarely undergo malignant transformation.

17. What infectious disorders commonly present with radicular pain and weakness?

Herpes zoster and Lyme disease. Both disorders are commonly seen in association with characteristic skin lesions.

18. What is the earliest objective manifestation of diabetic neuropathy?

Classically, this has been taught to be a decrease in vibratory sensation. However, a recent large multicenter study has indicated that the first manifestation is **decreased or absent tendoachilles reflexes**.

19. A patient presents with multiple neurofibromas and café-au-lait spots. What other tumors is this patient at risk for developing?

The patient has von Recklinghausen's disease and is therefore at increased risk for the development of tumors originating from the neural crest, including neuroblastomas, neuroganglionomas, and pheochromocytomas.

20. Describe the major theories concerning the etiology of diabetic neuropathy.

There are several major theories of the etiology of diabetic neuropathy, each supported by empirical evidence, though none unequivocally.

1. The first theory posits that peripheral nerves are **deprived of oxygen** due to changes in the vasa nervorum, alterations in erythrocyte deformability and oxygen-binding characteristics, and decreased oxygen permeability of the tissue. All of these changes are believed to be due to glycosylation of structural proteins induced by the hyperglycemia of diabetes. While histologic studies have lent support to this theory, it is interesting to note that peripheral nerves have relatively low oxygen requirements and that diabetes heightens their threshold of acute ischemic damage. It should be noted that ischemic lesions of nerves usually result in axonal disruption, not the demyelinating pattern often seen in diabetic neuropathy.

2. Another major theory with empirical support suggests that nerve damage may be due to **inflammatory infiltrates**, especially involving the vasa nervorum, with or without occlusion of the vessels. This theory is supported by the findings of perivascular lymphocytic infiltrates in nerve biopsies and may be particularly relevant to the genesis of proximal neuropathy and mononeuropathy multiplex.

3. The third theory relates to activation of the **polyol pathway** in nerves, which is triggered by the unregulated entrance of glucose into the nerve. As glucose enters the nerve faster than is needed to provide for its energy requirements, it accumulates and is converted to sorbitol by the enzyme aldose reductase. Once formed within the nerve, sorbitol is trapped there. How it ultimately affects the nerve is unknown, but it may decrease myoinositol concentration and Na^+/K^+-ATPase activity. Aldose reductase inhibitors are available for the treatment of diabetic neuropathy in several countries and have been shown to have beneficial effect on the progression of this condition. It is also worth noting that the major sites of end-organ damage in diabetes have activity in the polyol pathway.

4. A fourth putative pathway involves alteration of the metabolism of **essential fatty acids**, particularly the formation of γ-linolenic acid from linoleic acid which is decreased in diabetes. These essential fatty acids are components of membranes with important implication for their structure and function. They are also precursors of eicosanoids and are incorporated into many diacylglycerols. Deficiency or alteration in the balance of one or more essential fatty acids and/or essential fatty acid metabolites may have far-reaching effects on membrane stability and function, the generation of intracellular second messengers, and cholesterol transport—all of which impact on nerve function.

5. Finally, not all neuropathies seen in association with diabetes mellitus are necessarily due to the primary disease. These may be due to vitamin B_{12} deficiency, ethanol abuse (a possible etiology of diabetes mellitus), heavy metal intoxication, and chronic inflammatory demyelinating polyneuropathy (CIPD). The characteristic histologic finding of CIPD (onion bulb formation) is commonly seen in association with symmetric demyelinating polyneuropathy in insulin-dependent diabetes mellitus, and as both are believed to be autoimmune diseases, it is possible that the two could coexist in the same individual.

21. How is diabetic neuropathy treated?

The first step in treating diabetic neuropathy is to attain a euglycemic state if possible. Many patients experience remission of symptoms when glycemic control is established, and maintenance of euglycemia may be effective in preventing the development of autonomic and motor neuropathy in many patients.

The second arm of therapy includes nonnarcotic analgesics, tricyclic antidepressants, the anticonvulsants phenytoin and carbamazepine, the class IB antiarrhythmic mexiletine, topical capsaicin, and phenothiazines. In general, due to the lengthy duration of symptoms and the consequent need for long-term treatment, narcotic analgesics should be avoided because of the danger of addiction and their minimal impact on the patients' discomfort from this cause. All of these agents constitute symptomatic therapy. Pentoxifylline, however, has been used with some success on the premise that it would improve nerve ischemia.

In particularly severe and/or rapidly progressing cases, high-dose steroids (which play havoc with glycemic control) and intravenous IgG have been employed with success. Plasmapheresis has also been shown to terminate symptom progression, but its ability to regress established symptoms remains unclear. These measures may, if effective, treat the autonomic, motor, and sensory components of diabetic neuropathy and be disease-modifying.

Aldose reductase inhibitors are being used in other countries, and clinical evaluation of their effectiveness and safety is ongoing. These may prove helpful in treating the ranges of neuropathic complications seen in diabetes as well as preventing damage to other organ systems. Dietary supplementation with essential fatty acids (linoleic and γ-linolenic acids) may hold equal promise.

22. What is the natural course of painful diabetic neuropathy?

Simple paresthesias may respond to normalization of blood glucose levels within days to weeks. Otherwise, symptoms often gradually subside within 6–12 months. Other patients fail to improve or develop evidence of new nerve lesions. This should not be confused with the manifestations of diminished sensation or autonomic neuropathy, which do not spontaneously improve as a rule.

It has been shown that the prevalence of sensory neuropathy in the non-insulin-dependent diabetic population increases with the duration of illness and that both poor glycemic control and low serum insulin levels are independent risk factors in its genesis. Paradoxically, insulin use has also been identified as a risk for the development of distal symmetrical polyneuropathy. Similarly, male gender and increasing height may also be independent risk factors, although which of the two is actually the true prognostic sign is still uncertain.

23. What are the presenting signs and symptoms of sciatic neuropathy?

The vast majority of patients complain of weakness of the muscle groups innervated by the involved nerve (often the dorsi- and plantarflexors of the ankle). This is closely followed in frequency by complaints of numbness and paresthesias. The distal, burning, lancinating pain commonly associated with sciatic involvement is encountered less frequently. Clinically, nearly all patients have weakness and sensory loss (which may not become apparent until after the onset of weakness), and most will exhibit decreased or asymmetrical tendoachilles reflexes. While nerve conduction velocities are usually within normal limits, compound muscle action potentials are frequently diminished or unobtainable from the abductor hallucis, extensor digitorum brevis, and/or tibialis anterior. More than three-fourths of the patients show decreased or absent sensory nerve action potentials.

24. Which division of the sciatic nerve is most commonly involved in sciatic neuropathy?

Isolated involvement of the peroneal division is > 3 times as frequent as involvement of both the peroneal and sciatic divisions and > 10 times as frequent as isolated involvement of the sciatic division.

25. What is the natural course of sciatic neuropathy?

The natural course of this disorder is spontaneous improvement over up to 3 years. Continued improvement beyond this time is unlikely.

26. A lesion of which nerve would give rise to the following signs and symptoms: tenderness to palpation anterior to the medial aspect of the calcaneus, a positive Tinel sign, and weakness of the abductor digiti minimi quinti, and no abnormalities of cutaneous sensation. On electrophysiologic testing, a decreased compound muscle action potential is noted from the abductor digiti minimi quinti as well as fibrillation potentials. Plain film radiographs reveal a small anterior calcaneal spur.

The inferior calcaneal nerve. Note that the Tinel sign is variably present and that the nerve may theoretically be compressed between the origins of abductor hallucis and quadratus plantae, even in the absence of a demonstrable calcaneal spur.

27. What is myasthenia gravis?

Myasthenia gravis is a disorder characterized by progressive weakening of the involved muscles with continued effort. The extraocular muscles and the limb girdle muscles are frequently involved; thus patients may have difficulty following a moving object with their eyes or experience diplopia. Limb girdle weakness causes difficulty with rising from a chair, combing one's hair, etc. As the disease progresses, weakness of the respiratory musculature can impair ventilation with lethal effect. Patients may also experience difficulty speaking and be at risk for aspiration. Muscle mass and tone, deep tendon reflexes, and the sensory examination will generally be normal.

Myasthenia gravis is an autoimmune disease in which antibodies are formed to the acetylcholine receptors of the neuromuscular junction. However, antibody-negative myasthenia gravis occurs in about 10% of cases, and antibody titers do not correlate with the severity of disease or improvement after treatment with immunosuppressive agents. The precise mechanism of disease remains an enigma.

28. How is myasthenia gravis diagnosed?

Clinically based on observations of the characteristic signs, especially weakness which is improved on first awakening and worsens as the day progresses. The clinical diagnosis can be confirmed by the edrophonium test, in which the patient's strength improves when challenged with this short-acting acetylcholinesterase inhibitor. Electrophysiologic data consistent with myasthenia gravis include motor end-plate potentials of normal frequency but low amplitude and decrease of the compound muscle action potential on repetitive stimulation (Jolly test).

29. How is myasthenia gravis treated?

Symptomatic treatment is usually by anticholinesterase agents. Pyridostigmine is currently the drug of choice. Thymectomy remains an important component of treatment. In crises, corticosteroids, intravenous IgG, and plasmapheresis may be employed. Azathioprine and cyclosporine have also been found efficacious.

30. How may Eaton-Lambert syndrome be distinguished from myasthenia gravis?

In myasthenia gravis, motor end-plate potentials are decreased in amplitude and normal in frequency, but in Eaton-Lambert syndrome, they are normal in amplitude and decreased in frequency.

BIBLIOGRAPHY

1. Elliott KJ: Taxonomy and mechanisms of neuropathic pain. Semin Neurol 14:195–205, 1994.
2. Franklin GM, Shetterly SM, Cohen JA, et al: Risk factors for distal symmetric neuropathy in NIDDM: The San Luis Valley Diabetes Study. Diabetes Care 17:1172–1177, 1994.
3. Goldman SM, Funk J, Christensen V: Spinal stenosis: A common cause of podiatric symptoms. J Am Podiatr Assoc (In press).
4. Horrobin DF, Carmichael HA: Essential fatty acids in relation to diabetes. In Horrobin DF (ed): Treatment of Diabetic Neuropathy. New York, Churchill Livingstone, 1992.
5. James JS, Page JC: Painful diabetic peripheral neuropathy: A stepwise approach to treatment. J Am Podiatr Med Assoc 84:439–447, 1994.

6. Khella SA: Management of critically ill patients with myasthenia gravis, Guillain-Barre syndrome and inflammatory myopathies. In Mandell BF (ed): Acute Rheumatic and Immunological Diseases. New York, Marcel Dekker, 1994.
7. Krendel DA, Costigan DA, Hopkins LC: Successful treatment of neuropathies in patients with diabetes mellitus. Arch Neurol 52:1053–1061, 1993.
8. Mackin GA: Diagnosis of patients with peripheral nerve disease. Clin Podiatr Med Surg 11:545–569, 1994.
9. Mumenthaler M: Neurologic Differential Diagnosis, 2nd ed. New York, Thieme Verlag, 1992.
10. Oh SJ: Clinical Electromyography: Nerve Conduction Studies, 2nd ed. Philadelphia, Churchill Livingstone, 1993.
11. Park TA, Del Toro DR: Isolated inferior calcaneal neuropathy. Muscle Nerve 19:106–108, 1996.
12. Partanen J, Niskanen L, Lehtinen J, et al: Natural history of peripheral neuropathy in patients with non-insulin-dependent diabetes mellitus. N Engl J Med 333:89–93, 1995.
13. Suarez GA, Fealey RD, Camilleri M, Low PA: Idiopathic autonomic neuropathy: Clinical, neurophysiologic, and follow-up studies on 27 patients. Neurology 47:1675–1682, 1994.
14. Yeun EC, Olney RK, So YT: Sciatic neuropathy: Clinical and prognostic features in 73 patients. Neurology 44:1669–1674, 1994.
15. Younger DS, Rosoklija G: A differential diagnostic approach to progressive lower extremity weakness of neurogenic origin. Lower Extremity 1:125–131, 1994.

28. REFLEX SYMPATHETIC DYSTROPHY

Jennifer Fung-Schwartz, D.P.M., and Kelly Matthew-Gil, D.P.M.

1. What is the most common cause of reflex sympathetic dystrophy (RSD)?

Accidental trauma. Injury may be the result of fractures, dislocations or sprains, amputations, crush injuries, or even minor cuts of the toes or feet. Other etiologic factors include surgical procedures, diabetes mellitus, hemiparesis, venipuncture, infections, and neoplasms.

2. Who was the first to provide an accurate description of the signs and symptoms of RSD?

Mitchell in 1864 described conditions resembling RSD in Union soldiers with peripheral nerve injuries.

3. Who is responsible for coining the term *reflex sympathetic dystrophy*?

Evans in 1947.

4. What are the other names used in describing this condition?

Causalgia	Traumatic angiospasm
Sudeck's atrophy	Reflex neurovascular dystrophy
Algodystrophy	Complex regional pain syndrome
Acute bone atrophy	

5. Who coined the term *causalgia*?

Dunglingson coined the term to describe the burning pain syndrome that was originally described by Mitchell in gunshot victims.

6. What is the more current term that is used today?

Sympathetically maintained pain (SMP). Numerous terms have been applied to this syndrome, and most authors recognize these terms as being clinical variants of RSD. They are all thought to have the same underlying pathology in which the sympathetic nervous system continues to be overstimulated.

7. What is the pathogenesis of RSD?

The pathogenesis is unknown. Numerous theories have been postulated, but it is generally agreed that the sympathetic nervous system plays a vital role.

The "vicious cycle" theory proposed by Livingston states that the injury causes afferent painful stimuli to persist in the spinal cord, which in turn increases efferent sympathetic activity. Doupe proposed that abnormal synapses are formed between efferent sympathetic nerves and afferent sensory nerves, which discharge spontaneously. Roberts proposed that sympathetically maintained pain is caused by sensitization of WDR neurons in the spinal cord.

8. Do psychological factors contribute to the pathogenesis of RSD?

There is no evidence that predisposing psychological factors or a personality type contributes to the development of RSD. Currently, most authors agree that the sympathetic nervous system is sensitive to stress and that those people under considerable stress are likely to show sympathetically mediated physiologic reactions. The chronic pain also increases stress, which in turn increases sympathetically mediated physiologic reactions.

9. The diagnosis of RSD can be made when four cardinal clinical signs and symptoms are found. What are these findings?

1. Pain
2. Swelling
3. Stiffness
4. Skin discoloration

10. What techniques can be used to confirm the clinical diagnosis?

The diagnosis is usually a clinical one, but other diagnostic measures can aid in confirming the clinical diagnosis:

Plethysmography and venous blood gas measurement for determination of vasoconstriction.

Thermography or videothermogram to evaluate near-surface blood flow. A positive thermogram will show significant coolness in the affected extremity.

Xenon clearance or laser Doppler to measure peripheral blood flow.

Serologic tests, such as antinuclear antibody and rheumatoid factor (are usually negative).

Radiographic examination reveals patchy osteoporosis, which may progress to a diffuse ground-glass appearance.

Three-phase ^{99}Tc pyrophosphate bone scan, showing diffuse uptake in the blood flow, pool and delayed phase. In the delayed phase, periarticular uptake is noted in the affected part.

Other studies include electromyography and nerve conduction velocity studies, arteriography, and erythrocyte sedimentation rate. The results of these studies are negative.

11. Name the skin changes seen clinically with RSD.

1. Skin atrophy
2. Skin hyperpigmentation
3. Hyperhidrosis
4. Nail changes

12. Name the six criteria proposed by Genant for the diagnosis of RSD.

1. Pain and tenderness in the extremity
2. Soft-tissue swelling
3. Decreased motor function
4. Trophic skin changes
5. Vasomotor instability
6. Patchy osteoporosis

13. What is the differential diagnosis for RSD?

Tarsal tunnel syndrome
Raynaud's phenomenon
Diabetes and associated polyneuropathy
Disuse osteoporosis
Lupus erythematosus

14. If left untreated, RSD passes through three stages. What are they?

Stage 1—acute
Stage 2—dystrophic
Stage 3—atrophic

15. What are the signs and symptoms of Stage I?

Hyperalgesia, hyperesthesia, hyperpathia, localized edema, and pain that is aggravated by movement and emotional stress. The skin is warm, red, and dry toward the end of the stage, then becomes cyanotic, cold, and sweaty. This stage may last up to 6 months.

16. What are the signs and symptoms of Stage II?

Continuous burning, allodynia, hyperalgesia, and hyperpathia. The skin is often cool, pale gray, and cyanotic. Hair growth is decreased, and the nails are brittle. Muscle wasting causing limited joint mobility and radiographs showing spotty osteoporosis are significant.

17. What are the signs and symptoms of Stage III?

Irreversible marked tissue changes. The skin appears smooth, glossy, and pale or cyanotic. Skin temperature is decreased, with continued pain and muscle wasting. Significant diffuse bone atrophy is noted radiographically.

18. Name the two characteristic radiographic findings in RSD.

Although radiographic findings are nonspecific and vary depending on the stage of the syndrome, most authors agree that there are two radiographic findings that are characteristic of RSD.
1. Periarticular soft tissue swelling
2. Patchy osteoporosis

19. When bone demineralization is the predominant finding, RSD is frequently referred to as what?

Sudeck's atrophy

20. What is the proposed mechanism behind the characteristic osteoporosis seen in RSD?

The alteration of hemodynamics associated with abnormal sympathetic activity causes hyperemia, and it is this increase in blood flow to the bone that underlies the characteristic osteopenia.

21. Name four histologic findings on synovial biopsies that are characteristic for RSD.

These findings were described by Kozin for the first time in 1991:
1. Proliferation and disarray of synovial lining cells
2. Increased numbers of small blood vessels
3. Mild perivascular inflammatory infiltrate
4. Synovial edema

22. How is RSD treated?

Therapies are numerous, and results are varied. It is useful to start with physical therapy or exercises to improve mobility: active and passive range of motion exercises, paraffin baths or ice packs, massage, contrast baths (desensitization), biofeedback, and muscle re-education.

Edema is controlled by elevation.

Narcotic analgesics, NSAIDs, topical capsaicin, and transcutaneous electrical nerve stimulation (TENS) may be useful in the control of pain.

The sympathetic nervous system can be interrupted by sympathetic blocks, medication, or surgery. Surgical sympathectomy is reserved for patients who have undergone previous forms of sympathectomy with little or no results.

Calcitonin, intranasally or parenterally, may exert an effect through its anti-bone resorption effect or its analgesic effect.

Oral corticosteroids, usually prednisone (30–80 mg in various tapered doses), are used in patients who refuse or cannot tolerate invasive sympathetic blockade.

Tricyclic antidepressants and anxiolytics are used to treat depression and anxiety, which may result from this disorder.

23. What "treatment" is the most important diagnostic indicator of RSD?

Relief of pain and modifications of signs after a sympathetic blockade. Regional sympathetic blockade of the lower extremity may be achieved with a lumbar sympathetic block utilizing a local anesthetic. When properly performed, usually by an anesthesiologist, the response is prompt and dramatic.

24. How does the affected limb appear clinically after undergoing a sympathetic blockade?

• Vasodilatation resulting in increased temperature to the limb.
• Cyanosis and swelling often decrease over the next several hours.
• Function improves.

25. Some patients are hesitant to undergo the risks associated with an invasive sympathetic block. In this situation, which drug can be administered intravenously that will provide both diagnostic and prognostic information in patients with RSD?

Phentolamine. It is a short-acting alpha-adrenergic-blocking agent. Adverse effects include orthostatic hypotension, tachycardia, nasal stuffiness, nausea, vomiting, and diarrhea.

CONTROVERSY

26. Discuss the role of psychological factors in RSD.

An important aspect to be aware of when treating these patients is the possible psychological component. The question arises whether or not the sympathetic system is sensitive to stress.

Pro: According to Karsetter and Sherman, although RSD occurs among people of both sexes and ages, it appears particularly prevalent among teenage and young adult females who have passive personalities are are dominated by overbearing mothers. In Paks' review of 140 cases, psychiatric problems of emotional disturbance were believed to exist before the onset of the illness in 37% of cases. Julsrud, in 1980, stated that a background of vasomotor instability together with a hyperemotional temperament is a prerequisite of the symptoms of RSD.

Con: Haddox disputes this psychological component and states there is no objective evidence to support any assertion that these physiologic dysfunctions actually cause the disorder. He has found no evidence of an "RSD personality" or of predisposing psychological factors.

BIBLIOGRAPHY

1. Backonja MM: Reflex sympathetic dystrophy/sympathetically maintained pain/causalgia: The syndrome of neuropathic pain with dysautonomia. Semin Neurol 14:263–271, 1994.
2. Carlson T, Jacobs AM: Reflex sympathetic dystrophy syndrome. J Foot Surg 25:149–153, 1986.
3. Headley B: Historical perspective of causalgia: Management of sympathetically maintained pain. Phys Ther 67:1370–1374, 1987.
4. Karsetter KW, Sherman RA: Use of thermography for initial detection of early reflex sympathetic dystrophy. J Am Podiatr Med Assoc 81:198–205, 1991.
5. Kleinman D, Rosen RC, Cohen JM: Combined anesthetic and surgical treatment of reflex sympathetic dystrophy following a healed crush injury of the foot. J Foot Surg 29:55–58, 1990.
6. Kozin F: Reflex sympathetic dystrophy syndrome. Curr Opin Rheumatol 6:210–216, 1994.
7. Levine DZ: Burning pain in an extremity. Postgrad Med 90:175–185, 1991.
8. Mandel S, Rothrock RW: Sympathetic dystrophies. Postgrad Med 87:213–218, 1990.
9. Paice E: Reflex sympathetic dystrophy. BMJ 310:1645–1648, 1995.
10. Roberts WJ: A hypothesis on the basis for causalgia and related pains. Pain 24:297–311, 1986.
11. Rogers JN, Valley MA: Reflex sympathetic dystrophy. Clin Podiatr Med Surg 11:73–83, 1994.
12. Shelton RS, Lewis CW: Reflex sympathetic dystrophy: A review. J Acad Dermatol 22:513–520, 1990.
13. Turf RM, Bacardi BE: Causalgia: Clarification in terminology and a case presentation. J Foot Surg 25:284–295, 1986.
14. Van Wyngarden TM, Bleyaert AL: Reflex sympathetic dystrophy involving the foot. J Foot Surg 31:75–78, 1992.
15. Van Wyngarden TM, Bleyaert AL: Reflex sympathetic dystrophy: Objective clinical signs in diagnosis and treatment. J Am Podiatr Med Assoc 81:580–584, 1991.

29. PADDING, BRACING, AND ORTHODIGITA

Kendrick A. Whitney, D.P.M., and Alan K. Whitney, D.P.M.

1. Why should foot pads be beveled?
- Avoids an abrupt edge irritation
- Reduces pad displacement tendency
- Helps eliminate excessive bulk

2. The size of a pad aperture is determined by what two primary factors?
It should be (1) small enough to provide protection but (2) large enough to avoid encroachment.

3. What are the four general purposes of foot padding?
1. Protection of painful lesions and areas
2. Reduction of foot and toe malalignments
3. Rebalance of the foot and body
4. Substitution for missing, amputated parts

4. What was the cuboid pad designed to accomplish?
Following reduction of a subluxed calcaneocuboid joint (i.e., "cuboid syndrome") to prevent a resubluxation tendency.

5. Why should plantar pad apertures be elongated in a fore and aft direction?
To allow for the fore and aft "tracking mechanism," whereby during the contact phase of gait, the foot slides forward, while during the propulsive period, the foot moves backward over its supporting surface.

6. What is the heel valgus pad used for?
To counteract an existing tendency toward subtalar joint supination with excessive calcaneal inversion (i.e., recurrent lateral ankle sprain tendency) (see figure).

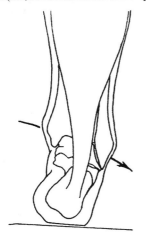 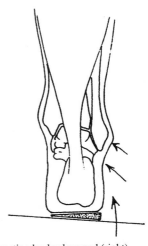

Lateral ankle sprain tendency (left) and counteracting heel valgus pad (right).

7. How do the height and density of a padding element relate?

In general, the density of a pad varies inversely with its needed height. In other words, a firmer or denser pad can be lower in height, whereas a softer, less dense pad must usually be higher or thicker to recruit similar forces.

8. What limits the effectiveness of a medial longitudinal pad cemented in the shoe?

A pad placed against the shoe counter is limited by the resistance offered by the counter. An ordinary medial shoe counter will not offer resistance comparable to that of the shoe with an extended, reinforced medial shoe counter (see figure).

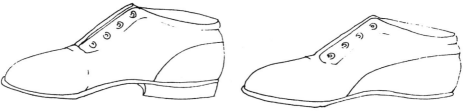

Usual heel counter (left) and extended reinforced medial shoe counter (right).

BRACING

9. What constitutes the primary weight-bearing structure(s) for the patella tendon-bearing brace (PTB)?

The majority of weightbearing is borne by the soft tissue of the leg, compressed by the properly fitted PTB. The patella tendon and medial tibial condyle account for only about 10% of the weight distribution.

10. Why should molded or prefabricated ankle–foot orthoses (AFOs) be fit so that the proximal edge of the orthosis is at least 1 inch below the neck of the fibula?

To prevent the possibility of compressing the common peroneal nerve (see figure).

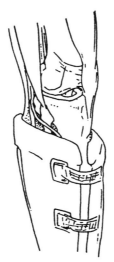

Common peroneal nerve passing below and around the neck of the fibula.

11. What is TRAFO? When should one be prescribed?

It is a tone-reducing ankle–foot orthosis and is well utilized for patients with a persistent hyperactive plantar grasp reflex. The TRAFO helps to maintain the digits in extension.

12. When should an articulated or posterior spring-type AFO be prescribed rather than the solid AFO?

The articulated or spring-type AFO allows for a more normal gait pattern by allowing dorsiflexion during the stance phase of gait, when complete restriction of ankle motion is not required.

13. What are the indications for a supramalleolar orthosis (SMO)?

An SMO may be used for cases of severe subtalar joint pronation with significant medial talar head displacement not controlled by foot orthoses (i.e., UCBL orthosis), yet not requiring a MAFO (molded ankle–foot orthosis). Some examples include a severe equinovalgus deformity, spastic cerebral palsy, tibialis posterior dysfunction, and milder ankle plantarflexion-type deformities associated with good postural control of proximal joints.

14. What are the indications for a PTB (patella-tendon bearing) AFO?

The PTN orthosis should be considered when a maximum reduction in weight-bearing is required, but a cast immobilization of the limb is not desired or recommended. Such indications may include diabetic foot complications, including neuropathic ulceration and Charcot arthropathy. PTB orthoses may also be used for heel pain syndromes, calcaneal fracture, postoperative ankle joint fusion, and avascular necrosis of the foot or ankle.

15. What is the Kirby Skive technique? How is it used to modify positive casts for making foot orthoses and molded AFOs?

The Kirby Skive involves a steep medial heel-wedge produced by angular deletion of the medial aspect of the positive heel cast (see figure). The varus wedge produced in the orthosis or MAFO increases the supination moment across the subtalar joint axis. This allows for significant pronation control for excessive pronation foot malalignments, such as the acquired adult flatfoot associated with posterior tibial dysfunction.

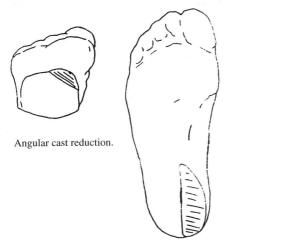

Angular cast reduction.

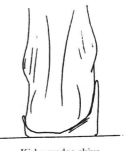

Kirby wedge skive.

16. What is the fundamental difference between the functional concept of the Whitman and Roberts foot orthoses?

The dynamic orthosis, devised by Royal Whitman, utilized the principle of foot resposturing through pain-avoidance. When the young patient allowed excessive foot pronation, the hard foot plate produced acute pain and subsequent withdrawal from the source of irritation. In contrast, Roberts Brace attempted to maintain neutral alignment of the subtalar joint by means of aggressive heel control.

ORTHODIGITA

17. In the typical lesser toe "buckle toe deformity," what is the sagittal plane relationship between the proximal, middle, and distal phalanges?

The middle phalanx is plantarflexed on the proximal phalanx, and the distal phalanx is dorsiflexed on the middle phalanx (see figure).

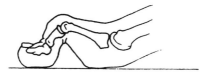

Buckletoe deformity.

18. List the more common etiologies for the digiti quinti adductovarus deformity.
- Tight, short, or pointed shoe toebox
- Foot pronation with forefoot abduction
- Abductory splay of fifth metatarsal
- Congenital origin of deformity

19. How does anterior body imbalance affect the position and tension of the lesser digits?

Anterior body displacement from its normal centralized posture induces a stabilizing increase in lesser digit contraction with a corresponding increase of digital flexor muscle tension.

20. Why should digital "crest pads" be tapered down in size from a medial to lateral direction?

The length of the lesser digits typically decreases lateralward, making the subdigital crest space smaller beneath the fourth toe than under the second toe. Therefore, a crest pad of uniform size is too small for the second toe space and too bulky for the fourth toe space (see figure).

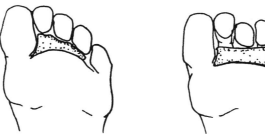

Tapered crest pad (left) and uniform thickness crest (right).

21. Describe the essential difference between mallet toe and hammer toe deformities.

The typical "mallet toe" deformity involves a plantarflexion deformity of the distal interphalangeal joint, whereas the classic "hammer toe" deformity involves a relatively fixed plantarflexion deformity of the proximal interphalangeal articulation (see figure).

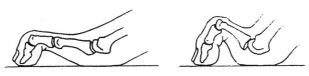

Mallet toe (left) and hammer toe (right).

22. Explain why digital deformities due to abnormal tendon insertion are so difficult to treat and require persistent retention of realignment.

The unbalanced deforming tendon forces tend to remain intact following realignment, making recurrence of the deformity likely.

23. In what situations is digital traction therapy contraindicated?

Acute joint pain

Joint inflammation

Joint infection

Joint neoplasm

Bone fragility

24. How does the relative length of the first metatarsal segment influence the development of the hallux abductovalgus deformity?

A relatively long first metatarsal segment and hallux tend to be abducted by the constraining effect of the footgear, which tends to push the hallux into the second toe space. A relatively short first segment tends to invite abnormal pronation, but hallux deformity is not necessarily invited.

BIBLIOGRAPHY

1. Budin HA: Principles and Practice of Orthodigita. New York, Strathmore Press, 1941.
2. Condie DN, Lamb J: Hip-knee-ankle-foot orthoses. In Biomechanical Basis of Orthotic Management. London, Butterworth-Heinemann Ltd., 1993.
3. Hennessey WJ, Johnson EW: Lower limb orthoses. In Physical Medicine and Rehabilitation. Philadelphia, W.B. Saunders, 1996.
4. Janisse DJ, Wertsch JJ, DelToro DR: Foot orthoses and prescription shoes. In Orthotics: Clinical Practice and Rehabilitation Technology. New York, Churchill Livingstone, 1995.
5. Kirby KA: The medial heel skive technique: Improving pronation control in foot orthoses. J Am Podiatr Assoc 82(4):000, 1992.
6. Trautman P: Lower limb orthoses. In Orthotics: Clinical Practice and Rehabilitation Technology. New York, Churchill Livingstone, 1995.
7. Whitney AK: Biomechanical Footwear Balancing. Philadelphia, Pennsylvania College of Podiatric Medicine, 1979.
8. Whitney AK, Whitney KA: Padding and Taping Therapy. In Principles and Practice of Podiatric Medicine. New York, Churchill Livingstone, 1990.
9. Whitney KA, Whitney AK: Orthodigita Techniques. In Principles and Practice of Podiatric Medicine, New York, Churchill Livingstone, 1990.
10. Whitney KA: Orthodigital evaluation and therapeutic management of digital deformity. In Hallux Valgus and Forefoot Surgery. New York, Churchill Livingstone, 1994.

30. REHABILITATION

Melvin B. Price, D.P.M., P.T., and Lisa Latham, P.T.

1. What is physical therapy?

Treatment by physical means. It is the profession that is concerned with health promotion through prevention of physical disabilities and with rehabilitation of persons disabled by pain, disease, or injury. Physical therapist are involved with evaluating patients and with treating them through the use of physical therapeutic measures as opposed to medication, surgery, or radiation.

2. Give examples of some physical therapy modalities.

Superficial heat (e.g., hot packs, whirlpools, paraffin baths)
Deep heat (e.g., ultrasound, diathermy)
Cryotherapy (e.g., ice or cold packs, contrast baths)
Electrotherapy (e.g., TENS, iontophoresis)
Exercise (e.g., active and passive range of motion, strength training)
Traction (e.g., cervical or lumbar traction)
Orthotics (e.g., braces, splints, canes)

3. What is ultrasound?

Therapeutic application of high-frequency sound waves that penetrate through tissue and cause an increase in tissue temperature to promote healing and reduce pain.

4. What ares some indications for ultrasound?

1. Contractures, joint capsule or adhesive scars
2. Chronic arthritis
3. Periarticular problems
4. Muscular problems
5. Neuromas
6. Sympathetic nervous system disorders
7. Plantar warts
8. Open wounds
9. Chronic systemic peripheral arterial disease

5. Are there contraindications to ultrasound?

1. Cancer
2. Tuberculosis
3. Psoriasis
4. Tissue being treated with radiation
5. Pacemaker (in area of pacemaker)
6. Pregnancy (over fetus)
7. Thrombophlebitis
8. Infected areas
9. Epiphyseal plate
10. Over orbits
11. Over spinal cord

6. What is transcutaneous nerve stimulation (TENS)?

This procedure involves applying controlled, low-voltage electrical pulses to the nervous system by passing electricity through the skin via electrodes. It is specifically designed for the treatment of pain.

7. How does TENS work?

1. It changes the sensitivity of peripheral receptors or free nerve endings responsible for the transduction of nociceptive stimuli.

2. It may block transmission of impulses in afferent nerves conveying nociceptive information (maybe by blocking K^+)

3. It may exert an effect on the autonomic nervous system through peripheral or central mechanisms.

4. "Gate theory." Large-diameter A-β afferents excite interneurons in the dorsal horn of the spinal column, producing inhibition of nociceptive input from smaller-diameter A-delta and C-fibers.

5. "Opiate theory." It may induce production or release of endogenous opiates, endorphins and enkephalins.

8. What is galvanic stimulation?

Galvanic stimulation is DC, or direct current—electrical current that flows in one direction for about 1 second or longer for the purpose of pain control.

9. What are the indications for galvanic stimulation?
• Absorption of medication (iontophoresis)
• Stimulation of denervated muscle

10. Are there contraindications to galvanic stimulation and iontophoresis?

Galvanic Stimulation	Iontophoresis
Pregnancy	All of the above and
Pacemakers	Lack of skin sensation
Cardiac disease	New skin tissue
Cancer	Allergies to medication
Thrombophlebitis	Concomitant use of oral medication that may
Over carotid sinus	negatively interact with ions introduced
Active hemorrhage	

11. What is phonophoresis?

Application of ultrasound through a medicated couplant used to drive medication into body tissues.

12. What is iontophoresis?

A treatment technique in which an electric current (continuous DC) is used to drive ions of various substances through the skin and into underlying tissues.

13. What is joint mobilization?

Specific passive movements to a joint, either oscillatory or sustained, to reduce pain and stiffness affecting movement and to restore normal joint motion. This passive movement is performed by the therapist at a speed slow enough that the patient can stop the movement. It may be applied with an oscillatory motion or sustained stretch intended to decrease pain or increase mobility.

14. When is joint mobilization used?

Following surgery, this technique is used to increase range of motion of a joint. Small movements, known as "joint play," must be present *before* gross movements such as dorsi- and plantarflexion can be attempted or achieved.

15. Once this "joint play" is achieved, what is a good technique to increase range of motion?

A good technique to employ is the contract–relax maneuver. The patient contracts against resistance in the *opposite* direction of the desired gain in range, and then holds this position for 5–10 sec before relaxing. During this relax phase, the therapist then increases the range by stretching in the desired direction. There will be little resistance to the stretch.

16. How does one grade muscle strength?

Grades for a manual muscle test are recorded as numerical scores ranging from 0–5, which denotes no activity to normal activity. The grade represents either a group of muscles performing the same action or individual muscles performing an isolated movement. These grades are based on several factors—the break test, active resistance, and application of resistance—according to the following scores:

0 (0)   No muscle activity
1 (T)   Detection of visible or palpable contractile activity
2 (P)   Completion of full range of motion (ROM) in the gravity-eliminated position
3 (F)   Completion of full ROM in the anti-gravity position
4 (G)   Completion of full ROM in the anti-gravity position with the patient able to tolerate strong resistance (the muscle will "give" or yield with maximal resistance)
5 (N)   Completion of full ROM in the anti-gravity position and no break against maximal resistance

Pluses (+) and minuses (–) may be used with F and P grades. F+ indicates completion of full ROM with the patient able to hold the end position against mild resistance. P– indicates that the patient can complete partial ROM in the gravity-eliminated position.

17. How can you tell if crutches are fitted properly?

1. With the patient standing, 2–3 fingerbreadths should separate the axilla and the axilla pad of the crutches, with crutches positioned 2 inches lateral to the patient and 4–6 inches anterior to the patient.

2. The handpieces should be positioned at greater trochanter, ulnar styloid process, or wrist crease with about 15–25 ° of elbow flexion.

During "fitting," make sure the patient's shoulders are not elevated or depressed, and make sure the patient is wearing shoes.

18. What is a three-point gait?

This requires bilateral ambulation aids or a walker and describes a "step-to" or "step-through" pattern. The walker or crutches and the non-weight-bearing extremity are advanced, and then the patient steps up to the walker or through the crutches. In a modification, the walker or crutches are advanced with the partial weight-bearing extremity, and then the full weight-bearing extremity is advanced.

19. A four-point gait?

This gait pattern describes alternate and reciprocal forward movement of the ambulation aid and the patient's opposite lower extremity—i.e., right crutch, left crutch, right foot.

20. A "swing-to" gait?

The crutches are moved forward simultaneously while the body weight is momentarily on both lower extremities. As weight is shifted onto the hands, both feet are brought forward until the feet are even or just slightly behind the crutches. The feet simultaneously "swing" to the forward position.

21. And a "swing-through" gait?

The crutches are brought forward as weight is momentarily borne on both lower extremities, followed by a shifting of weight to the hands. The legs then swing forward and *through* the crutches, landing on the floor ahead of the crutches.

22. How does an interferential current work?

An interferential current is set up so that two or more sinusoidal waves oscillating with slightly different frequencies are superimposed on an area of tissue. The electrodes must be positioned so that the two circuits cross each other on the skin: "a blending of alternating currents produces a constant or amplitude-modulated beat per second." In other words, the electrodes from the channels are set up in a criss-cross pattern so that the electrical stimulation output from each channel can "interfere" with the other.

23. What are the indications for using an interferential current?

1. Musculoskeletal disorders	5. AC indications
2. Vascular conditions	a. Pain management
3. Urogenital dysfunction	b. Edema reduction
4. Pain conditions	c. Muscle spasm

24. What is massage therapy?

Manipulations of the soft tissues of the body. As described by Gertrude Beard, an early pioneer in physical therapy, in 1952, "These manipulations are most effectively performed with the hands and are administered for the purpose of producing effects on the nervous, muscular, and respiratory systems and the local and general circulation of the blood and lymph." These manipulations are varied by the direction of the movement, amount of pressure applied, part of the hand used, actual motion that is performed, and the specific tissues of the body to which it is applied.

25. When is massage useful?

It is extremely useful in rehab following surgery. Friction massage is especially important in mobilization of the surgical scar and the prevention of adhesions.

26. What is biofeedback?

Objective information about movement, muscle activity, whole body balance, force, joint displacement, skin temperature, heart rate, blood pressure, or other physiologic events is amplified and displayed on an oscilloscope, blood pressure monitor, or other device so that the patient can learn to control these. The goal is to improve motor performance by facilitating motor learning.

27. When is the use of biofeedback appropriate?

• For generalized relaxation: for headaches, chronic pain, muscle spasms
• For improvement of motor control of appropriate activity: for substitution, elimination, or activation of specific muscle and reduction of spasticity, improvement of gait
• Increase awareness of weight-shifting
It is discontinued when the patient can voluntarily perform tasks.

28. Give an example of when biofeedback might be used?

Any time there is a tendon transfer of any type or when there is substitution of stance and swing phase muscles, biofeedback should be part of the rehab regimen.

29. What is a contrast bath?

Placement of one or more extremities alternately in very hot and very cold water. It is a "vascular exercise" that can increase superficial blood flow in the extremities and is believed to hasten healing. The baths begin with heat (105–110° F) and end with cold (59–69° F).

30. When are contrast baths used?

Contrast baths are used to increase superficial blood flow to treat athletic injuries, leg ulcers, strains, and sprains. It is especially useful in reflex sympathetic dystrophy, in breaking the pain and vascular shunting that occurs.

BIBLIOGRAPHY

1. Hecox B, Mehreteab TA, Weisberg J: Physical Agents. Norwalk, CT, Appleton & Lange, 1994.
2. Kisner C, Colby LA: Therapeutic Exercise, 3rd ed. Philadelphia, F.A. Davis, 1996.
3. O'Sullivan SB, Schmitz TJ: Physical Rehabilitation, 3rd ed. Philadelphia, F.A. Davis, 1994.
4. Scully R, Barnes ML: Physical Therapy, Philadelphia, J.B. Lippincott, 1989.

31. WOUND HEALING: PART I

Stephen Albert, D.P.M.

1. Name some nonlocal factors that influence wound healing.
Age, general health, nutritional status, and drug therapy.

2. Which nutrients should the clinician be concerned with in conjunction with wound healing?

Protein	Fats
Amino acids	Vitamins (A, B complex, C, D, E, and K)
Carbohydrates	Trace elements (zinc, iron, copper)

3. What two immune system cells play a major role in wound healing?
Macrophages and T-lymphocytes.

4. Which enhances wound healing, exposing the wound to air or providing a moist wound environment?
Moist wounds speed epithelialization.

5. What wound dressings provide moist wound healing?

1. Saline-soaked gauze
2. Transparent film
3. Occlusive wafer
4. Hydrogels
5. Calcium alginates
6. Nonadherent polyurethane foams
7. Absorptive dressings
8. Silver sulfadiazine creams

6. Describe the three basic phases of wound healing.

Phases	Events
1. Inflammation (substrate, lag)	Influx of platelets and leukocytes Release of cytokines and mediators Coagulation
2. Proliferative, fibroblastic (repair)	Re-epithelialization Angiogenesis Fibroplasia Wound contraction
3. Remodeling (maturation)	Deposition of matrix materials Collagen deposition/remodeling Return to preinjury state

7. What is a polypeptide growth factor?
An agent that promotes cell proliferation. Its action with an external receptor is thought to lead to intracellular changes preparing the cell for DNA synthesis and division. Other peptides in the same category include cytokines, interleukins, and colony-stimulating factors.

8. At what level does bacteria in a wound become associated with infection and delayed wound healing?
$> 10^5$ bacteria/gm of tissue.

9. Name some drugs that have a detrimental effect on wound healing.

Glucocorticosteroids	Retinoids
NSAIDs	Antineoplastic (chemotherapeutic) drugs

10. Name some topical agents that are cytotoxic to wound healing.

Chlorhexidine (Hibiclens)	Hydrogen peroxide
Povidone-iodine (Betadine)	Dakin's solution
Gentamicin sulfate	Acetic acid

11. What is a chronic wound?

A wound that has not healed in a timely fashion. Admittedly, it is an arbitrary and subjective definition. Chronic wounds commonly equate to ulcers (skin or dermal). Underlying causes include venous disease, arterial disease, pressure sores (decubitic), and neuropathic processes (e.g., diabetes mellitus, leprosy).

12. What is a keloid? How does it differ from a hypertrophic scar?

An abnormal wound response in a predisposed individual resulting in a fibrous growth of connective tissue in response to trauma, inflammation, surgery, or burns. Keloids are characterized by abundant deposition of collagen and glycoprotein. Keloids differ from hypertrophic scars by extending beyond the margin of the original wound.

13. Which groups are predisposed to keloid?

The incidence is higher in blacks and dark-skinned individuals. An incidence of 6–16% in the African-American population has been reported. Keloids have not been reported in albinos.

14. What is the most common lower-extremity ulcer?

Venous ulcers. Venous ulcers are characterized by copious drainage, an adherent fibrin base with a highly irregular edge, and location below the knee yet sparing the plantar foot.

15. List the signs and symptoms of venous insufficiency.

Chronic swelling	Pruritus
Aching, heavy tired feeling in lower extremities	Tenderness to palpation
Varicosities	Fibrotic, indurated, hyperpigmented skin

16. How are venous ulcers treated?

1. A compressive dressing to provide ambulatory and hemodynamic support. If this is not feasible, external venous pumps, bedrest, or strict leg elevation is recommended. However, bedrest is not only debilitating but costly.

2. Use of moist wound dressing as opposed to dry gauze or wet-to-dry dressings. Depending on the volume of wound exudate, the dressings are changed once or twice weekly, and the wound is gently cleansed and/or debrided as necessary.

17. What treatment is appropriate after healing of a venous ulcer?

1. Compression stockings usually ankle to knee
2. Antithrombotic therapy, if indicated
3. Glucocorticoid ointment as necessary for venous dermatitis

18. What are the indications for biopsy of lower-extremity ulcer?

• Atypical location and/or atypical signs and symptoms
• Unresponsiveness to traditional therapy

19. What are the critical factors leading to a pressure ulcer?

Prolonged pressure, shearing forces, friction, and moisture.

20. What are the stages of pressure ulcers and corresponding clinical signs as described by Shea?

Stage 1   An acute inflammatory response involving all epidermal layers. Accompanied by an irregular, ill-defined area of soft-tissue edema, induration, and heat.

Stage 2   An ulceration involving the underlying dermis to the subcutaneous tissue. There is an inflammatory and fibroblastic adipose response.

Stage 3   The ulcer extends into the subcutaneous adipose with extensive undermining and comprises a full-thickness defect.

Stage 4   Deeper penetration to deep fascia, muscle, and/or bone.

21. What are the characteristics of an arterial ulcer?

1. Absent to decreased pedal pulses
2. Commonly painful (however, this may be modified in the presence of peripheral neuropathy)—dependency alleviates the pain, elevation exacerbates it.
3. Dry necrotic ulcer with little exudate and irregular borders commonly superficial.
4. Usually located on digits or dorsum of the foot, although may occur elsewhere.
5. Surrounding tissues may exhibit coolness, purpuric or cyanotic color, and there may be shininess and/or tightness with hair loss.

22. What is considered to be the leading cause of diabetic foot lesions?

Peripheral neuropathy, which results in unrecognized trauma leading to ulceration, infection, and/or gangrene.

23. Describe Wagner's classification of diabetic foot ulceration.

Grade 0   Intact epidermis
Grade 1   Superficial ulcer (epidermal)
Grade 2   Ulcer involving the epidermis and dermis
Grade 3   More extensive ulcer involving soft tissue and bone
Grade 4   Local gangrene of toes or forefoot
Grade 5   Gangrene of entire foot

24. What are the visible characteristics of diabetic foot ulcers?

1. Usually located on submetatarsal head or at hallux
2. Round, punched-out ulcer with rim elevated from surrounding hyperkeratosis
3. Minimal drainage unless infected

25. How many bacterial species are usually isolated from diabetics with lower-extremity infection?

Two to five mixed aerobic-anaerobic flora.

26. What toe pressures in diabetics are associated with healing wounds?

> 55 mm Hg   Healing
45–55 mm Hg   Range of uncertainty
< 45 mm Hg   No wound healing

27. What considerations must be factored into reliance on the ankle brachial index in diabetics?

Medial arterial calcification with incompressible vessels will give artificially elevated pressures. Therefore, it has poor positive-predictive values. Toe pressures are not subject to artificial elevations.

28. What is the recurrence rate of diabetic ulcers when patients return to their own shoes? To "special" shoes?

83% and 17%, respectively.

29. When a diabetic foot infection does not respond to treatment, what steps should be taken?
Additional debridement and reculture.

30. How frequently does persistent, untreated ulceration in the diabetic foot lead to lower limb amputation?
84% of such cases result in lower-limb amputation, which is often followed by amputation of the opposite limb in ensuing years.

31. In diabetic feet, what two factors are most responsible for amputation?
Massive infection and gangrene.

32. Name several criteria that might indicate the need for hospitalization of a diabetic patient with a foot infection?

Febrile status	Deep infection
Sepsis	Ascending cellulitis
Leukocytosis	Coexisting peripheral arterial disease and ischemia

33. A diabetic foot ulcer that chronically recurs or remains resistant to treatment suggests what process?
Osteomyelitis. Clinical findings on examination of a diabetic foot ulcer that are suspicious for the presence of underlying osteomyelitis include visible bone at the ulcer base or the ability to probe to bone through the ulcer.

34. What are the radiographic features of chronic osteomyelitis?
1. Cortical erosions, intraosseous lysis, grossly remodeled bone
2. Size, shape, girth, contour, and/or architecture out of proportion to what would be expected normally
3. Loss of bone density, mixed with sclerosis
4. Periosteal reactions

35. Technetium bone scanning is highly sensitive for osteomyelitis. What are the components of a three-phase bone scan?

Angiogram phase	Allows a view of the radioisotope flowing through the vascular tree. It is performed in the first few minutes after radioisotope injection.
Blood pool phase	Views radioisotope accumulation in areas of hyperemia. It is performed usually within 5 minutes of injection.
Bone scan phase	Views radioisotope bound to those portions of bone with osteoblastic activity. It is performed approx. 2–4 hours after isotope injection.

BIBLIOGRAPHY

1. Albert SF, Mulder GD (eds): Wound Healing. Clin Podiatr Med Surg 8(4):788–929, 1991.
2. Boulton AJM: The pathogenesis of diabetic foot problems: An overview. Diabetic Med 13:51, 1996.
3. Edmonds ME, Blundell MP, Morris ME, et al: Improved survival of the diabetic foot: The role of a specialized foot clinic. Q J Med 60:763–771, 1986.
4. Joseph WS (ed): Infections in the Lower Extremity. Clin Podiatr Med Surg 7(3):441, 1990.
5. Nemith A (ed): Dermatol Clin 11(4): 1993.
6. Pecoraro RE, Reiber GE, Burgess EM: Pathways to diabetic limb amputation: Basis for prevention. Diabetes Care 13:513, 1990.
7. Rudolph R, Miller S (eds): Wound Healing. Clin Plastic Surg 7(3) 1990.
8. Yao JST, Pearch WH (ed): The Ischemic Extremity: Advances in Treatment. Norwalk, CT, Appleton & Lange, 1995.

32. WOUND HEALING: PART II

Gerit D. Mulder, D.P.M., M.S.

1. Determining the extent of contamination and distinguishing between contamination and infection in chronic wounds may sometimes be difficult. List seven established signs of infection.

1. Cellulitis
2. Purulent drainage
3. Wet gangrene
4. Persistently malodorous wound
5. Increased leukocytosis
6. Elevated body temperature
7. $> 10^5$ organisms/pgm of tissue

2. What is the difference between pressure reduction and pressure relief?

These terms are frequently used to describe the beneficial effects of devices on areas of tissue pressure. **Pressure relief** is defined as reducing the pressure below 35 mm Hg, while **pressure reduction** is defined as lowering the pressure down to, but not below, 35 mm Hg.

3. What is the National Pressure Ulcer Advisory Panel's definition for a Stage IV pressure ulcer?

A full-thickness skin loss with extensive destruction, tissue necrosis, or damage to muscle, bone, or supporting structures (e.g., tendon, joint capsule, etc.).

4. Why is a swab culture of a chronic wound a poor indicator of the "infecting" organisms? What is the alternative?

A swab culture reflects the organisms or contaminants present on a wound *surface* but is not necessarily an indicator of the organisms causing infection of the tissue. Ideally, one should culture a tissue biopsy. When this is not possible, the wound should be thoroughly flushed with sterile saline and water to remove all surface contaminants and debris, an area of the wound selected for swabbing (avoiding wound margins or intact skin), and a 30-second swab taken of a defined portion of the tissue. This will lead to results that more closely correlate with infecting pathogens.

5. Nutrients are important to wound healing. Below what level is serum albumin considered low? What are the results of protein deficiency?

Low serum albumin is defined as < 3.5 gm/dl. Results of deficiency include decreased or impaired wound healing, edema, impaired cellular immunity, decreased collagen synthesis, and decreased fibroblast proliferation.

6. When the skin layer containing melanocytes is damaged, the new skin may remain depigmented until new melanocytes migrate into the area. What is this layer of the skin called?

The stratum germinativum, or basal cell layer.

7. Why should bedridden patients *not* be positioned with the head of the bed at $> 30°$ angle for an extended period?

This position allows shearing forces to crimp and occlude blood flow to the sacral or ischial areas, thereby increasing the risk of pressure ulcer development in these areas.

8. Name five characteristics of venous ulcers.

Lipodermatosclerosis

Hemosiderin deposits (hyperpigmentation)

Location on medial lower leg (40%)

Pain sometimes relieved by elevation

Often associated with dermatitis

9. Why should Unna's boots be used with caution on patients with lower extremity neuropathy?

It is difficult to predict the amount of pressure applied to the leg with an Unna's boot. Insensate patients may not be able to feel pain from an Unna's boot that has been wrapped too tightly around the lower extremity, thereby resulting in decreased flow to the lower extremity.

10. What is the effect of persistent and extensive tissue maceration? What promotes extensive maceration?

Totally occlusive dressings and products that hold high amounts of exudate over the wound surface promote excessive maceration. Excessive maceration may result in decreased tissue tensile strength. Continued pressure and/or shear will result in greater tissue damage in the presence of decreased tensile strength and maceration.

11. Vascular disease and neuropathy may mask what early signs of infection in the diabetic?

Pain, erythema, and increased skin temperature.

12. Why is topical oxygen limited in its benefit to chronic wounds?

Topically applied oxygen penetrates open wounds to a depth of about 70 μm and cannot significantly elevate oxygen tensions in large wound areas. Topical oxygen cannot address many of the factors underlying tissue hypoxia and ischemia.

13. A 45-year-old woman has a venous ulcer located on the right medial malleolus, approx. 2.0 x 2.0 cm in size, superficial in depth, moderate in exudate, without signs or symptoms of infection, and with fragile periwound tissue. What treatment dressings, devices, and modalities should be used?

Any dressing that is nonadherent and absorbs exudate well may be considered, including foam wafer dressings, nonadherent woven dressings, and alginates. Adhesive dressings should be avoided on the surrounding fragile skin, as they may cause more damage when removed. Compression (e.g., stocking or wraps) needs to be applied over the lower extremity. If the wound requires daily dressing changes, wraps that may be easily removed or stockings can be considered.

14. What is the objective of "saucerizing" when debriding plantar diabetic ulcers?

Saucerization, or creating a "bowl," is intended to debride down to viable tissue while creating angled margins, thereby reducing pressure from "sharp" demarcated wound margins. This type of debridement also helps promote re-epithelialization.

15. The lower extremities of patients with chronic venous disease are frequently sensitive to topically applied agents. Name three common sensitizing agents found in wound care products and topicals.

Parabens, propylene glycols, wool alcohols.

16. What organism is most commonly responsible for necrotizing fasciitis? To which antibiotic is it sensitive?

Group A β-hemolytic streptococci are the infamous "flesh-eating bacteria," yet they are still sensitive to penicillin.

17. The epidemic strain of methicillin-resistant *Staphylococcus aureus* is resistant to the antibiotics gentamicin, erythromycin, and tetracycline, but not to one common antibiotic. Which one?

Vancomycin.

18. Which disease involves a collagen disorder (autoimmune response) and may cause excruciatingly painful ulcers on the lower extremity?

Raynaud's disease.

19. Mercurochrome is still misused on wounds. What are the potential problems, dangers, and disadvantages of using this product?

Mercurochrome is an organic mercuric salt containing fluorescein and alcohol. It is weakly antiseptic and bacteriostatic and has the lowest therapeutic index of most antiseptics. It may dry up wounds and impede healing. It is associated with contact dermatitis and the development of aplastic anemia. The alcohol component may cause pain, vasoconstriction, and tissue damage.

20. Chronic venous ulcers that are recalcitrant to treatment and have an unusual appearance, particularly a "cauliflower" appearance of the tissue in the wound and at the margins, should be biopsied. What pathology is one seeking?

An abnormal and/or cancerous growth, particularly squamous cell carcinoma. Squamous cell carcinoma is the carcinoma most frequently associated with long-standing venous ulcers.

21. A patient presents with a painful, rapidly developing cutaneous ulcer on his lower leg. The lesion has irregular borders with overhanging edges and a purplish discoloration of surrounding skin. What is this rare idiopathic skin disease?

Pyoderma gangrenosum. Lesions may develop anywhere on the body, but they are seen most commonly on the legs. Lesions may be single or multiple.

22. What are the most prevalent pathogens causing wound infection?

Pseudomonas aeruginosa and *Staphylococcus aureus*

23. What pathogen is most frequently associated with wound odor?

Pseudomonas aeruginosa

24. Epithelial skin replacements or partial-thickness skin grafts are frequently used on venous ulcers. Why are epidermal replacements limited in use on venous ulcers?

Epithelial replacements need a dermal layer to be effective. If the dermal layer has been damaged or is absent, as with most full-thickness wounds, an epithelial replacement will usually not take.

25. Numerous cofactors may impair healing in chronic wounds. Which cofactors result in insufficient oxygenation or perfusion of tissue?

Hypoxemia	Anemia
Hypoxia	Hypovolemia

CONTROVERSIES

26. Why is use of topical cytotoxic agents, such as Betadine or hydrogen peroxide, discouraged during wound healing?

The use of cytotoxic agents such as povidone-iodine (Betadine), hydrogen peroxide, and sodium hypochlorite on wounds has been controversial due to their alleged cytotoxic effects on fibroblasts and potential harm to viable tissue. When using these or other potentially cytotoxic agents, the clinician must weigh the advantages versus the disadvantages of the agents. While these agents may be diluted to noncytotoxic levels, there is no need for their use on clean, granulating wounds. The greatest damage comes from keeping high concentrations of the agents in prolonged contact with the wound, e.g., with wet-to-dry povidone–iodine soaks.

27. How compressive should compression dressings be? What types are preferable?

Many arguments exist concerning the type and amount of compression to be applied over lower extremities of patients with venous disease. In the absence of arterial disease or other medical problems that contraindicate compression, a range of 35–50 mm Hg at the ankle, decreasing as one progresses to the knee, is desirable.

Stockings offer predictable and reproducible amounts of compression but may not be practical on patients unable to apply them, when frequent dressing changes are necessary, or where the underlying dressing is bulky. Elastic wraps provide the poorest compression. Unna's boot may be difficult to tolerate. A four-layered compression technique usually offers the highest and most tolerable levels of compression.

BIBLIOGRAPHY

1. Brantigan CO, Senkowsky J: Group a beta hemolytic streptococcal necrotizing fasciitis. Wounds 7:262–268, 1995.
2. Kong F: Old favorites: Remedies from the past. Prim Intention 2:325–327, 1994.
3. Mulder GD, Fairchild PA, Jeter KF (eds): Clinician's Pocket Guide to Chronic Wound Repair, 3rd ed. Long Beach, Wound Healing Publ., 1995.
4. Perry C: Methicillin-resistant *Staphylococcus aureus*. Wound Care 5:1, 31–34, 1996.
5. Stotts NA, Wipke-Tevis D: Co-factors in impaired wound healing. Ostomy/Wound Manage 42:2, 44–54, 1996.

33. TUMORS AND MASSES

Peter Williams, D.P.M.

1. Are osteochondromas symptomatic?

Symptoms are related to the size and location of the tumor. Osteochondroma is the most common benign bone tumor. The lesion itself is asymptomatic and only causes pain or joint disruption if it is large enough or located near a joint. Certainly in the foot, this lesion becomes symptomatic fairly quickly because there are no deep locations or a large amount of muscle or fat. It is primarily located in the metaphysis of long bones.

2. When dealing with a high-grade Stage II sarcoma (fast-growing and malignant), correct systemic workup of the lesion is crucial. What is the appropriate order of workup?

No matter what type of lesion one is dealing with, nothing takes the place of a thorough **history and physical**. It should include a detailed family history, history of the lesion, social history (patient's vocation, activity level, age), and any other systemic diseases affecting the patient. It is then appropriate to **stage** the lesion radiographically, to find the anatomical location, size, borders, and evidence of metastasis. It is then logical to **diagnose**, primarily through findings from the radiographic studies and a biopsy, followed by **treatment**. Rushing through these steps or skipping one only sets up possible misdiagnosis and potential disaster for the patient. If one is concerned with a possible life-threatening tumor, these stages can still be utilized with the treating physician being an advocate for speed (i.e., pushing this patient to the front of the line in radiology, demanding quick medical consults, etc.).

3. What points need to be considered when biopsying a tumor?

a. Choice of needle biopsy or open biopsy
b. Will the biopsy alter the lesion?
c. Avoid contamination of adjacent tissue
d. Site of the biopsy

Biopsy is an important step in the management of bone and soft tissue tumors. An incorrect or inadequate biopsy can alter the specimen enough to make it difficult to determine the extent of the disease. The biopsy should be performed by the surgeon who will ultimately remove the lesion. The type, pathway, and method should all be well thought out, with surgical resection at a later date kept in mind. The biopsy should provide adequate tissue to determine the diagnosis and yet not contaminate any adjacent tissue or anatomical compartments.

4. Open biopsy is most commonly used for lesions that appear benign. True or false?

True. An open biopsy allows the surgeon to visualize the lesion and then decide whether to do an incisional or excisional biopsy. This choice depends on the size, location, and presumed nature (benign or malignant) of the lesion. Needle biopsy is slowly gaining favor in some circles, and its use is at least partially dependent on the experience of the pathologist and the location of the lesion.

5. Is the firmness of a tumor important when working one up?

No. Knowing whether a lesion is firm or soft has little benefit when working up a tumor. However, other aspects of the history and physical do provide valuable information. Whether the lesion is painful as well as the location (e.g., metaphysis or diaphysis, cortical or cancellous) are key aspects of the diagnosis. The age of the patient helps to narrow the possible diagnosis. Family history can contribute information such as the history of other similar lesions, occupational exposure, birth history, or trauma.

Age Distribution of Primary Osseous Tumors of the Foot

	BENIGN	MALIGNANT
Young (0–20 yrs)	Aneurysmal bone cyst Chondroblastoma Desmoplastic fibroma Enchondroma Giant cell tumor Neurolemmoma Osteoblastoma Osteochondroma Osteoid osteoma Osteoma Simple bone cyst	Adamantinoma Ewing's sarcoma Osteosarcoma
Middle group (20–50 yrs)	Aneurysmal bone cyst Chondroblastoma Chondromyxoid fi- broma Desmoplastic fibroma Giant cell tumor Hemangioma Lipoma Neurolemmoma Nonossifying fibroma Osteoblastoma Osteochondroma Osteoid osteoma Osteoma Simple bone cyst	Adamantinoma Chondrosarcoma Ewing's sarcoma Fibrosarcoma
Older group (50+ yrs)	Lipoma	Chondrosarcoma Fibrosarcoma Fibrous histiocytoma

6. Outline the stages for benign and malignant tumors.

Staging has prognostic implications and provides a rationale for treatment decisions.

Staging of Benign Tumors

STAGE	BEHAVIORAL CHARACTERISTICS
1	Static, healing spontaneously
2	Progressive growth
3	Locally aggressive, not limited by natural barriers

Staging of Malignant Tumors

STAGE	GRADE	SITE	METASTASIS
IA	Low	Intracompartmental	None
IB	Low	Extracompartmental	None
IIA	High	Intracompartmental	None
IIB	High	Extracompartmental	None
III	Any	Intra- or extracompartmental	Present

7. **When staging a lesion radiographically, which modality should be used as the *initial* radiographic diagnostic tool?**

Nothing should replace the **plain radiograph**. It reveals the location, extent of involvement, and sometimes diagnosis. It can also direct the clinician with regard to what diagnostic radiographic modality is needed next.

8. **How are MRI, CT and bone scan important for staging a lesion?**

They define the anatomy of the lesion. One must understand the extent of the boundaries of the lesion. This will help with biopsy planning, with making the diagnosis (though imaging usually will not make the diagnosis), and with finding possible metastasis.

9. **Why is the incision placement for a biopsy important?**

The biopsy placement needs to take into consideration that surgical resection of the entire lesion (or anatomical part) might follow, that one must not cause spreading of the tumor into an adjacent compartment or vasculature, and that an accurate biopsy will obviously expedite the correct treatment and an inadequate or incorrect biopsy could cause serious delay or misdiagnosis or no diagnosis.

10. **Once the diagnosis is known, how is the margin of resection defined for common bone tumors?**

Malignant meloma—wide or radical resection

Aneurysmal bone cyst—marginal resection with adjuvant or wide resection

Osteoid osteoma—marginal resection

Ewing's sarcoma—wide or radical resection

Lipoma—observation or marginal resection

11. **Which of the common bone tumors is considered benign *and* aggressive?**

Aneurysmal bone cyst is known for its great rate of growth, tremendous destruction of bone, and the clinical signs of pain and swelling. It can be located on any bone and on any site or location on the bone.

12. **Which bone tumor can reveal the following characteristics: often seen in the epiphyseal region of long bones, the foot can be the primary site, patient age is usually 20–40, and common symptoms are pain from weakened bone, local swelling, tenderness, and limited motion?**

Giant cell tumor

13. **Giant cell tumors are sometimes difficult to manage because of their juxta-articular location and aggressive nature. What aspects must the treating surgeon consider in deciding on the appropriate level of resection?**

1. Wide resection or marginal resection with adjuvant therapy
2. How to salvage the adjacent joint
3. The high recurrence rate
4. Supporting a weakened joint after surgical resection of the lesion

One must consider three other factors: (1) whether the bone involved is expendable; (2) whether complete destruction of involved bone has occurred; and (3) what is the host–tumor interaction (i.e., if the body has contained the tumor or not).

14. **What characteristics of the tumor are helpful in diagnosing a possible osteoid osteoma?**

- Clinical history that includes nighttime pain, localized pain, and relief with salicylates (although pain may be fairly constant and sometimes does not respond to aspirin or nonsteroidals).
- Positive three-phase bone scan. These lesions are quite vascular and respond to the three-phase bone scan very well.

- Center of the lesion is round and radiolucent and surrounded by varying amounts of reactive bone. Tomography or CT is needed to ascertain the geographic boundaries.
- History of intralesional curettage and now recurrence. It is difficult to remove the entire lesion with intralesional curettage, and it displays a high rate of recurrence with this method.

15. How does one differentiate between an osteoid osteoma and an osteoblastoma?

An **osteoid osteoma** has constant pain that is fairly localized and increases at night. It is sometimes alleviated by salicylates. They are localized in the bone and are usually 2 cm or smaller. **Osteoblastoma** is expansile and can cause cortical destruction. It causes less reactive bone formation and does not have the night pain and salicylate response that osteoid osteoma does. It also responds to intralesional curettage and bone grafting. En bloc marginal excision without biopsy is the treatment of choice for osteoid osteoma. It also displays the characteristic nidus on x-ray (which may or may not be obvious on plain film).

BIBLIOGRAPHY

1. Caporusso JM: Soft Tissue and Bone Tumors. Clin Podiatr Med Surg 10(4):1993 [entire volume].
2. Gould JS: Operative Foot Surgery. Philadelphia, W.B. Saunders, 1994.
3. Jahss MH (ed): Disorders of the Foot and Ankle, 2nd ed. Philadelphia, W.B. Saunders, 1991.

34. SOFT TISSUE TUMORS

M. Yvonne Tobar, D.P.M.

1. Name the most useful factors in discriminating a benign lesion from a malignant one.

The **age** of the patient and the **location** of the lesion. Sarcomas are very rare in the middle decades of life, between 20 and 60 years of age. Lesions in the heel were more often malignant than lesions in other areas of the foot and ankle in a study by Kirby.

2. What is the preferred treatment for ganglionic cysts?

Although a large number of ganglions resolve spontaneously, with an equal number being asymptomatic and requiring no therapy, conservative treatment results in recurrence in 50–75% of cases. It most commonly consists of aspiration of fluid (usually the same as synovial fluid that has been dialyzed) and injection of steroid.

Surgical excision is the most effective mode of therapy, but if done after aspiration, it should be delayed 4–6 weeks after recurrence to give the capsule time to regain strength and to decrease the chance of rupture on excision. Ruptured contents may elicit a foreign body reaction and make it more difficult to trace the stalk to its origin. Complete excision requires removal of the main cyst, stalk, subadjacent capsule of tendon sheath, and any underlying bony exostosis, which is commonly present. Compressive dressings with elastic wrap are advised for 2–3 weeks postoperatively.

3. Give the differential for periungual soft tissue masses.

Periungual fibroma	Dermatofibroma
Pyogenic granuloma	Ingrown toenail
Keloid	

4. What seven clinical characteristics are used to describe a soft tissue mass?

1. Location
2. Size
3. Shape
4. Color (e.g. flesh-colored, hyperpigmented, etc.)
5. Consistency (e.g., firm, soft, etc.)
6. Freely movable or fixed
7. Pulsatile (most commonly in hemangiomas)

5. A patient presents with a slowly growing, firm, round, elevated subcutaneous lesion and has a history of trauma or previous surgery. What lesion should be at the top of your differential?

An epidermal inclusion cyst. Among the most common lesions found on the foot, epidermal inclusion cysts represented 87.1% of epidermal tumors of 307,601 tumors and other lesions of the foot in Berlin's study. In the Kirby study, this cyst represented 9.7% of all tumors and was the most common lesion in zone 5 (toes), following only ganglion cysts and plantar fibromas in frequency. Treatment is incision and drainage, followed by excision of the capsule in its entirety.

6. What foot tumor is commonly seen in a patient with tuberous sclerosis?

Periungual fibroma (Koenen's tumor). This is a form of fibrous tumor seen in and around the nail bed and fold and is usually multiple in nature. Kothe described these tumors as being related to a case of tuberous sclerosis, and since then, they have been described as the most consistent lesion associated with tuberous sclerosis on the foot.

The lesions are digital, firm, flesh-colored tumors with a hyperkeratotic distal edge. They are asymptomatic unless they are large enough to cause shoe pressure, protruding from under the nail folds or subungually. Early lesions may appear as a ridge in the nail or as a "budding seed" accompanied by a ridging distal to the bud, disrupting the nail bed if large enough.

Treatment requires surgical excision, with common nail or nail matrix removal because of nail bed involvement. These have a high recurrence rate even after radical excision is performed.

7. What systemic conditions have been linked to plantar fibromatosis?

Alcoholism	Peyronie's disease
Epilepsy (long-term anti- convulsive therapy)	Coronary occlusion Syringomyelia

8. Discuss the controversy around surgical margins in plantar fibromatosis excision.

Some authors propose simple excision of isolated lesions. However, recent studies have found apparently normal fascia surrounding the lesions to be histologically abnormal, so the current therapeutic approaches usually taken are wide excision of smaller lesions to a total plantar fasciectomy for larger lesions. Some report a recurrence rate with lesional excision of 50–75%.

9. Why is the third interspace the most common site of neuroma formation?

Anatomy is the most likely cause. The lesion is a benign enlargement of the third common digital branch of the medial plantar nerve located between and often distal to the third and fourth metatarsal heads. It is frequently supplied by a communicating branch from the lateral plantar nerve as well.

10. What role do radiographs play in evaluating a Morton's neuroma?

Although the neuroma itself is not visible on x-rays, other pathologic conditions may be ruled out, and juxtaposition of the metatarsal heads, which may contribute to the neuroma etiology, will be seen.

11. How does a lipoma appear on MRI?

A well-circumscribed mass with the signal intensity of fat.

12. Which germ layers give rise to neoplasms?

Ectoderm originates tumors involving the skin and nerves, **endoderm** gives rise to glandular tumors, and **mesoderm** provides connective tissue, vascular, muscular, and bony masses.

13. Describe the clinical and histologic appearance of an eccrine poroma.

A slowly growing, solitary, painless, nonpigmented, superficial, pedunculated but partially flattened, smooth, soft lesion. Histologically, intertwined bundles of small cells having dark-staining nuclei from the epidermis to the cornium, involving the sweat gland. Often these are draining and granulating, clinically resembling pyogenic granuloma. Treatment is wide excision, with the pearly base also removed, extending subcutaneously 1/16-inch into normal tissue.

14. Which pseudotumor presents as a cobblestone appearance on the medial and lateral sides of the heels on weight-bearing, but disappears on digital pressure and non–weight-bearing?

Piezogenic pedal papules. *Piezo* comes from the Greek word meaning "pressure." Shelly and Rawnsley in 1968 described these very common incidental findings, seldom diagnosed because they are asymptomatic. These are dermatoceles, or herniations of fatty subcutaneous tissue into fibrotic connective tissue defects in the dermis. Because fat is normally well-vascularized and innervated, this could cause complaints of pain while standing, which is often the presenting symptom.

Piezogenic papules are more noticeable in obese individuals and are frequently seen in persons who complain of heel pain. Treatment with supportive heel cups or shoe cushioning usually relieves the herniations and pain, with instruction to avoid excessive periods of standing.

15. What is the origin of a ganglionic cyst?

It seems clear that their site of origin is the synovial tissue of diarthrodic joints and tendon sheaths, but their etiology is speculative, even though trauma seems to be the main precipitating factor. Jayson and Dixon, by elegant studies using arthrography and radiopaque dyes, state that through a valvular mechanism, synovial fluid is able to exit the joint or tendon sheath into the mass and not return. They found a definite common stalk with the joint. Clinically, the fact that the cyst increases in size on joint motion and will resorb if the joint is immobilized for a long enough period supports this theory.

16. Describe the etiology of a giant cell tumor of the tendon sheath.

Giant cell tumor, or pigmented villonodular synovitis, is theorized to be a benign inflammatory reaction to some unidentified agent, and, therefore, most feel this is not a true neoplasm.

17. How does a giant cell tumor present?

Giant cell tumor is insidious in onset and monoarticular, often marked by swelling and acute pain denoting pinching of the villi or nodules, accompanied by locking and interruption of joint motion. Exam reveals enlargement of the area with palpable, soft-to-firm, rubbery masses, irregular in shape, circumscribed, and movable. Joint fluid aspirate showing serosanguinous or yellow-brown fluid is the most consistently valuable diagnostic finding. Complete surgical synovectomy for the diffuse form, with local excision for the circumscribed form, is the treatment of choice. The high recurrence rate (20–50%) may be explained by attempts to shell out the lesion and leaving residual parts, rather than doing a wide excision.

18. What is the most common malignant lesion of the foot?

Synovial sarcoma. It was reported as 9% of all sarcomas, with 25% occurrence in the foot. It represents 56% of all sarcomas in the foot, the highest occurrence. The tumor arises from joint tissues, tendon sheaths, and bursae, and is mesenchymal in origin.

19. How does synovial sarcoma present? How is it treated?

Because synovial sarcomas are rare and slow growing, with an insidious onset, early diagnosis is difficult. It most commonly presents as a complaint of a mass, with tenderness and disability less frequent. Histologic examination is the only reliable means of diagnosis, with incisional biopsy causing the least surgical trauma. The lesions vary in gross appearance from solitary, well-defined nodules to irregular masses, without pathognomonic features, pale, creamy pink, fleshy masses with red and yellow mottled areas from hemorrhage and degeneration.

Enucleation of the lesion in error is often due to its characteristic growth, pushing the connective tissue around it into a pseudocapsule. Enucleation results in almost 100% recurrence. The treatment of choice, as with all soft-tissue masses, is incisional biopsy, not aspiration, followed by radical excision or amputation after histologic diagnosis. Metastasis to the pleura is the most frequent site of dispersion. Frequent spreading to lymph nodes may necessitate a regional dissection or amputation, even without the presence of palpable glands.

20. What is a benign nerve neoplasm of neuroectodermal origin, comprised of both Schwann cells and collagen fibers?

Neurilemmomas, also referred to as benign schwannomas. These are solitary, slow-growing, encapsulated tumors that develop below the perineurium, with trauma as a predisposing factor in lesion activation. They are extremely rare.

Presentation may consist of pain, numbness, paresthesias, hyperesthesias, or weakness of the affected part, with a positive Tinel's sign along the nerve course being common. Unlike a solitary neurofibroma, any nerve fibers involved with the lesion are compressed to one side of the rubbery, homogeneous mass, and if carefully dissected, the nerve of origin may be recognized. Careful longitudinal incision of the encapsulating perineurium may enable the surgeon to shell out the mass, resuturing the perineurium using the nerve sheath as a guide to prevent sensory-motor transposition. Healing of compressed nerve tissue may take up to 18 months after excision.

21. What are the two types of Kaposi's sarcoma and how do they present?

Kaposi's sarcoma has become a frequently encountered malignancy of the foot in recent times with the discovery of AIDS.

"Old world" Kaposi's affects people of Mediterranean and Jewish descent, with tribes of the Congo and Rwanda in Africa having the greatest number of cases reported. It was described by Kaposi in 1872 as primarily cutaneous, with lower extremity lesions being the most common. Visceral involvement of large vessels, pancreas, adrenals, testes, brain, and kidney has been reported in late-stage "old world" Kaposi's sarcoma.

North American Kaposi's sarcoma, seen among immunosuppressed individuals, usually presents as a painful, dark blue to violaceous macule, plaque, or nodule, with edema of the lower extremity indicating lymph node involvement. Individual lesions may coalesce to form plaques or tumors, eroding deeper and ulcerating normal tissue. Kaposi's sarcoma occurs 35 times more frequently in homosexual men than in heterosexual men of the same population.

BIBLIOGRAPHY

1. Berlin SJ: Statistical analysis of 307,601 tumors and other lesions of the foot. J Am Podiatr Med Assoc 85(11):1995.
2. Berlin SJ, et al: Kaposi's sarcoma of the foot. J Am Podiatr Med Assoc 79(7):1989.
3. Buggiani FP: Giant cell tumor of the tendon sheath. J Am Podiatr Assoc 71:166, 1981.
4. Burns AE: Plantar fibromatosis. J Am Podiatr Assoc 73:141, 1983.
5. David DR: Kaposi's sarcoma of the foot. J Am Podiatr Assoc 73:214, 1983.
6. Delgadillo, Arenson: Plantar fibromatosis: Surgical considerations with case histories. J Foot Surg 24(4):258, 1985.
7. Dockery GL: Painful piezogenic papules. J Am Podiatr Assoc 68:703, 1978.
8. Estersohn HS: Pyogenic granuloma. J Am Podiatr Assoc 73:297, 1983.
9. Feinstein M: Foot pathology associated with tuberous sclerosis and neurofibromatosis. J Am Podiatr Assoc 62:336, 1972.
10. Kerman BL: Lipoma of the foot. J Foot Surg 24:345, 1985.
11. Kirby EJ, Shereff MJ, Lewis MM: Soft-tissue tumors and tumor-like lesions of the foot. J Bone Joint Surg 71A(4):1989.
12. Miller T: Nodular fasciitis. J Am Podiatr Assoc 66:465, 1976.
13. Reale CD: Synovial sarcoma in the foot. J Foot Surg 24:162, 1985.
14. Salzman B: Periungual fibroma. J Am Podiatr Assoc 68:696, 1978.
15. Slavitt JA: Ganglions of the foot. J Am Podiatr Assoc 70:459, 1980.

35. MEDICAL EMERGENCIES

Maureen L. Caldwell, R.N., D.P.M.

COMPARTMENT SYNDROME

1. How many fascial compartments are found in the lower leg? What are they?

There are five fascial compartments in the lower leg: anterior, lateral, superficial posterior, deep posterior, and posterior tibial. The tibialis posterior muscle has its own compartment (see figure).

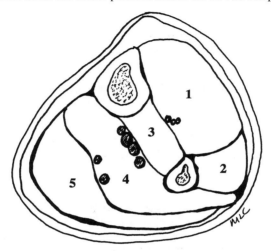

Fascial compartments of the lower leg. *1,* anterior; *2,* lateral; *3,* posterior tibial; *4,* deep posterior; *5,* superficial posterior.

2. List the classic signs of increased compartment pressure.

The classic signs of compartment syndrome are often referred to as the **5 Ps.**
- Pain out of proportion to the clinical situation
- Paresthesias in the nerves in the compartment
- Pain on passive stretch of muscles in the compartment
- Pallor
- Pulselessness

Some authors contradict the last two signs, stating that pallor and lack of pulse may not be evident even in severe cases. Other signs included are weakness of the muscle group and tenseness of the compartment.

3. What is an abnormal compartment pressure?

Normal pressure ranges between 0–8 mm Hg at rest but may increase to much higher levels temporarily during exercise with no sequelae. There is controversy about at which level of pressure damage occurs. It has been reported that capillary circulation stops at pressures ranging from 30 to as high as 55 mm Hg. However, pressure alone may not be the only factor. The length of time the pressure is sustained may also come into play. A compartment pressure of > 30 mm Hg should be considered abnormal but may not require surgical treatment. A pressure > 45 mm Hg usually requires surgical decompression.

4. What is the surgical treatment for compartment syndrome?
Fasciotomy or, as it may also be called, surgical decompression.

MALIGNANT HYPERTHERMIA

5. Define malignant hyperthermia.
This is a rare reaction experienced before, during, or after the administration of general anesthesia. The reaction involves a skeletal muscle abnormality in which the patient experiences severe muscle rigidity followed by hypercapnia, severely elevated body temperatures, hyperkalemia, heart arrhythmia, and end-organ failure. The reaction can be fatal within minutes if not recognized and treated promptly.

6. How frequently is malignant hyperthermia seen in the general population?
The incidence has been reported as high as 1:10,000 to as low as 1:200,000. It is an inherited trait.

7. Malignant hyperthermia is associated with certain triggering events. What are they?
• Inhaled agents such as halothane, isoflurane, enflurane, and desflurane
• Muscle relaxant succinylcholine
• Amide local anesthetics

8. Is there a safe inhaled anesthetic for patients with a susceptibility to malignant hypertension?
Nitrous oxide

9. What medication is used to treat malignant hypertension? At what dosage?
Dantrolene (Dantrium IV) is a fast-acting muscle relaxant that works by a different mechanism than other muscle relaxants. Its mechanism of action in malignant hypertension is unknown. The dosage of dantrolene begins at 2.5 mg/kg and is titrated to a maximum cumulative dose of 10 mg/kg or until symptoms resolve. For the average 70-kg person, up to 36 vials of dantrolene may be necessary. Since the introduction of dantrolene, the mortality rate from this condition has been reduced from 80% to < 10%.

PULMONARY EMBOLISM

10. Give the most common etiology of pulmonary embolism in the podiatric patient.
Deep vein thrombosis of the lower extremity.

11. Describe the common signs and symptoms of pulmonary embolism.
Hemoptysis
Chest pain
Shortness of breath
Decreased PO_2

12. What is the gold-standard diagnostic test for pulmonary embolism?

spinal CT
Pulmonary angiography is the definitive test for proving the presence of pulmonary embolism. Emboli as small as 0.5 mm may be demonstrated by this method. The biggest disadvantage of angiography is the invasive nature of the test.

13. How does pulmonary embolism affect the ventilation-perfusion scan (V/Q scan)?
In a pulmonary embolism, there is a mismatch between ventilation (V) and perfusion (Q). The oxygen is reaching the lung tissue, but due to the embolism, no blood is getting into the lung

tissue to pick up the oxygen. There is underperfusion in the embolic tissue and overperfusion in the normal lung tissue.

14. What is the first-line treatment for pulmonary embolism?

Heparin sulfate IV beginning with 5,000–10,000 U as a bolus followed by 1000–1500 U/hr (25 U/kg). Fibrinolytic therapy has not been proven to be effective to reduce the 2-week mortality rate, although it does more quickly normalize hemodynamic variables. Surgery is rarely indicated in pulmonary embolism.

ANAPHYLAXIS

15. What type of allergic reaction is anaphylaxis?

Type I antibody-mediated immediate hypersensitivity reaction.

16. Who first described anaphylaxis? What was their experiment?

Anaphylaxis comes from the Greek *ana*, meaning "away from," and *phylaxis*, meaning "protection." It was first described by Portier and Richet, who studied dogs and the effects of toxin extracted from the Mediterranean Sea anemone.

17. Is there a difference between anaphylaxis and an anaphylactoid reaction?

Anaphylactoid reaction is virtually indistinguishable from anaphylaxis and usually occurs in patients with a history of asthma. However, anaphylactoid reactions are not immunologically mediated.

18. What is the most common initiator of anaphylactic reaction?

Penicillin. The incidence of penicillin reaction is 15–40 out of every 100,000 persons treated.

19. Describe the pathophysiology of anaphylactic reactions.

Anaphylactic reactions are mediated by IgE antibodies, which bind to receptors on mast cells, causing these cells to release pharmacologically active substances, or mediators. There are three phases to the anaphylactic reaction:

1. **Sensitization Phase:** The antigen is first introduced to the patient, and IgE antibodies are formed and bind to the mast cells. No reaction takes place at this time.

2. **Activation Phase:** Subsequent re-exposure to the antigen triggers the mast cells to respond by releasing their contents.

3. **Effector Phase:** During this time, a complex response occurs as a result of the mediators released. The anaphylactic reaction occurs.

20. How do you recognize anaphylaxis?

Early Signs	Life-Threatening Signs
Lump in throat or hoarseness	Laryngeal edema
Generalized flush proceeding to urticaria	Hypotension
Angioedema	Hypoxia
Stridor	Cardiac arrhythmia
Mucus plugging	Convulsions
Wheezing	Circulatory collapse with cardiac arrest
Nausea and vomiting	

21. What is the initial treatment for an anaphylactic reaction?

Epinephrine, 0.3–0.5 ml subcutaneously of 1:1,000 solution or 3–5 ml of 1:10,000 solution, in severe life-threatening hypotension. Antihistamines may be helpful with early symptoms, but once systemic symptoms are present, antihistamines alone are not enough. As with any emergency situation, the establishment of airway, breathing, and circulation is vital.

CARDIAC EMERGENCIES

22. A patient in the clinic complains of severe substernal pressure pain. Give a differential diagnosis for chest pain.

Myocardial infarction	Pulmonary embolism
Angina	Cardiac arrhythmia
Aortic aneurysm	Pericarditis
Gastroesophageal reflux	Costochondritis

23. Which cardiac arrhythmia is the most lethal?
Ventricular fibrillation

24. What is the initial treatment for ventricular fibrillation?
Defibrillation is the most effective treatment for ventricular fibrillation. Begin with a non-synchronized precordial countershock beginning at 200 J, followed by 300 J and 400 J if not successful.

BURNS AND TRAUMA

25. What is the "rule of nines"?
The rule of nines is a system used to evaluate the percentage of body surface area involved with a burn injury. The body surface is divided into 11 areas, each equal to multiples of nine. For example, the anterior torso equals 18%, each arm is 9%, the genitalia equals 1% (see figure).

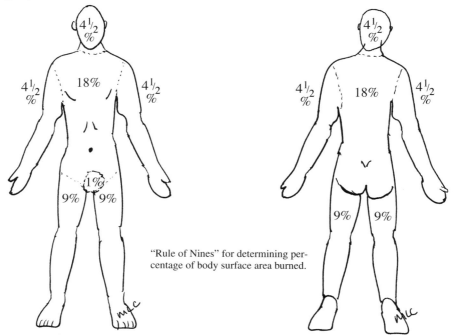

"Rule of Nines" for determining percentage of body surface area burned.

26. In replacing fluids lost from a burn, how is the fluid requirement calculated?
The total fluid can be determined by following the Parkland formula:
$$\% \text{ body area burned} \times \text{kg body weight} \times 4 \text{ ml}$$

Of this total, one-half is given in the first 8 hours, with one-fourth given in the next two 8-hour periods.

27. A patient has fallen from a 20-foot height and sustained a calcaneal fracture. What tests should you order on this patient?
1. Spine films to rule out vertebral compression fractures.
2. Urinalysis to rule out bladder tear.

28. A patient has sustained a gunshot wound to the left lower leg penetrating through the calf and into the tibia. What arteries could be compromised?
Posterior tibial, peroneal, and anterior tibial.

29. What are the clinical signs of arterial injury involving the lower extremity?
Diminished or absent pulses
Bruit over the injury
Brisk pulsatile bleeding from the wound
Tense, expanding or pulsatile hematoma
Pallor distal to the injury

DEMENTIA AND COMA

30. Give a differential diagnosis for the confused patient.
The mnemonic DEMENTIA can be used for the most common causes of confusion:
D = diabetes
E = elderly
M = medications
E = environmental (CO poisoning)
N = nutritional
T = trauma
I = infection
A = alcohol

31. What is the breath-to-compression ratio in one-person CPR versus two-person CPR?
One-person CPR = 1:15
Two-person CPR = 1:5

32. In an unresponsive patient, what two medications can be given safely to help determine the etiology?
1. Naloxone (Narcan)—to rule out narcotic sedation
2. Dextrose 50—to rule out a hypoglycemic reaction

33. How is naloxone (Narcan) administered?
Narcan can be given IV, IM, or SQ. IV administration is the most rapid, with an onset of 1–2 minutes. The dosage is 0.4 mg, which may be repeated every 2–3 minutes up to a maximum of 10 mg.

DIABETIC KETOACIDOSIS

34. Describe the pathophysiological events leading to diabetic ketoacidosis (DKA).
DKA is a starvation state initiated by lack of insulin. The flow chart on the next page gives the pathways of DKA.

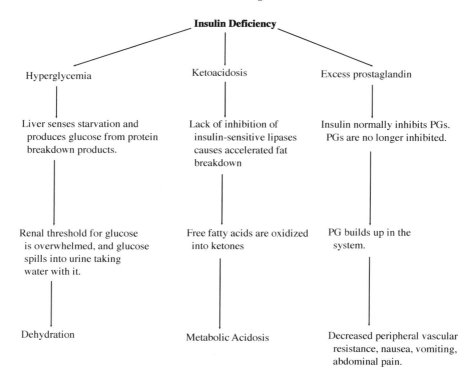

35. Which type of diabetics are more likely to develop DKA?

It is most common in type I, insulin-dependent diabetics and, in 20% of cases, occurs in newly diagnosed patients.

36. What are the early symptoms of DKA?

Polyuria	Altered mental status
Fatigue	Flushed appearance
Nausea and vomiting	Tachycardia
Abdominal pain	Fruity odor to the breath (Acetone smell)

37. What are the most common precipitating causes of DKA?

In 75% of cases of DKA, a precipitating underlying cause can be identified:
- Infection: May be only a minor infection. All sources of infection should be investigated.
- Noncompliance with insulin regimen: Failure of the patient to take scheduled insulin doses.
- Use of insulin pump: Patients do not have depot of long-acting insulin.
- Myocardial infarction
- Cerebral vascular accident

38. What are the goals of therapy for DKA?

- Replace fluids to correct dehydration
- Reduce glucose levels by administering IV insulin
- Correct acidosis
- Replace lost electrolytes, especially potassium
- Identify underlying cause

BIBLIOGRAPHY

1. Benjamini E, Leskowitz S: Immunology: A Short Course, 2nd ed. New York, Wiley-Liss, 1991, pp 241–259.
2. Fish L: Diabetic ketoacidosis. Postgrad Med 96(3):75–78, 1994.
3. Gerow G, et al: Compartment syndrome and shin splints. J Manip Physiol Ther 6(4):245–252, 1993.
4. Hayden J: Compartment syndromes. Postgrad Med 74(1):191–193, 1983.
5. Hill J: Anaphylaxis: Diagnosis and emergency care. Hosp Med (Oct) 16:16HH–16NN, 1981.
6. Kravis T, Warner C, Jacobs L: Emergency Medicine: A Comprehensive Review, 3rd ed. New York, Raven Press, 1993.
7. Malignant Hyperthermia Association of the United States: Malignant Hyperthermia. Knowing Your Role. Sherburne, NY, MHAUS Publications, 1996.
8. Matsen F: Compartmental syndromes. Hosp Pract 15:113–117, 1980.
9. Milione V, Kanat I: Burns: A review of the pathophysiology, treatment and complications of thermal injury. J Foot Surg 16(4):373–382, 1993.

36. POSTOPERATIVE COMPLICATIONS: LESSER METATARSALS

Morris A. Stribling, D.P.M.

1. In 1916 Meisenbach treated plantar lesions by what surgical technique?

Osteotomies 3 cm proximal to metatarsophalangeal joint; the distal fragments were displaced superiorly.

2. H.L. DuVries performed plantar condylectomies in 1953, which resulted in what complications? Why?

Loss of stabilizing function of plantar fascia and reduction of internal cubic content of the joint, which resulted in loss of tension in the plantar plate and a "floating toe."

3. M.R. Davidson described an osteoclasis similar to Meisenbach's in 1969. Where on the metatarsal was his osteoclasis performed? What complications can occur using this technique?

It was done at the distal neck, 90 degrees to the metatarsal shaft. Since the rationale is to allow nature to determine the exact amount of elevation by postoperative ambulation, the metatarsal can be dorsally displaced with excessive bone callus because of movement.

4. R.P. Jacoby described V-osteotomies in 1973 for correction of plantar calluses with fixation. What post-op complication can occur using this operative technique?

Painful transfer lesions and dorsally displaced metatarsals.

5. Elongated metatarsals corrected with a shortening osteotomy should be performed by what surgical techniques to avoid possible complications?

- Oblique osteotomy to the metatarsal head to avoid rotation
- Osteotomy in metaphyseal section promotes early union
- Non–weight-bearing until radiographic healing is noted to avoid delayed union

6. Where should skin incisions for metatarsal surgery be placed? Why?

Single metatarsal incision should be medial or lateral to the extensor tendon to prevent scar formation over tendons and limitation of motion. Multiple metatarsal surgery incisions in the interspaces will afford visibility and necessitate fewer incisions.

7. K-wire fixation in lesser metatarsal/PIPJ arthrodesis osteotomies should be in what position to avoid which postoperative complication?

- Avoid adjacent soft tissue impingement in interspace for pain and pin irritation
- K-wire should be placed into metatarsal head with metatarsal slightly plantar-flexed to avoid pin breakage and maintain rectus alignment

8. What is one of the most common postoperative complications following osteotomies of the central three metatarsals for painful plantar lesions?

Hatcher and Al found found an 18% recurrence rate and 39% transfer rate.

9. What type of painful skin lesions are commonly found on the plantar foot? What are their clinical differences?

- Callus: hyperkeratotic skin with continuous skin lines in an area of weight-bearing.
- Porokeratosis plantaris discreta: a type of plantar callus believed to be associated with malfunctioning eccrine glands. They have a white central nucleus, hyperhidrosis, and a yellow color.

• Hereditary calluses: non–weight-bearing, present in childhood, often with concomitant involvement of palmar and plantar skin.

10. What can cause delayed union in lesser metatarsal surgery?
• Motion at osteotomy site from unprotected weight-bearing
• Inadequate fixation or poor placement of osteotomy site

11. What clinical symptoms indicate a possible malunion?
• Prolonged swelling
• Deformity
• Pain and stiffness in the metatarsophalangeal joint

12. What radiographic evidence would you see with excessive motion at an osteotomy site?
Because of inadequate fixation, too much motion can cause "bony callus" formation. Bony callus is excess and irregular bone formation functioning to unite the bony ends. The process begins with hematoma formation, forming a scaffold for bone remodeling.

13. How would you treat a malunion if appropriately fixated?
Immobilization in a postoperative shoe for one month. If osteotomy was cylindric or unstable, there should be no weight bearing for 4–8 weeks and until radiographic evidence of healing is noted with cast application.

14. How would you treat a displaced fixation device (screw) in a lesser metatarsal osteotomy?
Remove the fixation device and fixate with .045 smooth K-wire.

15. What can cause a digital deformity after lesser metatarsal surgery?
• Wound contracture
• Total or partial metatarsal heal resection

16. What are the disadvantages of plantar condylectomy to remove plantar lesions?
Digits tend to float because of loss of stabilizing function of plantar fascia, and removal of condyles reduces the internal cubic content of the joint, resulting in loss of tension on the flexor plate.

17. What postoperative complications are common to midshaft fractures of lesser metatarsals?
Metatarsal shortening, angular displacement, and disruption of metatarsal parabola.

18. What is a Jones fracture? What post-op complications can occur from inadequate treatment?
A true Jones fracture is a transverse proximal fracture approximately 1.5 to 3.0 cm distal from the tuberosity of the fifth metatarsal. An avulsion fracture of the metatarsal base is commonly mistaken as a Jones fracture. Inadequate rigid fixation can lead to delayed or nonunion because these fractures are more disabling, slower to heal, and in some cases require bone grafts.

19. What is brachymetatarsia?
A congenital shortening of the metatarsal caused by premature closure of the growth plate due to heredity or trauma.

20. What are some common complications following surgical correction of brachymetatarsia?
1. Soft tissue correction involving V-Y skin plasty and Z lengthening of extensor tendon can lead to neurovascular damage.

2. Bony correction
  - Single metatarsal osteotomy with bone graft. Possible complications can be delay in incorporation and collapse at graft site.
  - Slide lengthening metatarsal osteotomies without grafting should be reserved for mild-to-moderate deformity. Possible complications could be non- or delayed union.
  - Distraction technique using an external fixator. Prolonged distraction can lead to vessel constriction and gangrene. Overlengthening can lead to metatarsophalangeal joints limitus.

21. Chronic joint pain in patients with Freiberg's disease after arthrotomy can be due to what?

Lack of subchondral drilling of erosed bone, lack of proper alignment intraoperatively and use of toe alignment device postoperatively, and/or lack of release of flexor plate intraoperatively.

22. Simple exostectomies for fifth metatarsal tailor's bunions can result in what postoperative complications?

  - Too little bone removed will cause reoccurrence and too much bone will lead to instability of the fifth ray
  - Disruption of loading and destabilization of the joint
  - Fracture of metatarsal head

23. Fifth metatarsal head resections for tailor's bunions lead to what postoperative complication?

Retraction of the fifth toe is a common complication following fifth metatarsal head resection. Lesser metatarsal implants and syndactylism can prevent this.

24. How long should a patient avoid weight-bearing after proximal fifth metatarsal osteotomies?

Six to eight weeks and after radiographic evidence of bone healing. Care must be taken not to fracture the lateral hinge.

25. Osteotomies for the correction of congenital metatarsus adductus must avoid damage to what osseous structure?

The growth plate.

BIBLIOGRAPHY

1. Addante JB, Kaufmann BA: The metatarsal osteotomy: a 10-year follow-up on the second, third, and fourth metatarsal osteotomies and a new approach to the fifth metatarsal osteotomy. J Foot Surg 16:92–96, 1977.
2. Buxbaum FD: Surgical correction of metatarsal-phalangeal joint dislocation and arthritis deformity: the partial head and plantar condylectomy. J Foot Surg 18:36–40, 1979.
3. Costa AJ: Delayed union in metatarsal osteotomies. J Foot Surg 16:127–131, 1977.
4. Durant J: Metatarsal head resection without transference of lesion. J Foot Surg 8:28, 1969.
5. DuVries HL: New approach to the treatment of intractable verruca plantaris (plantar wart). JAMA 152:1202–1203, 1953.
6. Fenton CF, Butlin WE: Displaced V-osteotomies. J Am Podiatry Assoc 72:150–152, 1982.
7. McGlamry ED, Banks A, Downey MS: Comprehensive Textbook of Foot Surgery, 2nd ed. Baltimore, Williams & Wilkins, 1992.
8. Meisenbach RO: Painful anterior arch of the foot: An operation for its relief by means of raising the arch. Am J Orthop Surg 14:206–211, 1916.
9. Reinherz RP, Toren OJ: Bone healing after adjacent metatarsal osteotomies. J Foot Surg 20:198–203, 1981.
10. Schweitzer DA, Lew H, Shuken J, et al: Central metatarsal shortening following osteotomy and its clinical significance. J Am Podiatry Assoc 72:6–10, 1982.
11. Skorecki J, Jacobs NA: Analysis of the vertical component of force in normal and pathological gait. J Biomech 58:11–34, 1972.
12. Thompson CT: Surgical treatment of disorders of the forepart of the foot. J Bone Joint Surg 46A:1119, 1964.
13. Walter JH, Pressman MM: External fixation in the treatment of metatarsal nonunions. J Am Podiatry Assoc 71:297–301, 1981.
14. Woolf WH: Eradication of the problem of plantar keratoma. J Am Podiatry Assoc 74:163–167, 1984.

37. GAIT ANALYSIS

Susan C. Warner, B.A., and R. Daryl Phillips, D.P.M.

1. What are the necessary prerequisites for performing a complete, basic gait examination?
- A clear, straight, flat pathway of at least 30 ft in length to allow 2–4 steps for speed-up and 2–4 steps for slow-down.
- Patient should be wearing shorts (preferably bicycling shorts).
- Patient barefoot.
- Ideally, males should be observed while shirtless and females should wear a swimsuit top or sports bra. A sleeveless, tightly-fitting tank top or T-shirt is acceptable, if necessary.
- Watch the patient from posterior, anterior, and lateral perspectives with the patient in stance and during gait.
- Know the patient's foot type. Always determine the basic biomechanical measurements of subtalar joint range of motion, neutral position, and forefoot-to-rearfoot relationship before analyzing gait.

2. What should the observer watch for during basic gait analysis?
Head tilt
Symmetric shoulder height
Symmetric ASIS and PSIS (anterior-superior/posterior-superior iliac spine) height
Knees functioning symmetrically in sagittal and frontal planes
Straight line of progression
Normal base of gait (number of cm between centers of heels upon stance)
Normal and symmetrical angle of gait (normal is 0–15° abducted)
Symmetric shoulder rotation
Level and symmetrically prominent scapulae
Symmetric arm swing with slight flexion of elbow at top of swing
Symmetric pelvic rotation
Symmetric step length
Normal heel-strike
Normal heel-lift (usually heel should lift about 60–70° from ground)
Normal toe-off

3. What is the difference between the terms *pronated/supinated* and *pronating/supinating*?
The terms *pronating* and *supinating* infer that subtalar joint motion is taking place either in the pronatory or supinatory direction, respectively. A *pronated* position of the foot means that the foot is abducted, dorsiflexed, and everted from its neutral position. A *supinated* foot is adducted, plantarflexed, and inverted from its neutral position.

4. When is the subtalar joint pronated and supinated during the gait cycle?
At **heel-strike**, the subtalar joint should be slightly supinated. However, immediately following heel-strike, the subtalar joint begins pronating and soon reaches approx. 4° of subtalar joint pronation. The midtarsal joint now becomes a mobile adapter and can adapt to variations in terrain more easily. Then, after the **contact** period is finished, the subtalar joint begins supinating. During **midstance**, the subtalar joint is supinating and reaches neutral position just before heel-lift. Throughout most of the **propulsive** period, the subtalar joint continues supinating and becomes supinated to approx. 4° to convert the foot into a rigid lever to prepare for toe-off. Just after **toe-off**, at the beginning of the swing phase, the subtalar joint pronates so that the foot can clear the ground. During **swing**, the subtalar joint again becomes supinated to prepare for the next heel-strike.

5. What indicators of pathologic gait should the observer listen for during gait analysis?

Forefoot slap: This may be due to physiologic or functional weakness of the anterior tibial muscle. It may also be due to the forefoot striking the ground prematurely, as is seen with such conditions as tight gastrocnemius/soleus muscles or tight hamstring muscles. A forefoot slap may also be seen in severe chronic pronation syndromes that cause the knee to be flexed at heel-strike.

Loud heel-strike (or heavy heel): This may be due to weakness of the gastrosoleus muscle complex. If the knee is extended as heel-strike takes place, a loud heel-strike may occur. Any syndrome that decreases shock absorption (e.g., cavus foot syndromes) can also cause this condition. The observer should always watch the legs and lower body for severe shock waves with each step taken by the patient.

6. What is the effect of a functional orthosis on subtalar joint motion during gait?

The subtalar joint is never just statically positioned in neutral during gait; it is either pronating or supinating. Some may think that an orthosis can hold one's subtalar joint in a constant neutral position. This is untrue, however, as orthoses function only to *limit* the degree and/or velocity of pronation or supination of the subtalar joint.

7. What are the phases of the gait cycle? How much of the gait cycle does each consume?

The **stance phase** lasts from heel-strike of one foot to toe-off of the same foot and takes up approx. 65% of the gait cycle. The stance phase is composed of two double-support periods which make up about 17% each and a single-support period which takes up the middle 30% of the stance phase. The **swing phase** makes up approx. 35% of the gait cycle and occurs between toe-off and the next heel-strike of the same foot.

8. Name the three periods of the stance phase and the percentage of time consumed by each.

Contact: This period begins with heel-strike of one foot and ends with forefoot loading of the same foot, which occurs at the same time as toe-off of the opposite foot. It consumes approx. 27% of the total stance phase.

Midstance: Midstance occurs between forefoot loading and heel-lift one foot. It makes up about 40% of the total stance phase.

Propulsion: The propulsive period starts with heel-lift and ends with toe-off. About 33% of the total stance phase is taken up by propulsion.

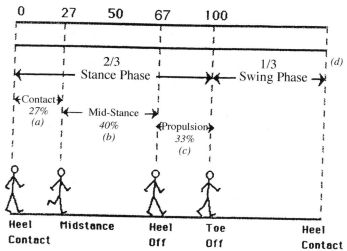

Phases of the gait cycle. (From Birrer RB, Dellacote MP, Grisafi PJ: Common Foot Problems in Primary Care. Philadelphia, Hanley & Belfus, 1992, with permission.)

9. How do extensor substitution, flexor substitution, and flexor stabilization differ?

Extensor substitution: The extensor digitorum longus fails to relax during the early contact period, which keeps the MTP joints dorsiflexed during contact while the flexor digitorum longus begins to fire. The long flexors and long extensors are never firing at the same time. In these patients, the lumbricales have lost the ability to stabilize the MTP joints. It may be seen in all types of syndromes in which the anterior tibial muscle does not adequately decelerate the velocity of forefoot strike. The toes slow to hit the ground and show hammering before contacting the ground.

Flexor substitution: The interossei have lost the ability to stabilize the MTP joints. Flexor substitution is usually seen during late stance phase in a patient with a supinated foot type. The condition is the result of a weak triceps surae, so the flexor hallucis longus and flexor digitorum longus fire longer than usual to assist the gastrosoleus complex in providing propulsion. The digits hammer during the propulsive period.

Flexor stabilization: This condition usually occurs in a patient with a pronated foot type. Again, the interossei have lost the ability to stabilize the MTP joints. The quadratus plantae loses its mechanical advantage and does not pull the flexor apparatus laterally as it should, thereby causing a varus rotation of the fourth and fifth digits and hammering of usually all of the lesser digits. Flexor stabilization is seen during the late stance phase of gait. It is the most common cause of hammertoes.

10. What aspects of gait should be observed to detect a possible limb-length discrepancy?

Head tilt: May tilt toward longer side if the patient compensates with a lateral spinal curvature or to the shorter side if not.

Shoulder height: Usually lower on the shorter side but may be lower on the longer side if the patient has a compensatory lateral spinal curvature.

Pelvic girth height: Higher on the long side.

Arm swing: The arm swing is greater on the short side to correlate with greater step length taken by the longer leg.

Step length: Greater on the long side.

Angle of gait: Greater on the long side due to increased pronation and therefore abduction of the foot on the pronated side.

Muscle mass and girth of calf and thigh muscles: May be increased on the pronated or longer side.

Genu recurvatum: May be present on the shorter side.

Genu flexion: May be present on the longer side.

Internal leg rotation: Greater on the pronated or longer side.

11. Why does one see a scissors-like gait in patients with spastic cerebral palsy?

Because of spasm of the adductor muscle groups, the knees are flexed, and the hips are adducted and internally rotated. Ankle equinus is often present. These patients usually have a supinated foot type and often develop a rigid pes cavus or even a clubfoot deformity. Ambulation has a wild and uncontrolled appearance. During gait, the patient may need to circumduct the leg to avoid knocking his or her knees together. There is gross instability and incoordination, with a wide base of gait during both stance and ambulation. The patient's arm swing is abducted away from the torso and is grossly exaggerated to help create balance. The patient also sways the upper torso from side-to-side for balance during gait.

12. When does a steppage gait occur and why?

A steppage gait is seen with paralysis of the anterior tibial muscle, so that patients are unable to dorsiflex the foot to clear the ground. The hips and spine extend and the body weight is leaned backward during swing to help the foot to clear the ground. The forefoot slaps the ground supinated at first and then pronates secondary to body weight. This type of gait is seen with polio and Charcot-Marie-Tooth disease, and it can be seen with either upper motor neuron or lower motor neuron disorders. A steppage gait is most commonly seen with peripheral nervous system disorders.

13. What is ataxia?

Ataxia is a staggering, unsteady type of gait. Patients have a drunken appearance during ambulation. They will likely be unable to heel or toe walk or to walk in tandem. Many need to hang onto the wall for support in order to ambulate.

14. What type of gait is seen with posterior column disease?

These patients exhibit ataxia and have a stomping gait. During stance and gait, there is a wide base of gait due to their loss of proprioception. This loss is most profound when the patient is asked to close his or her eyes, which removes visual feedback on the placement of the feet. This type of gait occurs in multiple sclerosis and other diseases that affect the posterior column and proprioception.

15. What kind of gait is seen with cerebellar disease?

Patients have a slightly broad-based gait and are ataxic both with their eyes open and closed. Thus, even if a patient is looking directly at his or her feet, he or she may not be able to place the feet in the correct position. If one asks these patients to walk, their gait might appear fairly normal at first, but if they are asked to turn suddenly while walking, stumbling and incoordination may occur.

16. Why is a broad-based gait sometimes seen during gait analysis?

There is a lack of lateral stability in patients who exhibit a wide-based gait. These patients widen their base of stance and gait in order to reduce this lateral instability and thus shift some of the instability forward into their line of progression. In this way, they can usually take their next step forward before losing their balance. A widened base of stance and gait is normal in young toddlers.

17. What different types of gait may be exhibited in patients affected by poliomyelitis? What foot type do these patients usually develop?

Most individuals develop a **pes cavus** eventually, and depending on the nerves and muscles affected by the disease, they can have a variety of pathologic gait types. The most commonly seen type is a steppage gait. Other types include calcaneal, genu recurvatum, flexed-knee, gluteus maximus, or gluteus medius gait.

18. Which type of gait is seen in patients with Parkinson's disease?

These individuals develop a loss of agility and a shuffling type of gait. There is great difficulty in initiating ambulation and in halting the gait cycle once it has begun. Gait commences with small, shuffling steps and then progresses with increasingly faster steps—i.e., a **festinating gait**. The observer may also notice stooped posture and a "pill-rolling" motion of the hands in these patients.

19. Describe the type of gait usually seen in Duchenne's muscular dystrophy.

A **Trendelenburg gait** with compensatory lordosis of the spine is usually seen in these patients. This is also known as a lurching or waddling type of gait. There is a weakness of the gluteus medius muscle, which causes the torso to shift toward the contralateral side during the swing phase. This shift helps to decrease the falling of the pelvis on the ipsilateral side. It is difficult for these patients to climb stairs or to rise from a sitting or squatting position (positive Gower's sign). Ankle equinus and equinovarus are common findings.

The lower-extremity muscles in Duchenne's muscular dystrophy seem to be unusually large and firm, but one should not be deceived by this finding. These muscles are actually very weak due to fat deposition within the muscle interstitium.

20. What is myelodysplasia? What types of foot deformity commonly occur as a result of it?

Myelodysplasia is a group of developmental deformities of the spinal cord, including spina bifida, spina bifida occulta, meningocele, myelomeningocele, and myelocele. Foot deformities that commonly develop are pes cavus, equinus, equinovarus, and severe forefoot valgus.

21. In a young child, is toe-walking normal?

A young child who toe-walks is most likely normal. Toe-walking occurs frequently in children and is considered normal up until about 2 years of age. However, the clinician should always first rule out upper motor neuron lesions in these children. If the child has > 20° of ankle joint dorsiflexion, then normal development will usually occur and he or she will likely eventually walk normally. If the child has 10–20° of ankle joint dorsiflexion, the clinician should consider prescribing a regimen of stretching exercises for the child. If there is < 10° of ankle dorsiflexion, then a more aggressive treatment program, such as serial casting, should be considered.

22. Is an in-toeing or pigeon-toed gait abnormal in a child?

A pigeon-toed gait is very common in children, but most grow out of this gait by early to mid-childhood. The clinician should nonetheless perform a thorough examination of young children to rule out hip subluxation and cerebral palsy. A lingering in-toeing type of gait is most commonly caused by internal femoral torsion, tibial torsion, forefoot valgus, or metatarsus adductus. When forefoot valgus is the cause of in-toeing, the subtalar joint is supinated and lateral instability is present. A child with a forefoot valgus may then turn his or her toes inward during gait so that he or she is subsequently falling forward into the line of progression instead of losing balance laterally. Theory suggests that these deformities may be caused by malpositioning of the fetus while in utero, by heredity, and by sleeping and sitting patterns that encourage the condition to linger.

23. What are the results of abnormal pronation during propulsion? When is this usually seen?

Overpronation or overuse syndrome with pronation occurring during propulsion causes fatigue of the muscles of the foot and leg. Arch fatigue and plantar fasciitis also often result. The muscles of the foot and leg attempt to recreate stability in the foot during propulsion because of the hypermobility of the bony structure of the foot. These patients often develop calluses secondary to shear forces and also often develop joint subluxations throughout the foot.

Pronation during propulsion can affect the knee, because during pronation there is internal rotation of the tibia, putting strain on the collateral ligaments of the knee. Abnormal pronation may also inhibit the normal motion of the sacroiliac joint on the side of the trailing leg during gait, which may produce fixation and symptoms at the sacroiliac joint. With pronation during propulsion, the spine leans toward the side of the trailing leg, instead of transferring weight smoothly to the leading leg. This may cause chronic strain of the lower back.

The clinician should always look for frontal plane abnormalities at the hip and knee and should also watch for an abductory twist at toe-off in these patients. During an abductory twist, the foot pivots on the lateral metatarsal head(s) while the rear foot swings inward toward the body's midline.

24. What are the results of any deformity that causes decreased shock absorption during ambulation?

Decreased shock absorption may eventually cause degenerative joint disease in the lower extremity and foot, as well as in the spinal column. Patients who have this kind of joint damage may therefore have a decreased ability to adapt to variable terrain while walking. In these patients, the normal amount of closed kinetic-chain pronation does not occur during the contact period. Any pes cavus deformity will usually cause this type of joint damage to some degree.

25. If an otherwise normal-looking patient's right foot is much more pronated than his or her left foot during stance and gait, what are the possible causes?

Tarsal coalition: A coalition occurs when there is a bridge between two or more bones of the tarsus, which results in limited motion. A coalition often eventually produces peroneal spastic flatfoot.

Posterior tibial tendon dysfunction: This is usually seen in an extreme pes planovalgus foot type. The posterior tibial tendon becomes irritated from overuse, and it may tear or rupture at its insertion into the navicular as a result of long-term stress in the area. The clinician should have these patients perform the single heel-rise test. If posterior tibial tendon dysfunction is present, the affected heel usually does not invert to the same degree as in the opposite foot.

Limb-length discrepancy: With a limb-length discrepancy, the subtalar joint pronates more on the longer side.

Vertical talus: Also known as rocker-bottom flatfoot or "persian slipper foot," this is a primary dislocation of the talonavicular joint. The navicular articulates with the dorsal aspect of the talus and thus sits in a plantarflexed, nearly vertical position.

Peroneal spastic flatfoot: This condition is a result of spasm of the peroneal muscles, which helps to splint or guard against pain by causing the foot to pronate.

Neurologic lesion: If the lesion affects only one side of the body, a unilateral flatfoot may be seen.

26. What is foot-drop?

Seen in the swing phase and early contact period, a foot-drop causes the foot to drop into an automatic equinovarus position secondary to gravity. This condition is due to a weak anterior tibial muscle. Heel contact may or may not occur after the initial ground contact by the forefoot.

27. Name some important etiologies of foot-drop.

Cerebrovascular accident	Poliomyelitis
Spinal cord lesion or tumor	Friedreich's ataxia
Trauma	Infection
Charcot-Marie-Tooth disease	Guillain-Barré syndrome
Refsum's disease	Dejerine-Sottas syndrome

28. What are some possible etiologies of ankle equinus?

Cerebral palsy	Spinal cord tumor/injury
Familial spastic diplegia	Charcot-Marie-Tooth disease
Clubfoot	Spinal muscular atrophy
Muscular dystrophy	(Kugelberg-Welander disease)

29. How is ankle equinus compensated for?

Sometimes there is no distal compensation for an equinus. This occurs in those patients who are true toe-walkers and who exhibit no heel contact with the ground. Compensation of this sort usually occurs with severe neuromuscular disease and is associated with an anterior cavus or a severe equinovarus foot type, but can also be seen in otherwise normal patients. In a true toe-walker, the subtalar joint remains supinated throughout the gait cycle. A true toe-walker may have no pain or associated symptoms because the heel never actually touches the ground.

In other individuals, compensation for an equinus may be fully distal to the ankle joint. In this case, dorsiflexion occurs at the oblique axis of the midtarsal joint and at the subtalar joint. These patients usually have a hypermobile pes planus and a maximally everted rearfoot with an inverted forefoot-to-rearfoot relationship.

Signs to watch for in individuals with proximal compensation are increased spinal lordosis secondary to increased internal leg rotation, genu valgum, and genu recurvatum or genu flexion. Pain and difficulties in these patients often arise when the heel actually contacts the ground.

Most people do not fit neatly into either of these categories and instead exhibit a mix of the two categories of compensation. They usually show varying degrees of compensation above and below the ankle joint.

30. Explain the windlass mechanism.

In 1954, J.H. Hicks first described this phenomenon completely. He noted that with passive extension of the hallux upon weight-bearing, the arch rises, the rearfoot inverts, the leg rotates laterally (or externally), and the plantar fascia becomes very taut. This maneuver is known today as the **Hubscher maneuver** or the **Jack test**.

Hicks found that the plantar fascia was indeed responsible in large part for raising and supporting the arch. He explained this phenomenon in terms of a **windlass**, where the cable which would wind around a spool is made up of the plantar fascia and the plantar pad, the drum (or spool) of the windlass is the metatarsal head, and the handle which winds the cable around the spool is the proximal phalanx. As the hallux is extended passively, the proximal phalanx puts tension on the cable (the plantar fascia and plantar pad). The plantar fascia, in turn, pulls its attachment to the calcaneus anterior. These actions together cause the bony arch of the foot to become higher and shorter in length, and thus, the arch rises.

31. Describe the normal time period in which genu varum and genu valgum are present in young children.

Bowlegs (**genu varum**) are normal in infancy and early childhood until about 2 years of age. After that, maximum valgus of the knees is usually reached by about age 3. Normal values are usually reached at around 6 or 7, although a genu valgum may be seen in some adolescents during puberty. Pathologic forms of genu varum, such as Blount's disease, rickets, and some forms of dysplasia must be ruled out.

32. Is genu recurvatum ever considered a normal finding?

Genu recurvatum is never considered to be a normal finding. This condition exists when the subtalar joint is unable to pronate enough so that the tibia can move forward during gait, and when the center of mass at the knee joint falls anterior to the knee so that the heel cannot lift from the ground. When treating patients who have an equinus with prescription orthotics, the podiatric physician should note that a genu recurvatum can result if too much control of the subtalar joint is attempted. Once this occurs, the patient can become very difficult to treat.

33. What etiologies of pes cavus must always be ruled out before a diagnosis of idiopathic pes cavus can be made?

Congenital

Spina bifida	Myelodysplasia	Cerebral palsy
Myelomeningocele	Muscular dystrophies	Charcot-Marie-Tooth disease
Friedreich's ataxia	Roussy-Lévy syndrome	Congenital syphilis
Congenital clubfoot	Syringomyelia	Dejerine-Sottas syndrome

Acquired

Poliomyelitis	Trauma
Spinal cord tumors	Plantar fibromatosis (lederhose syndrome)
Dystonia musculorum deformans	Infection (encephalitis)
Acquired syringomyelia	Hysteria (cerebral level)

34. How do global, local, anterior, and posterior pes cavus differ?

Anterior pes cavus occurs when the forefoot or any of its components is plantarflexed on the rearfoot. It is also known as anterior equinus or pseudoequinus. With the subtalar joint in neutral position and the talar declination angle brought to normal, the metatarsal heads would sit below the level of the ground with this type of foot.

Global and local pes cavus are subtypes of **anterior pes cavus**. With **anterior global**, all of the metatarsal heads lie below the surface of the ground. With **anterior local**, only a portion of the metatarsus is abnormally plantarflexed, so only some of the metatarsal heads would lie below the ground surface.

Posterior pes cavus, also called rearfoot cavus, usually exists along with an anterior cavus deformity and is usually not a separate entity in itself. This type of foot has a high calcaneal inclination angle, and usually plantarflexion of the forefoot on the rearfoot is also present with this foot type. A purely posterior pes cavus deformity is present only if the metatarsal heads sit at ground level, but the calcaneal inclination angle is still increased after the subtalar joint has been placed in neutral position and the talar declination angle has been brought to normal.

35. How does one differentiate between a functional and structural limb-length discrepancy?
    A **structural** inequality is caused by an anatomic shortening of bone on the affected side. A **functional** discrepancy is an increased or decreased length of the limb secondary to contracture at a joint or to axial deviation at a joint or joints. Often, individuals have a combination of these two deformities.
    With the patient standing, the clinician should see that the anterior-superior and posterior-superior iliac spine (ASIS and PSIS) are both low on the side that is affected. The discrepancy is structural if, when a heel-lift is placed under the shorter limb, the pelvis becomes level. If a limb-length discrepancy is functional, then the pelvis will become level only after the subtalar joint of the shorter side is placed in neutral position.

36. In what way are vertical talus and clubfoot similar?
    The two deformities both result in dislocation of the navicular. In clubfoot, the navicular is dislocated plantar and medial to the talus, while in the vertical talus, the navicular is positioned dorsal and lateral to the talus. In either of these deformities, the clinician should never address the equinus deformity first (either in serial casting or surgery), as this could result in a midtarsal breach, worsening of the rearfoot position, damage to the talus, or epiphyseal damage.

37. Name some of the possible etiologies of Haglund's deformity.

Pes cavus	Forefoot valgus
Fully or partially compensated	Idiopathic
rearfoot varus	Any deformity that produces an
Plantarflexed first ray	abductory twist at toe off

38. Describe some of the advanced systems currently used in gait analysis and their applications.
    Force plate: These systems measure the vertical and horizontal forces, reaction force, center of force, and velocity of force under the foot and find the moments of force around the three cardinal axes of the foot. These systems are used for determining abnormal force vectors in neuropathic patients and for calculating forces and moments across joints. The two types of force plates in use currently are the piezoelectric type (Kistler) and the strain gauge type (AMTI, Bertec, and several others).
    Pressure mats (Emed, F-scan): These portable in-shoe and platform capacitance mats have the capability to measure vertical pressures under the foot. With these systems, one can also track the movement of the center of pressure across the plantar surface of the foot.
    Pedobarograph: This system uses the critical light reflection system consisting of a microcomputer, a video camera, a plastic sheet with a pattern of tiny deformable bumps on its surface, and a side-illuminated transducer-mounted glass plate. When pressure is applied to the plastic sheet, the bumps flatten against the glass. The intensity of the light reflected and the pressure applied to the plastic sheet correlate directly (except at very high and at very low pressures).
    Videotaping: A videotape can be slowed down or stopped for closer inspection of certain aspects of gait. Some highly technical systems also use video camera(s) and computer programs to measure joint angles and joint motion velocities and accelerations (e.g., PEAK motion analysis system).

BIBLIOGRAPHY

1. Brown GP, Donatelli R, Catlin PA, Wooden MJ: The effect of two types of foot orthoses on rearfoot mechanics. J Orthop Sports Phys Ther 21:258–267, 1995.
2. Green DR, Carol A: Planal dominance. J Am Podiatr Med Assoc 74:98–103, 1984.
3. Hetherington VJ, Carnett J, Patterson BA: Motion of the first metatarsophalangeal joint. J Foot Surg 28:13–19, 1989.

4. Hicks JH: The mechanics of the foot: I. The joints. J Anat 87:345–357, 1953.
5. Hicks JH: The mechanics of the foot: II. The plantar aponeurosis and the arch. J Anat 88:25–31, 1954.
6. Kirby KA: Rotational equilibrium across the subtalar joint axis. J Am Podiatr Med Assoc 79:1–14, 1989.
7. Levens AS, Inman VT, Blosser JA: Transverse rotation of the segments of the lower extremity in locomotion. J Bone Joint Surg 30A:859–872, 1948.
8. Root ML, Orien WP, Weed JH, Hughes RJ (eds): Biomechanical Examination of the Foot: vol. I. Los Angeles, Clinical Biomechanics Corp., 1971.
9. Root ML, Orien WP, Weed JH (eds): Normal and Abnormal Function of the Foot: vol. II. Los Angeles, Clinical Biomechanics Corp., 1977.
10. Rose J, Gamble JG (eds): Human Walking, 2nd ed. Baltimore, Williams & Wilkins, 1994.
11. Sgarlato TE: The angle of gait. J Am Podiatr Assoc 55:645–650, 1965.
12. Stokes IAF, Hutton WC, Stott JRR: Forces acting on the metatarsals during normal walking. J Anat 129:579–590, 1979.
13. Sutherland DH, Olshen R, Cooper L, Woo SLY: The development of mature gait. J Bone Joint Surg 62A:336–353, 1980.
14. Sutherland DH: Gait Disorders in Childhood and Adolescence. Baltimore, Williams & Wilkins, 1984.
15. Valmassy RL: Biomechanical evaluation of the child. Clin Podiatr 1:563–579, 1984.

38. PODIATRIC PHARMACOLOGY

Vincent F. Giacalone, D.P.M., F.A.C.F.A.S.

1. Red-man (red-neck) syndrome can occur with the use of vancomycin. How is this syndrome manifested? How can it be avoided?

Red-man or red-neck syndrome consists of an erythematous or maculopapular rash or flushing of the face, neck, and upper torso along with associated pruritus. It may also occur with hypotension and angioedema. The event is stimulated by nonimmunologically-mediated rapid histamine release secondary to both the infusion rate and concentration of the IV vancomycin preparation.

The risk of a reaction can be reduced by infusing the solution over a 60-minute period and by limiting the concentration to 2.5–5 mg/ml of solution. In addition, administration of 1 gm every 12 hours is associated with fewer reactions than 500 mg every 6 hours.

2. Which nonsteroidal anti-inflammatory drugs (NSAIDs) are safer to use in patients with renal disease? Why?

To maintain normal glomerular filtration, the kidney depends on prostaglandin-mediated vasodilation. Many NSAIDs inhibit renal prostaglandin synthesis, thus stimulating acute renal failure.

For reasons that are not completely understood, aspirin and a nonsalicylate NSAID, sulindac (Clinoril), have only minimal effects on renal prostaglandin. One reason for sulindac's safety is that it may be converted to an inactive sulfone metabolite in the kidneys. These drugs should still be used with caution in patients with preexisting renal conditions.

3. Name the drugs that are contraindicated with concomitant use of the antifungal itraconazole.

Terfenadine (Seldane)   Cisapride (Propulsid)   Midazolam (Versed)
Astemizole (Hismanal)   Triazolam (Halcion)

Coadministration with digoxin, cyclosporine, tacrolimus, phenytoin, rifampin, H_2 antagonists, and warfarin should be used with caution. Itraconazole may result in increased plasma levels of digoxin or warfarin.

4. List several medications that may precipitate a gouty attack.

Salicylates	Thiazide diuretics	Others
Aspirin	Chlorothiazide	Methotrexate
Diflunisal	Hydrochlorothiazide	Nicotinic acid (niacin)
Salsalate	Metolazone	Ethambutol
Olsalazine		Levodopa
Sulfasalazine		

5. What is the effect of probenecid on penicillin and cephalosporin antibiotics?

Probenecid, at a dose of 500 mg four times a day, blocks the renal tubular excretion of penicillins and cephalosporins, thereby increasing the blood levels of these antibiotics.

6. Name the insulins in various categories and give the times of onset and durations of action for each category.

Category	Type	Onset (Hrs)	Peak (Hrs)	Duration (Hrs)
Short-acting	Regular, semilente	0.5–1	2–6	6–8
Intermediate-acting	NPH, lente	1–2	6–12	16–24
Long-acting	PZI, ultralente	4–8	14–20	24–36

7. A 42-year-old woman with a 17-year history of rheumatoid arthritis on long-term prednisone and NSAIDs is scheduled for surgery using general anesthesia. Is any alteration required in this patient's medication?

There are several published preoperative steroid adjustment regimens for patients on long-term steroid use. One of the most frequently cited indicates:

- The evening prior to surgery
  100 mg hydrocortisone IM or IV
- Just prior to surgery
  1. 100 mg hydrocortisone IM or IV *and*
  2. 0.5 hour preoperatively, start hydrocortisone via a continuous IV drip at 100 mg every 8 hours for 24 hours, or until the stress of the procedure has resolved.

For a similar patient undergoing a minor procedure under local anesthesia, it might be appropriate to administer 15 mg of prednisone orally early the morning of surgery, followed by 15 mg of prednisone later the same afternoon and the same dose the next afternoon.

Any of several algorithms may be used when considering surgery on this type of patient. The important factor is remembering to provide supplementation.

8. What medications are used to reverse warfarin (Coumadin) and heparin? What are the doses?

Warfarin: Vitamin K (phytonadione) is used to reverse the effects of warfarin. The antidote requires 24 hours to reach full effect. The usual dose is 5–10 mg orally, SC or IV. If an immediate hemostatic effect is required, transfusion with fresh frozen plasma at a dose of 10–20 ml/kg should be given.

Heparin: The anticoagulant effect of heparin disappears within several hours after discontinuation of the drug. Mild bleeding due to heparin can usually be controlled without the use of an antidote or antagonist. If life-threatening hemorrhage occurs, heparin's effect can be reversed by the *slow* IV infusion of protamine sulfate, usually 1 mg of protamine for every 100 U of heparin remaining in the patient, given at a *slow* rate of up to 50 mg/10 min.

9. Do warfarin and heparin function within the intrinsic or extrinsic pathways? Discuss their mechanisms of action.

Warfarin inhibits active coagulation factors of the *intrinsic* pathway. It inhibits the hepatic synthesis of vitamin-K-dependent factors and thereby interferes with fibrin formation and thrombus growth.

Heparin prevents the conversion of fibrinogen to fibrin in the presence of antithrombin III within the *extrinsic* pathway.

10. Name four amide and four ester type local anesthetic agents. How are they metabolized?

Esters	Amides
Procaine (Novacaine)	Lidocaine (Xylocaine)
Chloroprocaine (Nesacaine)	Mepivacaine (Carbocaine)
Tetracaine (Pontocaine)	Bupivacaine (Marcaine)
Hexylcaine (Cyclaine)	Etidocaine (Duranest)

Esters are metabolized through hydrolysis by plasma pseudocholinesterase. Amides are metabolized by hydrolysis in the liver. Caution should be taken when using an amide local anesthetic in patients with hepatic disease.

11. What is the mechanism of action of local anesthetics?

Local anesthetic agents prevent the generation and conduction of nerve impulses by reducing sodium permeability, increasing the electrical excitation threshold, slowing the nerve impulse propagation, and reducing the rate of rise of the action potential.

12. To provide adequate anesthesia to reduce a foot joint dislocation, you have injected a total of 27 ml of lidocaine 2% plain. Is this a safe dose to administer?

The toxic dose of lidocaine 2% plain is 15 ml.

Toxic Doses of Lidocaine and Bupivacaine

MEDICATION	STRENGTH	TOXIC DOSE
Lidocaine	1% plain	30 ml or 300 mg
Lidocaine	1% with epinephrine	50 ml or 500 mg
Bupivacaine	0.25% plain	70 ml or 175 mg
Bupivacaine	0.25% with epinephrine	90 ml or 225 mg

Lidocaine 1% plain is equal to 1000 mg/100 ml, and there is 10 mg/1 ml of solution. Simple multiplication reveals that 30 ml of solution contains 300 mg of lidocaine. If lidocaine 2% were used, the toxic amount in ml would be half (e.g., the toxic dose of lidocaine 2% plain is 15 ml).

13. A 47-year-old man has pain in his foot after removal of a wart. The patient is allergic to codeine. List several *oral* pain medications that can be used safely in this patient.

Aspirin   Propoxyphene (Darvon)
Acetaminophen   Pentazocine (Talwin)
NSAIDs

14. When should peak and trough levels for gentamicin be measured? What are the acceptable levels for each?

Loading dose: 5–7.5 mg/kg
Peak level: 6–10 µg/ml, drawn 30 min after complete infusion of a dose
Trough level" 0.5–2 µg/ml, drawn just before the next dose
Serum levels: Peak and trough levels should be assessed 24–48 hours after initiation of therapy, usually after the fourth dose.

15. How would you adjust the dose of vancomycin for a 50-year-old man with renal impairment?

Patients with renal impairment who receive vancomycin require a dose adjustment based on their creatinine clearance (CrCl) calculations:

Males

$$\frac{(140 - \text{age[yrs]}) \times \text{weight (kg)}}{\text{SCr (mg/dl)} \times 72} = \text{Estimated CrCl}$$

For example, a 70-kg, 50-year-old man with a serum creatinine (SCr) of 1.6 yields:

$$\frac{(140 - 50) \times 70}{(1.6 \times 72)} = 54.68 \text{ ml/min}$$

In this scenario, the estimated renal function is 54.7% of normal, and so the adjusted antibiotic dose should be 54.7% of the normal dose.

Females (multiply the equation by 0.85)

$$\frac{(140 - \text{age[yrs]}) \times \text{weight (kg)}}{\text{SCr (mg/dl)} \times 72} \times 0.85 = \text{Estimated CrCl}$$

For example, an 81-kg, 57-year-old woman with SCr of 3.3 yields:

$$\frac{(140 - 57) \times 81}{3.3 \times 72} \times 0.85 = 24.0 \text{ ml/min}$$

In this patient, the estimated renal function is 24.0% of normal, and so the adjusted antibiotic dose should be 24.0% of the normal dose.

16. Which IV antibiotics require dose adjustment in patients with renal impairment?

Erythromycin	Trimethoprim-sulfamethoxazole
Aminoglycosides	Penicillin and its derivatives
Vancomycin	Cephalosporins

17. A patient requires treatment of a *Pseudomonas* infection, but she is allergic to ciprofloxacin. List several alternative antibiotics.

Cefoperazone	Carbenicillin and ticarcillin
Ceftazidime	Mezlocillin, azlocillin, and piperacillin
Imipenem-cilastatin	Aztreonam
Tobramycin, amikacin, and gentamicin	Ticarcillin-clavulanic acid

18. State three ways in which to adjust an adult dose of medication for a 3-year-old child.

1. Clark's rule (for children > 1 yr):

$$\frac{\text{Weight of child (lbs)} \times \text{Adult dose}}{150} = \text{Child's dose}$$

2. Cowling's rule:

$$\frac{\text{Age (at next birthday)}}{24} = \% \text{ of adult dose}$$

3. Young's rule:

$$\frac{\text{Age}}{\text{Age} + 12} \times \text{Adult dose} = \text{Child's dose}$$

19. You performed a chemical matrixectomy on a 12-year-old girl earlier today, and her mother calls and states that she is in a fair amount of pain. What are your choices for an *oral* pain reliever for this patient?

Considering that the patient is 12-years-old, only a few oral pain relievers would be safe. Most pain medications are contraindicated in children under 12 years of age.

Analgesics: acetaminophen, codeine, meperidine

NSAID: ibuprofen, tolmentin

20. In a patient using ketorolac (Toradol), which class of drugs is contraindicated? Why?

Toradol is a potent NSAID, indicated for short-term use (up to 5 days) for severe and acute pain. Coadministration with aspirin and other NSAIDs will increase the risk of NSAID side effects and is strictly contraindicated.

21. Discuss the indications and contraindications for tramadol (Ultram). Why is it different from the NSAID class of medications?

Indications: Moderate to moderate-severe pain

Contraindications: Do not use in patients with known hypersensitivity to tramadol, those using hypnotics, other centrally acting analgesics, opioids, psychotropic drugs, or in acute intoxication states.

Tramadol is a centrally acting synthetic analgesic, while NSAIDs inhibit prostaglandin synthesis.

22. Name a soluble and an insoluble injectable steroid and give the duration of action of each (short or long acting).

Soluble: rapid onset and short duration
  1. Dexamethasone sodium phosphate (Decadron, Hexadrol)
  2. Betamethasone sodium (Celestone)

Insoluble: slow onset and long duration
  1. Dexamethasone acetate (Decadron-LA)
  2. Triamcinolone hexacetonide (Aristospan)

3. Triamcinolone diacetate (Aristicort, Kenacort)
4. Triamcinolone acetonide (Kenalog)
5. Methylprednisolone acetate (Depo-Medrol)

Insoluble steroids have a slow onset from 6–48 hrs and a long duration of several days to 2 weeks.

Combination
1. Betamethasone acetate and phosphate (Celestone, Soluspan)

23. A patient with a known seizure disorder begins to go into status epilepticus in your office. What is the drug of choice and the proper dosage to administer?

Diazepam (Valium) IV (preferred) or IM at a rate of no more than 5 mg/min is recommended in this situation. The usual adult dose is 5–10 mg, as required, repeated every 10–15 minutes to a maximum dose of 30 mg.

24. How does metformin (Glucophage) differ from the first- and second-generation oral hypoglycemic agents?

Metformin is an anti-hyperglycemic, not a hypoglycemic drug. It does not cause insulin release from the pancreas and will not cause hypoglycemia. It works primarily by increasing insulin action in peripheral tissues and reducing hepatic glucose output due to inhibition of gluconeogenesis. It may also reduce glucose absorption from the intestines.

The oral hypoglycemic agents work by stimulating insulin release from the pancreas. Via a complicated mechanism, they also allow circulating insulin to have a greater effect on peripheral tissues, resulting in a more effective utilization of insulin.

25. You prescribe ibuprofen for an inflammatory condition for a patient presently taking the medications Lanoxin, Lasix, Vasotec, and Coumadin. What, if any, is the concern with his existing medications?

Most NSAIDs are highly bound to protein-binding sites on serum albumin, as is warfarin (Coumadin). When taken concurrently, the NSAID will displace the warfarin and increase the amount of free warfarin in serum (serum concentration). As a result, the anticoagulant effects of warfarin are significantly increased, providing for a serious bleeding potential.

In addition, aspirin and most NSAIDs have antiplatelet action that can potentially contribute to excessive bleeding in anticoagulated patients. NSAIDs may precipitate a gastrointestinal hemorrhage with more serious complication in the anticoagulated patient.

There is no interaction between NSAIDs and digoxin (Lanoxin), furosemide (Lasix), and enalopril (Vasotec).

26. A 57-year-old man presents with an acute gouty attack. He has no drug allergies and is otherwise healthy. What medications can be used in treating this condition? What is the mechanism of action of each?

NSAIDs: The primary NSAID used in the treatment of gout is **indomethacin** (Indocin). Its primary mechanism of action is inhibition of prostaglandin synthesis, thereby inhibiting the inflammatory process.

Colchicine: Colchicine inhibits the migration of polymorphonuclear (PMN) leukocytes to the inflamed joint. This reduces the phagocytosis of urate crystals by the PMNs and thereby reduces the amount of lactic acid and inflammatory enzymes within the joint.

27. Name six penicillinase-resistant penicillins. Which are available as oral preparations?

Methicillin (Staphcillin, Azapen, Celbenin)
Nafcillin (Nafcil, Unipen, Naftopen, Nallpen)
Cloxacillin (Tegopen, Bactopen, Cloxipen)
Dicloxacillin (Dynapen, Pathocil, Diclocil, Veracillin)
Flucloxacillin (Floxapen, Heracillin, Flupen, Staphylex)

Oxacillin (Prostaphilin, Bactocill, Bristopen, Stapenor)
Oral preparations are available for nafcillin, oxacillin, cloxacillin, and dicloxacillin.

28. Can a patient who gives a history of penicillin allergy be placed on a cephalosporin?

An increased risk of allergic reaction exists with the cephalosporin antibiotics in patients known to be penicillin-allergic. One study places the risk at approx. 8.1%, compared to 1.9% in those with no penicillin allergy. Another study notes the rate of cross-reactivity in first- and second-generation cephalosporins to be 5.4–16.5%, although most consider the cross-reaction rate to be 3–7%.

Note that each generation of cephalosporins carries a different risk rate, with the third-generation cephalosporins having decidedly lower risk than the first- and second-generation cephalosporins. Conversely, other β-lactam antibiotics, such as imipenem-cilastatin, *do* cross-react in penicillin-allergic patients.

The monobactam **aztreonam** does not appear to cross-react and provides an excellent alternative in penicillin-allergic patients.[12]

29. A patient with long-standing peripheral vascular disease (PVD) has just been prescribed propranolol to help in controlling his hypertension. How might this affect his PVD?

Propranolol is a β-blocker. All β-antagonists reduce cardiac output and can precipitate or aggravate the symptoms of peripheral insufficiency in patients with arterial disease.

30. A 52-year-old diabetic patient seen in the emergency room is diagnosed as having gas gangrene. Your plan is for immediate surgical intervention. What antibiotics targeted at the gas-producing organisms can be given?

Clindamycin	Ceftriaxone
Metronidazole	Ticarcillin-clavulanic acid
Imipenem-cilastatin	Piperacillin, azlocillin, and mezlocillin
Cefoxitin	Ampicillin-sulbactam
Cefotaxime	Piperacillin-tazobactam
Ceftizoxime	Natural penicillin

It is generally accepted that clindamycin, metronidazole, and imipenem-cilastatin are the preferred choices.

31. The culture and sensitivity report on your patient with a postoperative infection indicates methicillin-resistant *Staphylococcus aureus*. What is your drug of choice and the recommended dose?

Vancomycin is the drug of choice. The usual IV dose in adults with normal renal function is 1 gm every 12 hours, infused over a 60-minute period.

32. How is the blood level of vancomycin monitored? What is the appropriate blood level?

Vancomycin is monitored by obtaining peak and trough levels. The desirable range for therapeutic peak levels is 20–40 μg/ml and for trough levels is 5–10 μg/ml.

Ototoxicity is the most serious potential adverse effect of vancomycin. However, it has primarily been noted in patients with peak blood levels > 80–100 μg/ml.

33. Following a first metatarsal cuneiform fusion, a 53-year-old woman is diagnosed with a pulmonary embolism. What would be an appropriate medication for this condition? What dosage?

Heparin is the drug of choice. The preferred heparin schedule is the continuous method. Give 10,000–15,000 units of heparin by bolus, followed by 1000–2000 units every hour. Heparin dosing should be monitored by the partial thromboplastin time (PPT) and should be kept between 1.5–2.5 times normal.

34. List several medications used to treat chronic gout, and explain their mechanisms of action.

1. *Probenecid:* Inhibits renal tubular absorption of urate, thereby increasing its renal excretion.

2. *Sulfinpyrazone:* Inhibits renal tubular absorption of urate, thereby increasing its renal excretion.

3. *Allopurinol:* Inhibits xanthine oxidase, which is an enzyme necessary for the conversion of xanthine to uric acid.

35. You are about to make the first osteotomy for an Austin procedure on a healthy 34-year-old man, when the anesthesiologist asks you to stop the procedure. The patient's body temperature is rising rapidly. What might this condition be? How should you treat it?

The disorder is malignant hyperthermia. Dantrolene sodium (Dantrium) is the drug of choice. An initial dose of 1–2 mg/kg IV push is given and may be repeated every 5–10 minutes until symptoms are reversed or a maximum of 10 mg/kg is reached.

36. A 28-year-old construction worker presents 8 hours after stepping on a rusty nail while working on a muddy job site. He is otherwise healthy and does not remember ever receiving a tetanus injection. What, if anything, would you give this patient to cover for tetanus?

Assuming that the patient was never immunized, he should be given 250 U of tetanus immune globin IM and 0.5 ml of tetanus toxoid IM. If a patient has been previously immunized and presents with a dirty wound, he should receive 0.5 ml of tetanus toxoid IM.

37. A 32-year-old healthy woman with onychomycosis previously developed an allergic reaction to Sporonox. What should you consider when selecting another oral agent?

An important question to ask this patient is if she is presently using birth control pills or if she is pregnant. Griseofulvin (Fulvicin) may increase the metabolism of estrogen within oral contraceptives, resulting in an unwanted pregnancy. In addition, griseofulvin, terbinafine (Lamisil), and ketoconazole (Nizoral) are contraindicated in pregnancy due to their teratogenic effects.

38. A 67-year-old man with a history of congestive heart failure and penicillin allergy presents with an abscess and localized cellulitis of the hallux. His medication list includes digoxin (Lanoxin), furosemide (Lasix), and terfenadine (Seldane). You perform an incision and drainage and prescribe clarithromycin due to his penicillin allergy. Is this a good choice in this patient?

Clarithromycin is contraindicated in patients receiving terfenadine who have a preexisting cardiac abnormality (arrhythmia, bradycardia, QT-prolongation, ischemic heart disease, etc.) or electrolyte disturbances. The result can be cardiotoxicity, arrhythmia, or death.

39. A 54-year-old obese man is scheduled for an Achilles tendon repair after an acute tear. He has a history of deep vein thrombosis and phlebitis. What medication might you use prophylactically to help prevent this problem postoperatively?

Minidose heparin is most frequently employed as a prophylaxis at doses of 5000 units SC every 8–12 hours, started at least 2 hours preoperatively and continued until ambulatory.

40. Which is the only insulin that may be given via an IV solution?

Regular insulin. This is because regular insulin is a true solution and not a suspension, as are all the other insulin preparations.

41. What is the difference between Percodan and Percocet?

Percodan contains oxycodone and aspirin. **Percocet** contains oxycodone and acetaminophen.

42. A patient on clindamycin develops pseudomembranous colitis. What is the drug of choice to treat this condition?

Vancomycin is the drug of choice, although metronidazole is also effective.

43. You have prescribed ciprofloxacin to a 56-year-old patient. He is basically healthy, except for a gastric ulcer, for which he uses Maalox occasionally, and a history of migraine headaches. What instructions should you give this patient regarding the dosage and its administration?

Ingestion of ciprofloxacin within 2 hours after a dose of 30 ml of an antacid reduces the bioavailability of ciprofloxacin to 18–25% compared to that administered alone. Similar reduction in absorption rates of ciprofloxacin have been noted with the use of calcium and iron products. However, the administration of ciprofloxacin 2 hours *before* or 6 hours *after* an antacid, iron, or calcium product does not interfere with absorption.

44. A patient has just been diagnosed with early Lyme disease. What is the drug of choice and dosage?

In the early days, Lyme disease was treated with oral tetracycline, penicillin, or erythromycin, but recent studies have led to the use of other antibiotics with greater sensitivities to *Borrellia burgdorferi.*

For early Lyme disease, oral **doxycycline**, 100 mg twice daily, or **amoxicillin,** 500 mg four times daily, each for 10–30 days, is generally an effective medication. Children and pregnant women should not use doxycycline (or tetracycline), and those allergic to penicillin should be prescribed erythromycin, 250 mg three times daily for 10–30 days.

In the later stages of disease, patients with Lyme **arthritis** should be prescribed doxycycline, 100 mg twice daily for 30 days, or amoxicillin, plus probenecid, 500 mg each four times daily for 30 days. Another alternative is ceftriaxone, 2 gm IV once daily for 14 days.

Neurologic manifestations require ceftriaxone, 2 gm IV once daily, or cefotaxime, 2 gm IV three times daily, both for 14–30 days. Those with penicillin and/or cephalosporin allergy may use doxycycline, 200 mg twice daily for 30 days, or vancomycin, 1 gm twice daily for 14–30 days.

In one study, cefuroxime was found to be as effective with fewer side effects than doxycycline. However, doxycycline appears to be the mainstay of treatment at this point, although newer and more effective agents are being investigated.

45. List several antibiotics that can be used in a patient with *Enterococcus* infection.

Amoxicillin   Imipenem (Primaxin)
Amoxicillin-clavulanic acid (Augmentin)   Ampicillin alone or with an aminoglycoside
Vancomycin

46. Your clinical diagnosis on a 32-year-old female with an itchy rash is tinea pedis. You prescribe oxiconazole 1% cream. What instructions for daily application and length of time for its use should you provide her?

Oxiconazole has been shown to produce a greater than 90% improvement in the clinical signs and symptoms of tinea pedis as compared with baseline when applied twice a day for a 1-month period.

BIBLIOGRAPHY

1. Bailie GR, Neal D: Vancomycin ototoxicity and nephrotoxicity: A review. Med Toxicol Adverse Drug Exp 3:376, 1988.
2. Ciabattoni G, Boss AH, Patrignani P: Effects of sulindac on renal and extrarenal eicosanoid synthesis. Clin Pharmacol Ther 41:380, 1987.
3. DeFronzo RA, Goodman AM: Efficacy of metformin in patients with non-insulin-dependent diabetes mellitus. N Engl J Med 333:541, 1995.
4. Edson RS, Terrell CL: The aminoglycosides. Mayo Clin Proc 66:1158, 1991.
5. Furst DE: Clinically important interactions of nonsteroidal antiinflammatory drugs with other medications. J Rheumatol 15(suppl 17):58, 1988.
6. Gronert A: Malignant hyperthermia. Anesthesiology 53:396, 1980.
7. Lin RY: A perspective on penicillin allergy. Arch Med 152:930, 1992.

8. Nix DE, Watson WA, Handy L: The effect of sucralfate pretreatment on the pharamacokinetics of ciprofloxacin. Pharmacotherapy 9:377, 1989.
9. Petz LD: Immunologic cross reactivity between penicillin and cephalosporin: A review. J Infect Dis 137:S74, 1978.
10. Polk RE, Healy DP, et al: Vancomycin and the red-man syndrome: Pharmacodynamics of histamine release. J Infect Dis 157:502, 1988.
11. Saxon A, Beall GN, Rohr AS, Adelman DC: Immediate hypersensitivity reactions to beta-lactam antibiotics. Ann Intern Med 107:204, 1987.
12. Sigal LH: Summary of the Fifth International Congress on Lyme Borreliosis. Arthritis Rheum 37:10, 1994.
13. Steere AC: Lyme disease. N Engl J Med 321:586, 1989.
14. Symposium on Antimicrobial Agents, pts I–VII. Mayo Clin Proc Oct 1991–Mar 1992.
15. Yaster M, Deshpande JK: Management of pediatric pain with opioid analgesics. J Pediatr 113:421, 1988.

39. SURGICAL APPROACHES TO THE FOOT

Lawrence B. Harkless, D.P.M., and Kim Felder-Johnson, D.P.M.

1. What is the best approach to remove an osteochondroma located in the central-most medial aspect of the nail bed?

A medial approach through the nail bed after simple avulsion of the nail.

2. What is the best approach to a myxoid cyst dorsum of the third distal interphalangeal joint (DIPJ)?

Two semi-elliptical dorsal transverse incisions encompassing the lesion. This approach provides excellent exposure to the joint, which is often involved.

3. What is the approach for removal of nail groove corn lateral aspect of the fifth toe?

Two dorsal linear semi-elliptical incisions encompassing the lesion and part of the nail plate.

4. What are two approaches for a partial first ray amputation, and which one is best?

1. Dorsal medial racquet incision creating a side-to-side flap.

2. A medial incision on the first metatarsal curving dorsally over the hallux, creating a medial-to-lateral flap.

The medial incision provides better exposure to the plantar structures and deep central space. In addition, this incision provides a better flap to cover areas of skin loss, especially in an infection and gangrene.

5. What are the approaches to the first metatarsophalangeal joint (MTPJ)?

1. Dorsal linear
2. Medial

6. What are the landmarks for each approach?

For the dorsal linear approach, most medial aspects of the EHL tendon and most dorsal medial aspects of the metatarsal head. The point halfway between these two landmarks is where the incision should be placed.

For the medial approach, a point bisecting the medial aspect of the first metatarsal head should be ascertained, and this usually corresponds to the superior margin of the abductor hallucis tendon. The incision should be extended distally and proximally along this margin.

7. What are the advantages of a dorsal vs. medial incision?

The dorsal incision allows exposure to the first web space, obviating the need for a second incision to perform a sesamoidectomy or lateral release. This avoids a scar on the dorsal aspect of the foot and is therefore often more cosmetically pleasing to the patient. The skin on the medial aspect of the first MTPJ at the junction between dorsal and plantar skin usually produces a scar that is almost invisible.

8. A 35-year-old male sustained a fracture to the tibial sesamoid that has remained painful despite a reasonable course of conservative treatment. What are the approaches for excision, and which is preferred?

1. Medial, along the superior border of the abductor hallucis.
2. Plantar, directly over the sesamoid.

The medial approach avoids placing a scar on the plantar aspect of the foot.

9. What are the two approaches to a partial fifth ray amputation?

1. Dorsal racquet-shaped incision creating a side-to-side flap.

2. A lateral incision on the fifth metatarsal, curving dorsally over the fifth and creating a lateral-to-medial flap.

10. Which one is best?

The lateral incision provides better exposure as well as a better flap to cover areas of skin loss, especially as a result of infection or gangrene.

11. What is the most widely used approach to correcting a mallet toe and why? What are the landmarks for the approach?

A transverse semi-elliptical incision encompassing the lesion. This approach provides the best exposure, allows for shortening, and provides stability. The landmark is the highest point at the DIPJ upon flexion.

12. What approach for first metatarsal cuneiform joint fusion provides the best exposure and what vital structures should be isolated or avoided?

A medial approach provides the best exposure. It facilitates the exposure to the joint, which is very deep, and allows for easy placement of screws. The medial branch of the medial dorsal cutaneous nerve obliques dorsally over the first metatarsal cuneiform joint, which should be identified and retracted.

13. What are the approaches for heel spur excision?

1. Medial linear incision inferior aspect of the heel from the porta pedis distally (Duvries approach).

2. Transverse plantar incision distal to the weightbearing surface.

3. A curved incision beginning distal to the porta pedis.

14. Some of the earliest treatments for ingrown toenails included soft tissue procedures, including the Cotting and the DuVries. Describe these procedures for soft tissue correction of ingrown toenails.

The Cotting procedure, reported in 1873, was one of the earliest treatments for ingrown toenails. This procedure was described as an open wound incision measuring one inch long by three-fourths of an inch wide that removed all the diseased tissue with a large piece of proud flesh, skin deep from one side of the toe. No portion of the nail was removed, and the wound was treated until healing occurred in approximately four weeks. Cotting based this procedure on the theory that scar formation would draw the soft tissue away from the nail, relieving all pressure.

DuVries described a soft tissue wedge resection for the side of the toe. A triangular section of tissue was excised through two semi-elliptical incisions extending along the side of the toe. The margins of the ellipse were coapted and maintained with suture pulling the nail lip and nail groove down. The theory behind this procedure is that by removing the wedge of tissue and pulling the nail groove down, pressure is relieved from the border of the toenail.

15. What are the incisional approaches to a Morton's neuroma?

The dorsal approach has the greatest advantage of early ambulation because the incision is on a non-weightbearing surface. Healing may occur sooner than on the plantar surface. The disadvantage is the difficulty that may be encountered trying to reach the nerve deep within the interspace. The deep transverse intermetatarsal ligament needs to be incised to reach the deep proximal nerve and distal digital branches.

The advantage of the web-splitting incision is exposure of the bifurcation of the common nerve into the digital branches. The exposure allows for visualization and separation of the vascular structures from the nerves. The disadvantage is the technical difficulty required because of the interface of the digits and the poor visibility of the proximal portion of the common digital nerve or proximal neuroma.

The plantar longitudinal approach has the best exposure of all the incisions. It allows for complete visibility of the nerve and vascular structures. This approach also allows for the choice of incising the deep transverse metatarsal ligament or leaving it intact. The greatest disadvantage is the potential for a painful plantar scar on a weightbearing surface and a longer healing course. Careful placement of the incision between the metatarsal heads is key in trying to avoid this complication.

The plantar transverse incision is made distal to the metatarsal heads within the sulcus area proximal to the interdigital folds. This incision allows for early ambulation, good visibility, and easy access to the neuroma. The incision through the plantar skin may result in longer healing, but the placement on a non-weightbearing surface aids in decreasing the risk of a painful plantar scar.

17. What are some advantages and disadvantages to the different incisional approaches to correction of a digital deformity?

Hammertoe and clawtoe deformities are typically performed through dorsal linear or elliptical incisions. The linear incision is usually appropriate in the absence of a dorsal corn. In the presence of dorsal lesions, the elliptical approach is usually used to allow for excision of the lesion. Either approach can result in complications with contracture or cosmesis if incisions are inappropriately placed or if made too long or wide. If there is a concern of cosmesis and a dorsal scar, a medial or lateral longitudinal approach may be used. The concern with this approach is risk of compromise to the digital vasculature and difficulty with exposure.

The transverse elliptical approach is most commonly used in correction of a mallet toe but can also be used with the other digital deformities. Appropriate placement and measurement of the width of the ellipse is necessary to avoid soft tissue contracture or compromise of the vasculature. This approach may provide less exposure to the joint depending on placement of the incision and the size of the digit.

18. What is the stepwise approach to the correction of a digital deformity?

A digital deformity is first reduced by a resectional arthroplasty of the head of the proximal phalanx. The Kelikian pushup test should be performed to assess if the deformity is reduced in the sagittal plane to the level of the normal lesser toes. If the remaining stump of proximal phalanx remains dorsiflexed, the soft tissue (extensor capsule, hood and wing mechanism, and EDL tendon) at the MTPJ should be released.

The foot should then be loaded to simulate weightbearing to assess reduction of the deformity. If the deformity persists at the MTPJ, a plantar plate release should be performed. Then it is again loaded, and, if the deformity remains, the toe should be stabilized with 0.045 K-wire. The intent is to stabilize the toe for 4–6 weeks to allow soft tissue fibrosis, which should allow the toe to remain in a rectus alignment.

19. List the incisional approaches for a panmetatarsal head resection and who described them.

- The three incisional dorsal longitudinal approach (Larmon, 1951). The first incision is located over the dorsal medial aspect of the first MTPJ. The second incision is between the second and third metatarsal heads, and the third incision is between the fourth and fifth metatarsal heads.
- Five dorsal linear incisions over each metatarsal head (Hodor and Dobbs, JAPMA, 1983).
- Dorsal transverse (Clayton, 1960).
- Plantar transverse (Hoffman, 1912).
- Plantar elliptical (Fowler, 1959).

20. Which panmetatarsal head approach provides the best exposure for severe digital contractures with dorsal dislocation of the lesser metatarsal phalangeal joints?

The plantar transverse ellipse approach provides the best exposure to the metatarsal heads when the toes are dorsally dislocated. The metatarsal heads are more prominent plantarly, which makes excision through a dorsal approach very difficult, especially if osteoporosis is present.

This approach allows for excision of redundant skin and allows tightening of the plantar skin, which in turn provides more digital stability and alignment.

21. What approach should be utilized for exposure to the sinus tarsi?

An oblique incision is centered over the sinus tarsi from 1 cm distal and posterior to the tip of the lateral malleolus and extending anterior and distal to the region of the second cuneiform.

22. What are the indications for such an approach?

Subtalar fusion, arthroereisis procedure, grice, and sinus tarsi arthralgia.

23. What are the landmarks for the dorsal medial approach to the medial column of the foot?

The inferior aspect of the medial malleolus, the height of the talonavicular joint dorsally, and the first metatarsal base distally. A dot placed on each area with the points connected should provide an outline for the incision with a slight curve dorsally.

24. What are the indications and advantages for such an approach?

Medial column fusions (talonavicular joint, navicular cuneiform joint, and the first metatarsal cuneiform joint). An advantage is that it avoids the venous network of vessels if placed to plantar and hastens the exposure.

25. What is the best approach for a Lisfranc fracture dislocation?

Three dorsal linear incisions:
1. A linear incision on the medial aspect of the first metatarsal cuneiform joint.
2. A dorsal longitudinal incision between the second and third metatarsal base centered over the tarso/metatarsal joints.
3. A dorsal incision over the fourth and fifth metatarsal base.
This approach provides the best exposure.

26. What approach should be used for a deep central space infection?

A Loeffler and Ballard approach. The incision begins plantarly between the first and second metatarsal heads and curves laterally in the central arch and extends proximally into the tarsal tunnel. This approach allows for visualization of all the deep structures of the foot that originate in the leg. Infection follows the path of least resistance; hence the tendons should be followed proximally to ensure all infection has been eradicated.

27. Describe the approach for syndactyly of the fourth and fifth toes with recurrent heloma molle.

With a marking pen, outline on the fifth toe from the base of the web just dorsal to the midline to the level of the DIPJ. The incision will extend plantarward to the base of the web along the fifth toe. Place the fifth and fourth toes together in their corrected position to transfer the marking. Excise the skin along the outline. Close the incision with combination vertical mattress and simple sutures, dorsally and plantarly.

28. Describe the approach for a condylectomy of the lateral aspect of the base of the proximal phalanx fourth toe for a recalcitrant soft corn.

A dorsal lateral linear incision beginning at the distal third of the proximal phalanx, extending proximally to the metatarsal phalangeal joint. The incision is deepened down to bone. A linear incision is made into the capsule. The capsule is freed laterally from the proximal phalanx base. The condyle is removed with a double action bone forcep.

29. Describe the approach for Haglund's deformity with enthesophyte and insertional degeneration of the Achilles tendon.

A slightly curved, L-shaped incision beginning 1 cm proximal to the superior lateral margins of the calcaneus lateral to the Achilles tendon. The incision curves medially at its insertion to end at the most medial margin of the tendinous insertion. After following this approach, incise the subcutaneous tissue. Identify and retract the sural nerve laterally. Incise the periosteum in a linear fashion and reflect subperiosteally to expose the eminence. Resect the posterior superior tuberosity of the calcaneus with an osteotome with the cut oriented obliquely from anterior superior to posterior inferior. A concavity should be created. A linear incision is made into the tendon's central aspect from the most superior aspect of the calcaneus distally to its insertion. The tendon is retracted medially and laterally and the enthesophyte excised. The tendon should be inspected for degenerative changes at its insertion. If changes are noted, the tendon should be detached and all degenerative changes excised. The tendon should be reattached with a suture anchor of choice.

30. Describe the approaches for hallux interphalangeal (IP) sesamoid excision.

A longitudinal plantar approach with the incision centered over the plantar aspect of the hallux IP joint. Subcutaneous tissue is incised, exposing the flexor hallucis longus (FHL). A linear incision is made centrally within the FHL. The tendon is retracted medially and laterally, exposing the sesamoid at the level of the central plantar aspect of the head of the proximal phalanx between the condyles.

A linear incision on the medial inferior aspect of the hallux IP joint is centered at the hallux IP joint at the inferior aspect of the proximal phalanx. The incision is deepened down to the level of the capsule, and the capsule is incised linearly. The flexor tendon is identified and retracted plantarly, the hallux is plantar flexed, and the sesamoid should be noted superior at the head of the proximal phalanx between the condyles. The bone is completely excised. The most difficult part of removal is release of the most distal lateral superior aspect. This can be facilitated by the use of a small, curved scissor. A rongeur can also be used to tear the attachment since the sesamoid usually fits well in the jaws of the rongeur.

31. Describe the approach for a Dwyer calcaneal osteotomy.

The landmarks for the approach are the peroneal tubercle and the superior margin of the calcaneus in the central aspect of the bone and in the inferior aspect of the calcaneus. These points should be conducted to create an oblique incision beginning 2 cm proximal to the superior aspect of the calcaneus, extending distally through the central body of the calcaneus proximal to the peroneal tubercle, and ending in the inferior aspect of the calcaneus. The subcutaneous tissue is incised linearly. The sural nerve should be identified and retracted. A linear cut is made into the periosteum. The periosteum is reflected with a key elevator. The closing wedge osteotomy is then performed with the apex medial, and the medial cortex is left intact. It should be noted that the shape of the calcaneus medially is concave, and the cut should be made three-quarters of the way through the calcaneus; the remainder of the osteotomy is feathered. The osteotomy is then closed and fixated with staples or a screw.

32. Describe the approach for interpositional arthroplasty, second metatarsophalangeal joint, for degenerative joint disease.

A dorsal longitudinal incision is made over the second metatarsophalangeal joint with the incision centered over the joint. The subcutaneous tissue is incised, exposing the extensor tendons. The extensor tendon is freed along the medial margin and retracted laterally, exposing the capsule of the metatarsophalangeal joint. A U-shaped capsulotomy is performed with the base proximal. The capsule is freed, exposing the metatarsophalangeal joint. A partial metatarsal head resection is performed, leaving the plantar condyles intact. A capsule is sutured with two Keith needles and interposed between the remaining head of the metatarsal and the proximal phalanx base. The needles are then pulled through the plantar aspect of the foot to adequately interpose the soft tissue and sutured on a button with appropriate soft tissue cushioning.

INDEX

Page numbers in **boldface type** indicate complete chapters.